Dental Materials: Latest Advances and Prospects

Dental Materials: Latest Advances and Prospects

Editor

Vittorio Checchi

MDPI • Basel • Beijing • Wuhan • Barcelona • Belgrade • Manchester • Tokyo • Cluj • Tianjin

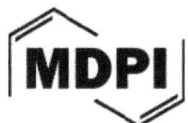

Editor
Vittorio Checchi
University of Modena and
Reggio Emilia
Italy

Editorial Office
MDPI
St. Alban-Anlage 66
4052 Basel, Switzerland

This is a reprint of articles from the Special Issue published online in the open access journal *Applied Sciences* (ISSN 2076-3417) (available at: https://www.mdpi.com/journal/applsci/special_issues/Advanced_Dental_Materials).

For citation purposes, cite each article independently as indicated on the article page online and as indicated below:

LastName, A.A.; LastName, B.B.; LastName, C.C. Article Title. *Journal Name* **Year**, *Volume Number*, Page Range.

ISBN 978-3-0365-6364-0 (Hbk)
ISBN 978-3-0365-6365-7 (PDF)

Cover image courtesy of Vittorio Checchi

© 2023 by the authors. Articles in this book are Open Access and distributed under the Creative Commons Attribution (CC BY) license, which allows users to download, copy and build upon published articles, as long as the author and publisher are properly credited, which ensures maximum dissemination and a wider impact of our publications.
The book as a whole is distributed by MDPI under the terms and conditions of the Creative Commons license CC BY-NC-ND.

Contents

About the Editor ix

Vittorio Checchi
Special Issue on Dental Materials: Latest Advances and Prospects
Reprinted from: *Appl. Sci.* 2022, 12, 8833, doi:10.3390/app12178833 1

Alberto Murri Dello Diago, Milena Cadenaro, Rossana Ricchiuto, Federico Banchelli, Enrico Spinas, Vittorio Checchi and Luca Giannetti
Hypersensitivity in Molar Incisor Hypomineralization: Superficial Infiltration Treatment
Reprinted from: *Appl. Sci.* 2021, 11, 1823, doi:10.3390/app11041823 5

Luigi Generali, Francesco Cavani, Federico Franceschetti, Paolo Sassatelli, Luciano Giardino, Chiara Pirani, et al.
Calcium Hydroxide Removal Using Four Different Irrigation Systems: A Quantitative Evaluation by Scanning Electron Microscopy
Reprinted from: *Appl. Sci.* 2022, 12, 271, doi:10.3390/app12010271 13

Sorana-Maria Bucur, Luminița Ligia Vaida, Cristian Doru Olteanu and Vittorio Checchi
A Brief Review on Micro-Implants and Their Use in Orthodontics and Dentofacial Orthopaedics
Reprinted from: *Appl. Sci.* 2021, 11, 10719, doi:10.3390/app112210719 23

Celia Tobar, Verónica Rodríguez, Carlos Lopez-Suarez, Jesús Peláez, Jorge Cortés-Bretón Brinckmann and María J. Suárez
Effect of Digital Technologies on the Marginal Accuracy of Conventional and Cantilever Co–Cr Posterior-Fixed Partial Dentures Frameworks
Reprinted from: *Appl. Sci.* 2021, 11, 2988, doi:10.3390/app11072988 39

Nicola De Angelis, Luca Solimei, Claudio Pasquale, Lorenzo Alvito, Alberto Lagazzo and Fabrizio Barberis
Mechanical Properties and Corrosion Resistance of TiAl6V4 Alloy Produced with SLM Technique and Used for Customized Mesh in Bone Augmentations
Reprinted from: *Appl. Sci.* 2021, 11, 5622, doi:10.3390/app11125622 51

Arturo Sanchez-Perez, Nuria Cano-Millá, María José Moya Villaescusa, José María Montoya Carralero and Carlos Navarro Cuellar
Effect of Photofunctionalization with 6 W or 85 W UVC on the Degree of Wettability of RBM Titanium in Relation to the Irradiation Time
Reprinted from: *Appl. Sci.* 2021, 11, 5427, doi:10.3390/app11125427 63

Andrea Maria Chisnoiu, Marioara Moldovan, Codruta Sarosi, Radu Marcel Chisnoiu, Doina Iulia Rotaru, Ada Gabriela Delean, et al.
Marginal Adaptation Assessment for Two Composite Layering Techniques Using Dye Penetration, AFM, SEM and FTIR: An In-Vitro Comparative Study
Reprinted from: *Appl. Sci.* 2021, 11, 5657, doi:10.3390/app11125657 73

Shanshan Liang, Hongqiang Ye and Fusong Yuan
Changes in Crystal Phase, Morphology, and Flexural Strength of As-Sintered Translucent Monolithic Zirconia Ceramic Modified by Femtosecond Laser
Reprinted from: *Appl. Sci.* 2021, 11, 6925, doi:10.3390/app11156925 87

Marco Farronato, Davide Farronato, Francesco Inchingolo, Laura Grassi, Valentina Lanteri and Cinzia Maspero
Evaluation of Dental Surface after De-Bonding Orthodontic Bracket Bonded with a Novel Fluorescent Composite: In Vitro Comparative Study
Reprinted from: *Appl. Sci.* **2021**, *11*, 6354, doi:10.3390/app11146354 99

Young-Sam Kim, Young-Min Park, Saverio Cosola, Abanob Riad, Enrica Giammarinaro, Ugo Covani and Simone Marconcini
Retrospective Analysis on Inferior Third Molar Position by Means of Orthopantomography or CBCT: Periapical Band-Like Radiolucent Sign
Reprinted from: *Appl. Sci.* **2021**, *11*, 6389, doi:10.3390/app11146389 109

Daniel Moreinos, Ronald Wigler, Yuval Geffen, Sharon Akrish and Shaul Lin
Healing Capacity of Bone Surrounding Biofilm-Infected and Non-Infected Gutta-Percha: A Study of Rat Calvaria
Reprinted from: *Appl. Sci.* **2021**, *11*, 6710, doi:10.3390/app11156710 121

Fadis F. Murzakhanov, Peter O. Grishin, Margarita A. Goldberg, Boris V. Yavkin, Georgy V. Mamin, Sergei B. Orlinskii, et al.
Radiation-Induced Stable Radicals in Calcium Phosphates: Results of Multifrequency EPR, EDNMR, ESEEM, and ENDOR Studies
Reprinted from: *Appl. Sci.* **2021**, *11*, 7727, doi:10.3390/app11167727 131

Sorana Maria Bucur, Anamaria Bud, Adrian Gligor, Alexandru Vlasa, Dorin Ioan Cocoș and Eugen Silviu Bud
Observational Study Regarding Two Bonding Systems and the Challenges of Their Use in Orthodontics: An In Vitro Evaluation
Reprinted from: *Appl. Sci.* **2021**, *11*, 7091, doi:10.3390/app11157091 145

Joo-Seong Kim, Tae-Sik Jang, Suk-Young Kim and Won-Pyo Lee
Octacalcium Phosphate Bone Substitute (Bontree®): From Basic Research to Clinical Case Study
Reprinted from: *Appl. Sci.* **2021**, *11*, 7921, doi:10.3390/app11177921 155

Arata Ito, Hideki Kitaura, Haruki Sugisawa, Takahiro Noguchi, Fumitoshi Ohori and Itaru Mizoguchi
Titanium Nitride Plating Reduces Nickel Ion Release from Orthodontic Wire
Reprinted from: *Appl. Sci.* **2021**, *11*, 9745, doi:10.3390/app11209745 169

Anna Lehmann, Kacper Nijakowski, Michalina Nowakowska, Patryk Woś, Maria Misiaszek and Anna Surdacka
Influence of Selected Restorative Materials on the Environmental pH: In Vitro Comparative Study
Reprinted from: *Appl. Sci.* **2021**, *11*, 11975, doi:10.3390/app112411975 183

Lucia Memè, Enrico M. Strappa, Riccardo Monterubbianesi, Fabrizio Bambini and Stefano Mummolo
SEM and FT-MIR Analysis of Human Demineralized Dentin Matrix: An In Vitro Study
Reprinted from: *Appl. Sci.* **2022**, *12*, 1480, doi:10.3390/app12031480 195

Peter van der Schoor, Markus Schlee and Hai-Bo Wen
Prospective Pilot Study of Immediately Provisionalized Restorations of Trabecular Metal-Enhanced Titanium Dental Implants: A 5-Year Follow-Up Report
Reprinted from: *Appl. Sci.* **2022**, *12*, 942, doi:10.3390/app12030942 207

Sorina-Mihaela Solomon, Irina-Georgeta Sufaru, Silvia Teslaru, Cristina Mihaela Ghiciuc and Celina Silvia Stafie
Finding the Perfect Membrane: Current Knowledge on Barrier Membranes in Regenerative Procedures: A Descriptive Review
Reprinted from: *Appl. Sci.* **2022**, *12*, 1042, doi:10.3390/app12031042 . . . . **217**

About the Editor

Vittorio Checchi

Vittorio Checchi is an Associate Professor of Restorative Dentistry, University of Modena & Reggio Emilia, Italy. He is the Head of the Restorative Dentistry Department of the Dental and Maxillo-Facial Unit of the CHIMOMO Department at the University of Modena & Reggio Emilia (Italy). He graduated with honors in Dentistry at the University of Bologna (Italy) in 2006. He was adjunct professor at the University of Bologna (Italy) from 2007 to 2009. He attended the Postdoctoral Externship Program at the Dental School of Columbia University in New York (USA) in 2009. He received his PhD in "Biomedical technologies applied to dental sciences" at the Second University of Naples (Italy) in 2010. He was Assistant Professor at the Dental School of the University of Trieste (Italy) from 2012 to 2017. He was Assistant Professor at the Dental School of the University of Modena & Reggio Emilia (Italy) from 2019 to 2022. He is a lecturer in the Master of Aesthetic Restorative and Prosthetic Dentistry at the University of Bologna from 2016 to today.

He is the author of 94 scientific papers published in national and international journals, with an H-Index of 19.

http://personale.unimore.it/Rubrica/dettaglio/vchecchi

Editorial

Special Issue on Dental Materials: Latest Advances and Prospects

Vittorio Checchi

Department of Surgery, Medicine, Dentistry and Morphological Sciences, University of Modena & Reggio Emilia, 41125 Modena, Italy; vittorio.checchi@unimore.it; Tel.: +39-0594224763

Citation: Checchi, V. Special Issue on Dental Materials: Latest Advances and Prospects. *Appl. Sci.* **2022**, *12*, 8833. https://doi.org/10.3390/app12178833

Received: 29 August 2022
Accepted: 30 August 2022
Published: 2 September 2022

Publisher's Note: MDPI stays neutral with regard to jurisdictional claims in published maps and institutional affiliations.

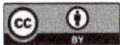

Copyright: © 2022 by the author. Licensee MDPI, Basel, Switzerland. This article is an open access article distributed under the terms and conditions of the Creative Commons Attribution (CC BY) license (https:// creativecommons.org/licenses/by/ 4.0/).

Most fields of dentistry are closely related to newly developed materials, and all clinical improvements often follow or, in any case, go hand in hand with the creation and development of innovative and higher-performing materials, instruments, and equipment. Thanks to contemporary dental material applications, the effectiveness of clinical dentistry has made remarkable advances. In recent years, new materials have been developed and proposed in each field of dentistry: prosthesis, restorative dentistry, endodontics, implantology, and orthodontics. Unfortunately, as often happens, this productive challenge is not always accompanied by valid scientific research, and consequently, the clinician finds at his disposal materials that are not necessarily better than the previous ones.

The aim of this Special Issue was to collect high-quality research articles, clinical studies, review articles, and case reports focused on the latest advances and prospects of dental materials.

A total of 19 papers (17 research papers and 2 review papers) are presented in this successful Special Issue.

Murri Dello Diago et al. [1] evaluated the efficacy of erosion–infiltration treatments with resin in children with a strong hypersensitivity and also developed a minimally invasive diagnostic–therapeutic pathway for young MIH patients. All patients reported lower sensitivity values at the end of the treatment. The authors concluded that the treatment of erosion infiltration with resin is a minimally invasive preventive treatment that significantly improves the problem of hypersensitivity in permanent molars with MIH.

Lehmann et al. [2] aimed to assess how selected restorative materials influence the environmental pH. The initial pH levels were significantly lower for glass ionomer cements compared to composites. With time, the pH increased for samples with glass ionomer cements, whereas it decreased for samples with composites. In the end, all materials were in the pH range between 5.3 and 6.0. The authors concluded that, immediately after application, restorative materials decrease the environmental pH, especially light-cured glass ionomer cements. For glass ionomers, within two weeks, the pH increased to levels comparable with composites.

Chisnoiu et al. [3] compared the effect of two different layering techniques of the dental composite in reducing the marginal microleakage when a brand-new material is used. Some better results were obtained for the oblique layering technique, but the differences from the other method have not been statistically validated.

Liang et al. [4], with an in vitro study, evaluated the changes in surface morphology and flexural strength of translucent monolithic zirconia surfaces treated with femtosecond laser technology. The surface roughness after femtosecond laser treatment was significantly improved compared with the negative control group and the group that received the airborne particle abrasion treatment. In comparison with the airborne particle abrasion group, the flexural strength of the group that received the femtosecond laser treatment was significantly improved. The femtosecond laser approach using appropriate parameters seemed to enhance the roughness of the zirconia without reducing its flexural strength.

Tobar et al. [5] evaluated the effect of different manufacturing techniques and pontic design on the vertical marginal fit of cobalt–chromium (Co–Cr) posterior fixed partial denture (FPD) frameworks. The vertical marginal discrepancy values of all FPDs were below 50 µm. No differences were found among intermediate pontic groups or cantilevered groups. Likewise, when differences in a marginal discrepancy between both framework designs were analyzed, no differences were observed. The analyzed digital technologies demonstrated a high precision of fit on Co–Cr frameworks and on both pontic designs.

Generali et al. [6] compared conventional endodontic needle irrigation, passive ultrasonic irrigation, apical negative pressure irrigation, and mechanical activation to remove calcium hydroxide from single straight root canals. Eighty-four mandibular premolars were prepared in a crown-down manner up to size #40. Considering the whole canal, all instruments showed better performance than conventional endodontic needle irrigation in removing calcium hydroxide. Passive Ultrasonic Irrigation and Mechanical Activation could remove a significantly higher amount of calcium hydroxide than Apical Negative Pressure Irrigation. Passive Ultrasonic Irrigation and Mechanical Activation have been able to remove more calcium hydroxide than Apical Negative Pressure Irrigation.

Moreinos et al. [7] aimed to evaluate the healing capacity of bony lesions around biofilm-infected and non-infected gutta-percha (GP) points. This study showed that bone healing is possible around both sterile and infected GP points. This contradicts the claim that some root canal treatments fail because of non-microbial factors, including extruded root canal filling materials, which may cause foreign body reactions. The healing observed suggests that overextension should not be considered an indication for endodontic surgery.

In their descriptive review, Solomon et al. [8] presented a synthesis of the types of barrier membranes available and their characteristics, as well as future trends in the development of barrier membranes along with some allergological aspects of membrane use.

De Angelis et al. [9] investigated the material used for titanium meshes. Specific test samples were obtained from two different manufacturers with two different shapes: surfaces without perforations and with calibrated perforations. The authors concluded that a normal masticatory load cannot modify the device and that chemical action in the case of exposure does not create macroscopic and microscopic alterations of the surface.

Kim et al. [10] evaluated the effect of a commercialized octacalcium phosphate (OCP)-based synthetic bone substitute material in vitro, in vivo, and in clinical cases. Compared with a commercial biphasic calcium phosphate ceramic (MBCP+TM), OCP suppressed RANKL and increased ALP activity. An animal model showed that 1.0 mm OCP granules had a higher new bone formation ability than 0.5 mm OCP granules. Moreover, eight implants placed in the three patients showed a 100% success rate after 1 year of functional loading. This basic research and clinical application showed the safety and efficacy of OCP for bone regeneration.

Sanchez-Perez et al. [11] studied how photoactivation with ultraviolet C light can reverse the effects derived from biological aging by restoring a hydrophilic surface. Power proved to be the most important factor, and the best hydrophilicity result was obtained with a power of 85 W for 60 min at a wavelength of 254 nm.

Van der Schoor et al. [12] described 5-year survival results and crestal bone level changes around immediately provisionalized Trabecular Metal Dental Implants. Clinical evaluations with radiographs were conducted at 1 month, 3 months, 6 months, and 1 to 5 years. In total, 30 patients (37 implants) were treated. There was one implant failure; cumulative survival at 5 years was 97.2%. After the initial bone loss of 0.40 mm in the first 6 months, there were no statistically significant changes in the crestal bone level over time up to 5 years of follow-up.

In their systematic review, Bucur et al. [13] reviewed the literature and evaluated the failure rates and factors that affect the stability and success of temporary anchorage devices used as orthodontic anchorage. Although all articles included in this meta-analysis reported success rates of greater than 80%, the factors determining success rates were inconsistent between the studies analyzed, making it difficult to reach conclusions.

Ito et al. [14] examined whether plating of orthodontic wire with titanium nitride could prevent the leaching of metal ions from the wire on immersion in acid. Results indicated that titanium nitride plating of orthodontic wire significantly suppressed the elution of metal ions on immersion in acid.

Bucur et al. [15] analyzed and identified a methodology for the improvement in the shear bond strength of orthodontic brackets bonded with two orthodontic adhesive systems under various enamel conditions (dry, moistened with water, and moistened with saliva). While clinically acceptable shear bond strengths were obtained for all studied groups, in the case of water contamination, it is preferable to use Fuji Ortho LC instead of Transbond Plus.

Farronato et al. [16] compared the effect of fluorescent and conventional non-fluorescent composites on dental surfaces and composite remnants by in vitro de-bonding tests. The use of fluorescent composite could significantly improve the quality of de-bonding by reducing the quantity of composite residuals and visible enamel damage, while reducing the time needed for successful procedure performance.

Memè et al. [17] investigated the effect of different times of demineralization on the chemical composition and the surface morphology of dentinal particles. Extracted teeth were divided into five groups based on demineralization time with 12% EDTA. Fourier-Transform Mid-Infrared spectroscopy analysis showed a progressive reduction in the concentration in the specimens ($T0 > T2 > T5 > T10 > T60$). A Scanning Electron Microscopy examination showed that increasing the times of demineralization resulted in a smoother surface of the dentin particles and a higher number of dentinal tubules.

Murzakhanov et al. [18] presented the results of a study of radiation-induced defects in various synthetic calcium phosphate powder materials (hydroxyapatite and octacalcium phosphate) by electron paramagnetic resonance spectroscopy at the X, Q, and W-bands (9, 34, and 95 GHz for the microwave frequencies, respectively). It was shown that in addition to the classical electron paramagnetic resonance techniques, other experimental approaches such as ELDOR-detected NMR, electron spin echo envelope modulation, and electron–nuclear double resonance can be used to analyze the electron–nuclear interactions of CP powders.

Finally, Kim et al. [19] stated that when the root of an impacted inferior third molar is impacted in the lingual cortical plate, a periapical band-like radiolucent sign may appear in the orthopantomography image. This could be useful for the prediction of root position and surgical risks.

Although submissions for this Special Issue have been closed, more in-depth research in the field is being collected in a new Special Issue: "Dental Materials: Latest Advances and Prospects–Volume II" (https://www.mdpi.com/journal/applsci/special_issues/Advanced_Dental_Materials_II).

Funding: This research received no external funding.

Acknowledgments: Thanks to all the authors and peer reviewers for their valuable contributions to this Special Issue "Dental Materials: Latest Advances and Prospects". I would also like to express my gratitude to all the staff and people involved in this Special Issue.

Conflicts of Interest: The author declares no conflict of interest.

References

1. Murri Dello Diago, A.; Cadenaro, M.; Ricchiuto, R.; Banchelli, F.; Spinas, E.; Checchi, V.; Giannetti, L. Hypersensitivity in Molar Incisor Hypomineralization: Superficial Infiltration Treatment. *Appl. Sci.* **2021**, *11*, 1823. [CrossRef]
2. Lehmann, A.; Nijakowski, K.; Nowakowska, M.; Woś, P.; Misiaszek, M.; Surdacka, A. Influence of Selected Restorative Materials on the Environmental pH: In Vitro Comparative Study. *Appl. Sci.* **2021**, *11*, 11975. [CrossRef]
3. Chisnoiu, A.M.; Moldovan, M.; Sarosi, C.; Chisnoiu, R.M.; Rotaru, D.I.; Delean, A.G.; Pastrav, O.; Muntean, A.; Petean, I.; Tudoran, L.B.; et al. Marginal Adaptation Assessment for Two Composite Layering Techniques Using Dye Penetration, AFM, SEM and FTIR: An In-Vitro Comparative Study. *Appl. Sci.* **2021**, *11*, 5657. [CrossRef]
4. Liang, S.; Ye, H.; Yuan, F. Changes in Crystal Phase, Morphology, and Flexural Strength of As-Sintered Translucent Monolithic Zirconia Ceramic Modified by Femtosecond Laser. *Appl. Sci.* **2021**, *11*, 6925. [CrossRef]

5. Tobar, C.; Rodríguez, V.; Lopez-Suarez, C.; Peláez, J.; Brinckmann, J.C.-B.; Suárez, M.J. Effect of Digital Technologies on the Marginal Accuracy of Conventional and Cantilever Co–Cr Posterior-Fixed Partial Dentures Frameworks. *Appl. Sci.* **2021**, *11*, 2988. [CrossRef]
6. Generali, L.; Cavani, F.; Franceschetti, F.; Sassatelli, P.; Giardino, L.; Pirani, C.; Iacono, F.; Bertoldi, C.; Angerame, D.; Checchi, V.; et al. Calcium Hydroxide Removal Using Four Different Irrigation Systems: A Quantitative Evaluation by Scanning Electron Microscopy. *Appl. Sci.* **2022**, *12*, 271. [CrossRef]
7. Moreinos, D.; Wigler, R.; Geffen, Y.; Akrish, S.; Lin, S. Healing Capacity of Bone Surrounding Biofilm-Infected and Non-Infected Gutta-Percha: A Study of Rat Calvaria. *Appl. Sci.* **2021**, *11*, 6710. [CrossRef]
8. Solomon, S.-M.; Sufaru, I.-G.; Teslaru, S.; Ghiciuc, C.M.; Stafie, C.S. Finding the Perfect Membrane: Current Knowledge on Barrier Membranes in Regenerative Procedures: A Descriptive Review. *Appl. Sci.* **2022**, *12*, 1042. [CrossRef]
9. De Angelis, N.; Solimei, L.; Pasquale, C.; Alvito, L.; Lagazzo, A.; Barberis, F. Mechanical Properties and Corrosion Resistance of TiAl6V4 Alloy Produced with SLM Technique and Used for Customized Mesh in Bone Augmentations. *Appl. Sci.* **2021**, *11*, 5622. [CrossRef]
10. Kim, J.-S.; Jang, T.-S.; Kim, S.-Y.; Lee, W.-P. Octacalcium Phosphate Bone Substitute (Bontree®): From Basic Research to Clinical Case Study. *Appl. Sci.* **2021**, *11*, 7921. [CrossRef]
11. Sanchez-Perez, A.; Cano-Millá, N.; Moya Villaescusa, M.J.; Montoya Carralero, J.M.; Navarro Cuellar, C. Effect of Photofunctionalization with 6 W or 85 W UVC on the Degree of Wettability of RBM Titanium in Relation to the Irradiation Time. *Appl. Sci.* **2021**, *11*, 5427. [CrossRef]
12. van der Schoor, P.; Schlee, M.; Wen, H.-B. Prospective Pilot Study of Immediately Provisionalized Restorations of Trabecular Metal-Enhanced Titanium Dental Implants: A 5-Year Follow-Up Report. *Appl. Sci.* **2022**, *12*, 942. [CrossRef]
13. Bucur, S.-M.; Vaida, L.L.; Olteanu, C.D.; Checchi, V. A Brief Review on Micro-Implants and Their Use in Orthodontics and Dentofacial Orthopaedics. *Appl. Sci.* **2021**, *11*, 10719. [CrossRef]
14. Ito, A.; Kitaura, H.; Sugisawa, H.; Noguchi, T.; Ohori, F.; Mizoguchi, I. Titanium Nitride Plating Reduces Nickel Ion Release from Orthodontic Wire. *Appl. Sci.* **2021**, *11*, 9745. [CrossRef]
15. Bucur, S.M.; Bud, A.; Gligor, A.; Vlasa, A.; Cocoș, D.I.; Bud, E.S. Observational Study Regarding Two Bonding Systems and the Challenges of Their Use in Orthodontics: An In Vitro Evaluation. *Appl. Sci.* **2021**, *11*, 7091. [CrossRef]
16. Farronato, M.; Farronato, D.; Inchingolo, F.; Grassi, L.; Lanteri, V.; Maspero, C. Evaluation of Dental Surface after De-Bonding Orthodontic Bracket Bonded with a Novel Fluorescent Composite: In Vitro Comparative Study. *Appl. Sci.* **2021**, *11*, 6354. [CrossRef]
17. Memè, L.; Strappa, E.M.; Monterubbianesi, R.; Bambini, F.; Mummolo, S. SEM and FT-MIR Analysis of Human Demineralized Dentin Matrix: An In Vitro Study. *Appl. Sci.* **2022**, *12*, 1480. [CrossRef]
18. Murzakhanov, F.F.; Grishin, P.O.; Goldberg, M.A.; Yavkin, B.V.; Mamin, G.V.; Orlinskii, S.B.; Fedotov, A.Y.; Petrakova, N.V.; Antuzevics, A.; Gafurov, M.R.; et al. Radiation-Induced Stable Radicals in Calcium Phosphates: Results of Multifrequency EPR, EDNMR, ESEEM, and ENDOR Studies. *Appl. Sci.* **2021**, *11*, 7727. [CrossRef]
19. Kim, Y.-S.; Park, Y.-M.; Cosola, S.; Riad, A.; Giammarinaro, E.; Covani, U.; Marconcini, S. Retrospective Analysis on Inferior Third Molar Position by Means of Orthopantomography or CBCT: Periapical Band-Like Radiolucent Sign. *Appl. Sci.* **2021**, *11*, 6389. [CrossRef]

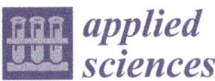

Article

Hypersensitivity in Molar Incisor Hypomineralization: Superficial Infiltration Treatment

Alberto Murri Dello Diago [1,*], Milena Cadenaro [2], Rossana Ricchiuto [1], Federico Banchelli [1], Enrico Spinas [3], Vittorio Checchi [1] and Luca Giannetti [1]

[1] Department of Surgery, Medicine, Dentistry and Morphological Sciences related to Transplant, Oncology and Regenerative Medicine, University of Modena and Reggio Emilia, 41125 Modena, Italy; rossana.ricchiuto@gmail.com (R.R.); federico.banchelli@unimore.it (F.B.); vittorio.checchi@unimore.it (V.C.); luca.giannetti@unimore.it (L.G.)
[2] Institute for Maternal and Child Health-IRCCS "Burlo Garofolo", University of Trieste, 34137 Trieste, Italy; mcadenaro@units.it
[3] Department of Surgical Sciences, University of Cagliari, 09124 Cagliari, Italy; enricospinas@tiscali.it
* Correspondence: alberto.murridellodiago@gmail.com; Tel.: +393-288-288-121

Abstract: To date, there are no standardized protocols available in the literature for hypersensitivity treatment in molar incisor hypomineralization (MIH) patients. The aim of this study was to evaluate the efficacy of erosion–infiltration treatments with resin in children with a strong hypersensitivity and also to develop a minimally invasive diagnostic–therapeutic pathway for young MIH patients. Patients with clinical signs of MIH were enrolled according to international guidelines. A total of 42 patients (8–14 years old) with sensitivity of at least one molar and patients with post eruptive enamel fractures, but without dentin involvement or cavitated carious lesions were selected. A single superficial infiltration treatment with ICON (DMG, Germany) was performed with a modified etching technique. Sensitivity was tested with the Schiff Scale and Wong Baker Face Scale and was repeated at 12 months follow-up. All patients reported lower sensitivity values at the end of the treatment. Significant differences of sensitivity according to the Schiff scale were reported between T0 and all subsequent follow-ups, $p < 0.05$. The treatment of erosion infiltration with ICON resin is a minimally invasive preventive treatment that significantly improves the problem of hypersensitivity in permanent molars with MIH.

Keywords: MIH; hypersensitivity; enamel infiltration; hypomineralization

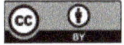

1. Introduction

In 2001, Weerheijm proposed the term molar incisor hypomineralization (MIH) to define a qualitative defect of the enamel from a systemic origin, which can affect 1 to all 4 of the permanent molars and can also involve the permanent incisors [1].

The prevalence of different MIH defects varies according to geographical areas, from 2.4% to 44% [2–4]. Clinically, tooth enamel affected by MIH is hypomineralized and opaque with a porous appearance and it is either white, yellow or brown in color [5–7].

In studies conducted with a polarized light microscope [8–11], the enamel defect appeared so porous that immediately after tooth eruption fractures or cracks under the action of masticatory forces (post-eruptive enamel breakdown-PEB) could occur [12].

The different composition of the enamel affected by MIH and its altered crystalline structure are the cause of the main clinical issues reported by the affected patients. The high hypersensitivity of these elements is therefore the reason for the poor quality of life during the daily oral maintenance procedures and during the consumption of food and cold drinks.

The treatment of teeth affected by MIH should be a minimally invasive procedure that aims to protect, strengthen and preserve dental structure. Numerous therapeutic alternatives have been proposed over time for the treatment of MIH-affected teeth [13,14], but the clinical management of these conditions is very demanding and difficult to learn for generic dentists, who often adopt less conservative treatments [15].

The scientific community exclusively proposes non-specific treatments based on fluoride and/or casein mineralizers or desensitizing pastes, in order to reduce hypersensitivity [16,17]. However, there are no studies available defining guidelines for this condition.

The aim of this study is to propose a precise and standardized protocol for the improvement of hypersensitivity in patients with MIH through a superficial resin infiltration technique.

2. Materials and Methods

This study was approved by the Ethics Committee of the Area Vasta Emilia Nord, Emilia Romagna, Italy (EC Prot. # 307/2018/OSS/AOUMO).

All patients' parents/legal guardians read and signed an informed consent for participation in the study and authorization for treatment.

Sixty-seven pediatric patients (6 to 14 years old) were selected from the Department of Pediatric Dentistry, University of Modena and Reggio Emilia. The recruitment period lasted 3 months. Patients were assessed by a dental expert in restorative treatments (A.M.D.D.) and subjects who presented visual enamel defects of permanent molars due to MIH, according to the diagnostic criteria proposed by the European Academy of Pediatric Dentistry (EAPD) in 2010 [18], were considered for study inclusion. Patients with sensitivity of at least one of the molars affected by MIH, or with post eruptive enamel fractures, but without dentin involvement or cavitated carious lesions were approached (Figure 1).

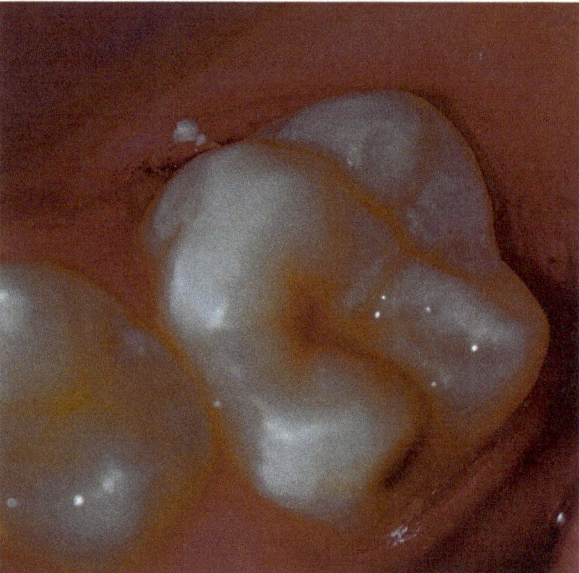

Figure 1. Clinical view of enamel defects of permanent molars due to molar incisor hypomineralization (MIH).

Bitewing examinations were performed to exclude interproximal carious lesions. Twenty-five patients were excluded due to lesions with dentin involvement or cavitated and interproximal caries.

The patient was asked to respond to a questionnaire regarding the selected tooth's sensitivity, both prior to and following the treatment. The patients' parents or legal guardians were asked to respond to questions regarding time of gestation, maternal health during gestation, child's weight at delivery, complications during childbirth, diseases in early childhood, breastfeeding, antibiotics assumption during the first two years of life, administration of fluoride-based tablets, and family history of MIH. All information was recorded by an operator and stored in a dedicated database.

Before treatment, the following parameters were recorded into a dedicated Excel spreadsheet: plaque accumulation evaluated by the full mouth plaque score (FMPS) [19], periodontal status with the Löe and Silness gingival index (GI) [20], and bleeding on probing (BoP) with the caton bleeding score [21].

Sensitivity was determined by the examiner using the Schiff cold air sensitivity scale (SCASS), measured by responses to a thermal, cold air jet stimulus (0 = subject does not respond to stimulus, 3 = subject responds to stimulus, considers stimulus to be painful, and requests discontinuation of the stimulus) [22]. Sensitivity to tactile stimulation (during oral hygiene and eating ice cream) with patients' response to the intensity of pain was registered according to the Wong–Baker faces scale (WBFS) for pediatric patients (0 = no pain, 10 = intense pain) [23].

All measurements of clinical parameters were repeated at baseline (T0), immediately after treatment (T1), one week (T2), one month (T3), and twelve months (T4) after treatment.

The superficial infiltration technique was performed with ICON (DMG, Hamburg, Germany) [14,24,25], an infiltration system that appears to be extremally useful in the treatment of initial caries and enamel alterations. Manufacturer instructions were followed, with the exception of the etching phase, and carried out with orthophosphoric acid rather than with hydrochloric acid, given the greater porosity of the tissue and the high hypersensitivity of the patient. This technique allows, after an initial erosion phase of the most superficial enamel layer, to infiltrate the porosity system of the defect with a low viscosity resin. The procedure included no anesthesia, rubber dam isolation followed by affected tooth cleaning and removal of any cleaning residue with water spray, 30 s of etching with 37% orthophosphoric acid, 30 s of drying with Icon Dry, 3 min of infiltration with Icon Infiltration, and 40 s of light curing. The application of Icon Infiltration should be repeated for 1 min, followed by 40 s of light curing and final polishing.

At each follow-up visit, an objective examination was carried out to assess plaque accumulation and gingival status. The patient was then asked to assign a value from 0 to 10 on the WBFS scale representative of sensitivity, and the operator repeated the Schiff test.

Data were evaluated and expressed as absolute frequencies and percentages, based on the numerical or categorical nature of the variables. Furthermore, a comparative assessment was made between the "post" data and the "pre" data, for each post-intervention time-point, using statistical inferential tests for paired data (Wilcoxon signed-rank test or similar, after evaluation of the distribution of data), with 95% confidence level.

3. Results

A total of 42 patients were recruited into the study; 22 females and 20 males, aged between 8 and 14 years old. They all presented only one tooth with sensitivity; therefore, there was no need to choose between more than one sensitive tooth to be included into the study. No patients have been lost at the 12 months follow-up recall.

Most of the patients (51%) had been treated with antibiotic treatment during the first few months of life due to respiratory problems. Moreover, 76% were born prematurely and/or had problems during childbirth.

Considering the pre-treatment questionnaires completed by the patients' parents/legal guardians, the possible etiological relationship proposed in the literature is confirmed (Table 1).

Table 1. Pre-treatment questionnaires on etiological causes.

Etiology Causes	
Born prematurely/problem during childbirth	76%
Fluoride intake	13%
Asthma	28.60%
Bronchitis	33.40%
Pneumonia	15%
Respiratory tract infections	31.90%
Celiac disease	26%

All inflammation indices were not repeated immediately after treatment (T1) as they were not different from T0. The inflammation index drastically reduced following a decreasing trend from the first follow-up. Oral hygiene significantly improved with the absence of plaque in 85.7% of patients after 12 months of treatment, with a disappearance of gingival inflammation in 81% of cases. Gingival bleeding persisted only in two patients at all controls, while the remaining 40 showed negative BoP.

The Wong–Baker faces scale during daily hygiene (Figure 2) recorded between 4 and 6 at T0 in 81% of cases, and between 0 and 2 after 12 months in all patients showing a 100% improvement.

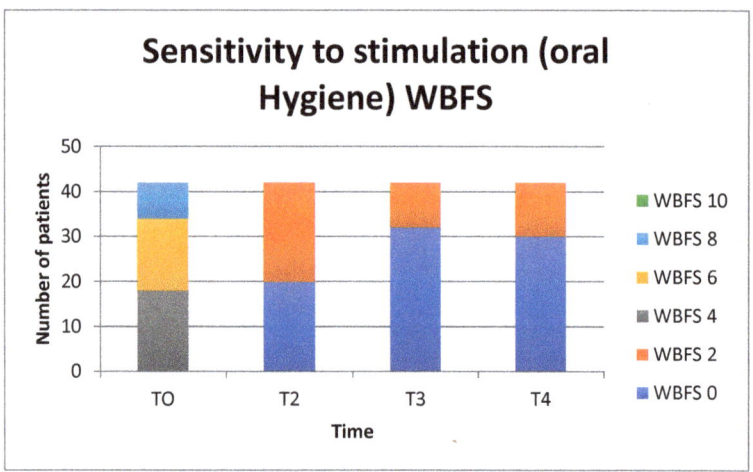

Figure 2. Wong–Baker faces scale (WBFS) sensitivity test to oral hygiene stimulation.

The face scale, referring to the consumption of ice cream (Figure 3), recorded values at T0 of up to 10 in 14% of cases and 8 in 38%; at T4 only two children continued to record a value of 4, while all the others indicated scores of 0–2, with a 95% improvement.

Significant differences of sensitivity according to the SCASS scale (Figure 4) were reported between T0 and all subsequent follow-ups, $p < 0.05$.

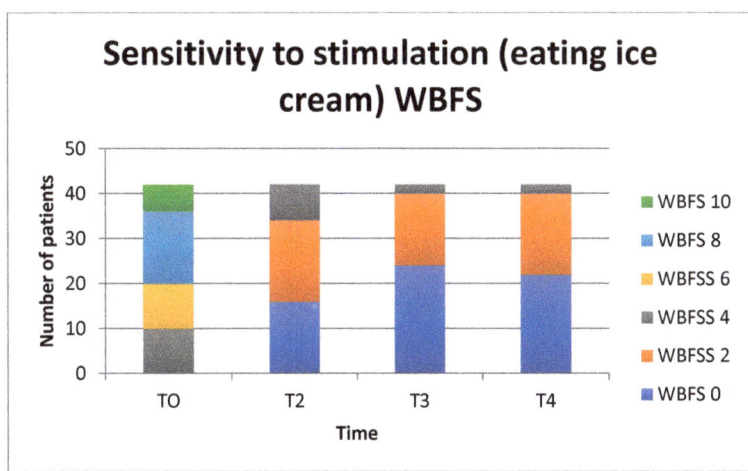

Figure 3. WBFS sensitivity test eating ice cream.

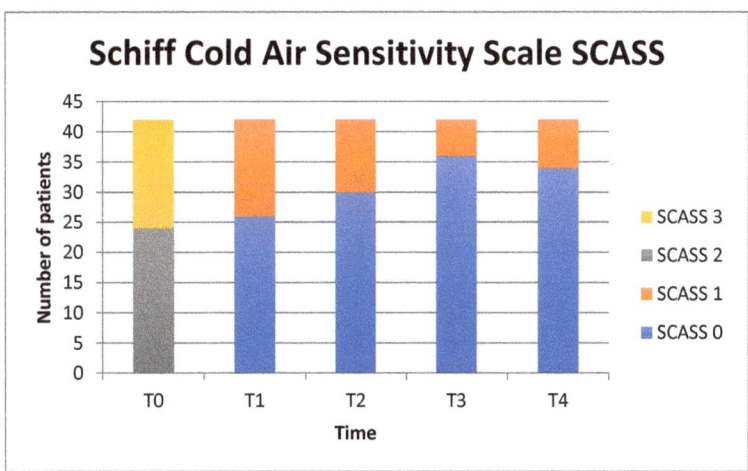

Figure 4. SCASS sensitivity test.

4. Discussion

The aim of MIH treatment is to protect, strengthen and preserve the tooth structure when not previously compromised by post eruptive fractures and/or carious lesions. When the pathological scenario is complicated by hypersensitivity to thermal stimuli, the first form of prevention by the clinician is to alleviate the hypersensitivity, in order to facilitate better oral hygiene and reduce the risk of dental caries as much as possible. The choice of preventive treatment is not univocal and the most recent literature examines the use of remineralizers [26]. According to Restrepo, it is evident that the topical application of fluoride varnish does not improve enamel remineralization with MIH and does not consider hypersensitivity [27]. A very recent paper on the use of Casein phosphopeptide-amorphous calcium phosphate nanocomplex (CPP-ACP), an optimal remineralizing and anti-cariogen agent, for the treatment of MIH teeth showed to be effective and safe in bleaching teeth with enamel white opacities but didn't provide significant data regarding hypersensitivity [28]. Ozgul instead published encouraging results on the treatment of hypersensitivity with casein, but with a short follow-up [16]. In a research by Pasini et al., a positive follow-up at 120 days was reported in patients with MIH molar hypersensitivity treated with casein, but the described procedure required repeated applications [29].

Recently a new desensitizing paste has been developed, based on Pro-Argin technology, made of 8% arginine and calcium carbonate for the treatment of dentinal hypersensitivity. Bekes et al. tested sensitivity after 8 weeks of application, but the results did not favor the product with scientific evidence [17]. The data report an improvement of the mechanical characteristics of the enamel of anterior teeth with MIH after the application of a resin infiltration system, suggesting that this technique could be a valid alternative for hypersensitivity to thermal stimuli due to occlusion of porosity [30,31].

The results of this study are important preliminary data to define a new minimally invasive approach protocol for permanent molars with hypersensitivity. This study shows a significant reduction in hypersensitivity in MIH molars already after one single infiltration with resin. The proposed protocol foresees a single application of resin infiltration, and the reported results do not contradict its effectiveness even in daily home hygiene procedures or during the consumption of cold foods [31].

Sensitivity decreased drastically immediately after the treatment and the improvement trend in the following months suggests a stabilization of the resin within the inter-prismatic gaps, even under the action of the masticatory load.

In all patients, an improvement in the SCASS value was obtained compared to that registered before the treatment. The hypothesis is that having started from very high sensitivity values, they also experience minimal sensory changes that will stabilize over time. In only six patients the stimulus was still perceived after one month, but not as painful as prior to treatment.

Questionnaires of patient treatment evaluation revealed a 100% patient satisfaction.

5. Conclusions

The study conducted, despite the small number of patients, provides useful and statistically significant preliminary data. Larger studies with extended follow-up will be useful for reinforcing these results. Furthermore, this non-invasive treatment could be repeated in patients with persistent sensitivity stimulus, and its efficacy should be investigated.

Author Contributions: Conceptualization, M.C. and L.G.; methodology, A.M.D.D. and R.R.; validation, E.S., V.C. and L.G.; formal analysis, E.S. and A.M.D.D.; investigation, A.M.D.D., R.R. and F.B.; data curation, F.B.; writing—original draft preparation, A.M.D.D., R.R. and F.B.; writing—review and editing, M.C., E.S., V.C. and L.G.; visualization, M.C. and V.C.; supervision, E.S. and L.G.; project administration, A.M.D.D. and L.G. All authors have read and agreed to the published version of the manuscript.

Funding: This research received no external funding.

Institutional Review Board Statement: The study was conducted according to the guidelines of the Declaration of Helsinki, and approved by the Ethics Committee of the Area Vasta Emilia Nord, Emilia Romagna, Italy (EC Prot. # 307/2018/OSS/AOUMO).

Conflicts of Interest: The authors declare no conflict of interest.

References

1. Weerhrijm, K. Molar Incisor Hypomineralisation (MIH). *Eur. J. Paediatr. Dent.* **2003**, *3*, 114–120.
2. Tirlet, G.; Chabouis, H.F.; Attal, J.P. Infiltration, a new therapy for masking enamel white spots: A 19- month follow-up case series. *Eur. J. Esthet. Dent.* **2013**, *8*, 180–190. [PubMed]
3. Steffen, R.; Krämer, N.; Bekes, K. The Würzburg MIH concept: The MIH treatment need index (MIH TNI): A new index to assess and plan treatment in patients with molar incisior hypomineralisation (MIH). *Eur. Arch. Paediatr. Dent.* **2017**, *18*, 355–361. [CrossRef] [PubMed]
4. Hartsock, L.A.; Burnheimer, J.; Modesto, A.; Vieira, A.R. A Snapshot of the Prevalence of Molar Incisor Hypomineralization and Fluorosis in Pittsburgh, Pennsylvania, USA. *Pediatr. Dent.* **2020**, *42*, 36–40. [PubMed]
5. Jälevik, B. Prevalence and Diagnosis of Molar-Incisor-Hypomineralisation (MIH): A systematic review. *Eur. Arch. Paediatr. Dent.* **2010**, *11*, 59–64. [CrossRef]

6. Jälevik, B.; Norén, J.G. Enamel hypomineralization of permanent first molars: A morphological study and survey of possible aetiological factors. *Int. J. Paediatr. Dent.* **2000**, *10*, 278–289. [CrossRef]
7. Apponi, R.; Presti, S.; Spinas, E.; Giannetti, L. Biological genetic and aetiology aspects in molar incisor hypomineralization. *J. Biol. Regul. Homeost. Agents* **2020**, *34*, 1219–1222.
8. Da Costa-Silva, C.M.; Ambrosano, G.M.; Jeremias, F.; De Souza, J.F.; Mialhe, F.L. Increase in severity of molar- incisor hypomineralization and its relationship with the colour of enamel opacity: A prospective cohort study. *Int. J. Paediatr. Dent.* **2011**, *21*, 333–341. [CrossRef]
9. Denis, M.; Atlan, A.; Vennat, E.; Tirlet, G.; Attal, J.P. White defects on enamel: Diagnosis and anatomopathology: Two essential factors for proper treatment (part 1). *Int. Orthod.* **2013**, *11*, 139–165. [CrossRef]
10. Farah, R.A.; Monk, B.C.; Swain, M.V.; Drummond, B.K. Protein content of molar-incisor hypomineralisation enamel. *J. Dent.* **2010**, *38*, 591–596. [CrossRef]
11. Crombie, F.A.; Manton, D.J.; Palamara, J.E.; Zalizniak, I.; Cochrane, N.J.; Reynolds, E.C. Characterisation of developmentally hypomineralised human enamel. *J. Dent.* **2013**, *41*, 611–618. [CrossRef]
12. Bullio Fragelli, C.M.; Jeremias, F.; Feltrin de Souza, J.; Paschoal, M.A.; de Cássia Loiola Cordeiro, R.; Santos-Pinto, L. Longitudinal Evaluation of the Structural Integrity of Teeth Affected by Molar Incisor Hypomineralisation. *Caries Res.* **2015**, *49*, 378–383. [CrossRef]
13. Giannetti, L.; Murri Dello Diago, A.; Corciolani, E.; Spinas, E. Deep infiltration for the treatment of hypomineralized enamel lesions in a patient with molar incisor hypomineralization: A clinical case. *J. Biol. Regul. Homeost. Agents* **2018**, *32*, 751–754.
14. Giannetti, L.; Murri Dello Diago, A.; Silingardi, G.; Spinas, E. Superficial infiltration to treat white hypomineralized defects of enamel: Clinical trial with 12-month follow-up. *J. Biol. Regul. Homeost. Agents* **2018**, *32*, 1335–1338. [PubMed]
15. Giannetti, L.; Bartoli, G.; Banchelli, F.; Spinas, E.; Murri Dello Diago, A. MIH: A survey amongst dental practitioners in Modena and Reggio Emilia districts. *Dent. Cadmos* **2018**, *86*, 172–180. [CrossRef]
16. Ozgül, B.M.; Saat, S.; Sönmez, H.; Oz, F.T. Clinical evaluation of desensitizing treatment for incisor teeth affected by molar-incisor hypomineralization. *J. Clin. Pediatr. Dent.* **2013**, *38*, 101–105. [CrossRef] [PubMed]
17. Bekes, K.; Heinzelmann, K.; Lettner, S.; Schaller, H.G. Efficacy of desensitizing products containing 8% arginine and calcium carbonate for hypersensitivity relief in MIH-affected molars: An 8-week clinical study. *Clin. Oral. Investig.* **2017**, *21*, 2311–2317. [CrossRef]
18. Lygidakis, N.A.; Wong, F.; Jälevik, B.; Vierrou, A.M.; Alaluusua, S.; Espelid, I. Best Clinical Practice Guidance for clinicians dealing with children presenting with Molar-Incisor-Hypomineralisation (MIH). *Eur. Arch. Paediatr. Dent.* **2010**, *11*, 75–81. [CrossRef] [PubMed]
19. Bentley, C.D.; Disney, J.A. A comparison of partial and full mouth scoring of plaque and gingivitis in oral hygiene studies. *J. Clin. Periodontol.* **1995**, *22*, 131–135. [CrossRef]
20. Loe, H.; Silness, J. Periodontal disease in pregnancy I. Prevalence and severity. *Acta Odontol. Scand.* **1963**, *21*, 533–551. [CrossRef] [PubMed]
21. O'Leary, T.J.; Drake, R.B.; Naylor, J.E. The plaque control record. *J. Periodontol.* **1972**, *43*, 38. [CrossRef]
22. Schiff, T.; Delgado, E.; Zhang, Y.P.; Cummins, D.; De Vizio, W.; Mateo, L.R. Clinical evaluation of the efficacy of an in-office desensitizing paste containing 8% arginine and calcium carbonate in providing instant and lasting relief of dentin hypersensitivity. *Am. J. Dent.* **2009**, *22*, 8a–15a. [PubMed]
23. Wong, D.L.; Baker, C.M. Pain in children: Comparison of assessment scales. *Pediatr. Nurs.* **1988**, *14*, 9–17. [PubMed]
24. Attal, J.P.; Atlan, A.; Denis, M.; Vennat, E.; Tirlet, G. White spots on enamel: Treatment protocol by superficial or deep infiltration (part 2). *Int. Orthod.* **2014**, *12*, 1–31. [CrossRef]
25. Jia, L.; Stawarczyk, B.; Schmidlin, P.R.; Attin, T.; Wiegand, A. Effect of caries infiltrant application on shear bond strength of different adhesive systems to sound and demineralized enamel. *J. Adhes. Dent.* **2012**, *14*, 569–574. [PubMed]
26. Ghanim, A.; Silva, M.J.; Elfrink, M.E.C.; Lygidakis, N.A.; Marino, R.J.; Weerheijm, K.L.; Manton, D.J. Molar incisor hypomineralisation (MIH) training manualfor clinical field surveys and practice. *Eur. Arch. Paediatr. Dent.* **2017**, *18*, 225–242. [CrossRef]
27. Restrepo, M.; Jeremias, F.; Santos-Pinto, L.; Cordeiro, R.C.; Zuanon, A.C. Effect of Fluoride Varnish on Enamel Remineralization in Anterior Teeth with Molar Incisor Hypomineralization. *J. Clin. Pediatr. Dent.* **2016**, *40*, 207–210. [CrossRef]
28. Mastroberardino, S.; Campus, G.; Strohmenger, L.; Villa, A.; Cagetti, M.G. An Innovative Approach to Treat Incisors Hypomineralization (MIH): A Combined Use of Casein Phosphopeptide- Amorphous Calcium Phosphate and Hydrogen Peroxide-A Case Report. *Case Rep. Dent.* **2012**, *2012*, 379593. [CrossRef] [PubMed]
29. Pasini, M.; Giuca, M.R.; Scatena, M.; Gatto, R.; Caruso, S. Molar incisor hypomineralization treatment with casein phosphopeptide and amorphous calcium phosphate in children. *Minerva Stomatol.* **2018**, *67*, 20–25. [PubMed]
30. Paris, S.; Schwendicke, F.; Seddig, S.; Müller, W.D.; Dörfer, C.; Meyer-Lueckel, H. Micro-hardness and mineral loss of enamel lesions after infiltration with various resins: Influence of infiltrant composition and application frequency in vitro. *J. Dent.* **2013**, *41*, 543–548. [CrossRef]
31. Taher, N.M.; Alkhamis, H.A.; Dowaidi, S.M. The influence of resin infiltration system on enamel microhardness and surface roughness: An in vitro study. *Saudi Dent. J.* **2012**, *24*, 79–84. [CrossRef] [PubMed]

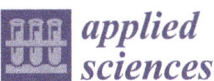

Article

Calcium Hydroxide Removal Using Four Different Irrigation Systems: A Quantitative Evaluation by Scanning Electron Microscopy

Luigi Generali [1,*], Francesco Cavani [2], Federico Franceschetti [1], Paolo Sassatelli [3], Luciano Giardino [4], Chiara Pirani [5], Francesco Iacono [5], Carlo Bertoldi [1], Daniele Angerame [6], Vittorio Checchi [1] and Eugenio Pedullà [7]

1. Department of Surgery, Medicine, Dentistry and Morphological Sciences with Transplant Surgery, Oncology and Regenerative Medicine Relevance (CHIMOMO), University of Modena and Reggio Emilia, 41124 Modena, Italy; federicofranceschetti.ita@gmail.com (F.F.); carlo.bertoldi@unimore.it (C.B.); vittorio.checchi@unimore.it (V.C.)
2. Section of Human Morphology, Department of Biomedical, Metabolic and Neural Science, University of Modena and Reggio Emilia, 41124 Modena, Italy; francesco.cavani@unimore.it
3. Product Engineer, Beckett Thermal Solution, 41043 Formigine, Italy; paolo.sassatelli@beckettthermal.com
4. Independent Researcher, 88900 Crotone, Italy; lucianogiardino057@gmail.com
5. Private Practice, 40122 Bologna, Italy; chiara.pirani4@unibo.it (C.P.); francesco.iacono@hotmail.it (F.I.)
6. Clinical Department of Medical, Surgical and Health Sciences, University of Trieste, 34149 Trieste, Italy; d.angerame@fmc.units.it
7. Department of General Surgery and Surgical-Medical Specialties, University of Catania, 95123 Catania, Italy; eugeniopedulla@gmail.com
* Correspondence: luigi.generali@unimore.it; Tel.: +39-059-4224324

Abstract: This study compares conventional endodontic needle irrigation, passive ultrasonic irrigation, apical negative pressure irrigation, and mechanical activation to remove calcium hydroxide from single straight root canals. Eighty-four mandibular premolars were prepared in a crown-down manner up to size #40. Two teeth represented a negative control, and another two served as a positive control. Calcium hydroxide paste was placed inside root canals. The remaining eighty samples were analyzed based on the activation techniques, and the cleanliness of the canals was quantified using Fiji's software on 500× magnified SEM backscattered electron micrographs. Considering the whole canal, all instruments showed better performance than conventional endodontic needle irrigation in removing calcium hydroxide ($p < 0.05$). Irrisafe and XP-endo Finisher could remove a significantly higher amount of calcium hydroxide than Endovac ($p < 0.05$). Irrisafe and XP-endo Finisher have been able to remove more calcium hydroxide than EndoVac.

Keywords: apical negative pressure irrigation; calcium hydroxide removal; intracanal medicament; mechanical activation; ultrasonic activation

1. Introduction

The prevention and eradication of bacteria from tooth cavities still represents one of the major concerns of root canal treatment. Among the materials proposed as intracanal medicament, calcium hydroxide ($Ca(OH)_2$) (CH) has been widely studied for its antimicrobial efficacy, and the benefits of its use are well documented [1–4]. On the other hand, the dressing material has to be removed entirely before root canal filling [5,6], since various research studies have shown that CH residues on dentin walls can compromise the canal seal by promoting micro-leakage between the sealer and gutta-percha, hindering the penetration of the sealer inside dentinal tubules and interacting with the setting of some sealers [7–9]. Moreover, different studies have identified an additional issue, which is the difficulty to completely remove CH from the apical third of the canals [7,10–12]. Despite the various protocols and techniques that have been proposed [13–16], studies have shown that instrumentation and irrigation are unable to clean completely the whole root canal system from CH [17,18]. The most commonly described root canal cleansing method is the use of a master apical file inserted until the working length (WL) and in conjunction with the abundant irrigation of sodium hypochlorite (NaOCl) and EDTA [19]. However, a recent review reported that the ultrasonic activation of irrigants seems more effective for removing CH than other techniques [9]. Kourti and Pantelidou [20] demonstrated that the use of the EndoVac (Kerr Endo, Orange County, CA, USA), an irrigation system using apical negative pressure that sucks the irrigants employing a microcannula placed at the WL, improved CH removal with respect to ultrasonic activation and conventional endodontic needle irrigation. Recently, XP-endo Finisher (FKG Dentaire SA, La Chaux de Fonds, Switzerland) has been developed to improve the efficacy of the final irrigation procedure. XP-endo Finisher exhibits a reduced core size (#25), zero taper, and the peculiar heat-treated NiTi alloy named MaxWire (Martensite-Austenite-electropolish-fileX) [21] that allows the instrument a great flexibility, leading to the removal of debris from hard-to-reach regions while limiting the damage on dentine at the same time. Moreover, the rotational movement can potentially produce agitation of the irrigant solutions, so it was suggested as a final step of disinfection procedures. The first published articles [22–24] confirmed the XP-endo Finisher's superior effectiveness in cleaning the dentin walls compared to the conventional technique.

This study was aimed to evaluate quantitatively the residual amount of CH, comparing the effect of four irrigation systems: conventional endodontic needle irrigation, Irrisafe (Satelec Acteon Group, Merignac, France), EndoVac and XP-endo Finisher, by means of scanning electron microscopy equipped with an environmental-dispersive X-ray detector (SEM-EDX). The null hypothesis tested was the absence of a difference in the amount of CH removal between the four different irrigation systems employed in root canal cleaning.

2. Materials and Methods

2.1. Root Canal Instrumentation

One hundred and forty-seven mandibular single-rooted premolars were withdrawn from a pool of extracted teeth. After radiographical examination of teeth in a mesiodistal and buccolingual direction, only teeth with a single straight canal were selected. Teeth with previous root canal treatment, calcifications, apical curvature, immature apices, or resorptions were discarded. A total of eighty-four teeth were included in the study. The specimens were stored in distilled water for no longer than 15 days before the experiment. The crowns were partially removed with a size 701 high-speed fissure bur (Komet Italia, Milano, Italy) under water irrigation to standardized root lengths at 18 mm. After access cavity preparation, a #10 K-file (Dentsply Maillefer, Ballaigues, Switzerland) was introduced into the canal until its tip emerged at the apical foramen, which was observed under a microscope at 10× magnification (OPMI PICO; Carl Zeiss Meditec Inc., Jena, Germany), and the WL was determined subtracting 1 mm from the measurement. To reproduce in vivo conditions, the apex was sealed with cyanoacrylate [25]. Each tooth was instrumented in a crown-down manner by using the ProTaper Gold rotary system (Dentsply Maillefer, Ballaigues, Switzerland) to size 40 at the WL. After each instrument change, the root canal was rinsed with 1 mL 5% of NaOCl (Niclor, Ogna, Muggiò, Italy) with a side vented needle (27-gauge) inserted on a syringe (Max-i-Probe, Dentsply Rinn, Elgin, IL, USA) introduced before the binding point but at a distance greater than 2 mm from the WL. The final rinse after instrumentation was performed with 1 mL 5% NaOCl and subsequently 1 mL 17% EDTA (Ogna), which were both left in place for 1 min, and with 5 mL of sterile water (Baxter, Roma, Italy) delivered with a 27-gauge side-vented needle (Max-i-Probe). Sterile paper points (ProTaper Gold paper points F4, Dentsply Maillefer, Ballaigues, Switzerland) were employed to dry the root canals. As a negative control, two teeth were used that did not undergo any further treatment. CH paste (Calxyl®, OCO präparate, Dirmstein, Germany) was placed inside root canals with a size #30 lentulo spiral (Dentsply Maillefer, Ballaigues, Switzerland) and sterile paper points. The access cavities were filled with cotton and a temporary filling material (Cavit, 3M ESPE, Seefeld, Germany). Two radiographs of all teeth were taken in mesiodistal and bucco-lingual directions to verify the complete filling of all canals with CH paste. The lingual and buccal surfaces were marked with a longitudinal groove each, that was made with a diamond disk without penetrating the canal to facilitate the subsequent split in two halves (Figure 1A). Then, the specimens were kept at 37 °C at 100% humidity for a month in a Heracell VIOS 250i incubator (Thermo Scientific, Waltham, MA, USA).

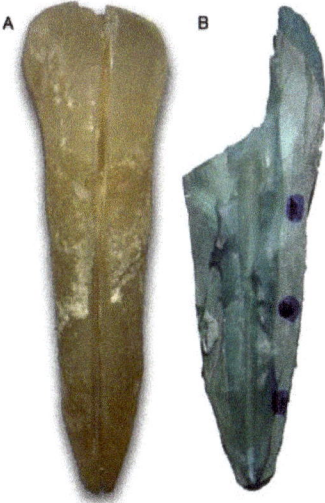

Figure 1. (**A**) Buccal surface with the longitudinal groove made with a diamond disk. (**B**) A split half of a sample ready for SEM analysis.

2.2. Retreatment Procedures

After removal of the temporary fillings, two teeth did not undergo any further treatment and were used as positive controls. The remaining eighty teeth were subdivided into four experimental groups (n = 20) according to the systems used: conventional endodontic needle irrigation group (CENI), Irrisafe group (IS), EndoVac group (EV), and XP-endo Finisher group (XPF). The specimens were fixed in a tube stand and placed in a thermostatic bath heated to 37 °C to simulate the body temperature. In all groups, a master apical file ProTaper Universal size 40 at WL was used to remove the CH, and then, different techniques were applied.

The subsequent irrigation steps were performed after leaving the samples in the thermostatic bath for at least 20 min.

In the CENI group, irrigation was performed with a syringe with a 27-gauge side-vented needle placed 2 mm from the WL with 3 mL of 5% NaOCl left in place for 60 s, which was followed by 3 mL of 17% EDTA for 60 s and 5 mL of sterile water. No additional agitation of irrigants was performed.

In the IS group, the same irrigation protocol as in the CENI group was used, but ultrasonic activation of NaOCl and EDTA were obtained with the P5 Newtron (Satelec) mounting a stainless steel non-cutting 25 tip (Irrisafe, Satelec), which was inserted 2 mm from the WL for 1 min for each irrigant.

NaOCl was delivered with the master delivery tip in the EV group and simultaneously aspirated by using the macrocannula for 30 s with an up-and-down movement from a point where it started to bind to a point just below the canal orifice. NaOCl was left in place for 60 s. After this, three cycles of microirrigation were performed by inserting the microcannula at the WL for 6 s, then at 2 mm from the WL for 6 s, and eventually at WL for another 6 s. This was done until a total of 30 s was reached for each cycle. At the end of cycles, the microcannula completely aspirated the irrigant from within the canal. The first and third cycles were performed by using 5% NaOCl, whereas the second cycle used 17% EDTA.

In the XPF group, the same irrigation protocol as in the CENI group was used, but NaOCl and EDTA were activated using the XP-endo Finisher file. The file, mounted on an endodontic motor (X-Smart Plus, Dentsply Maillefer, Tulsa, OK, USA) rotated at a speed of 800 rpm and 1 N cm torque, and it was cooled down with ethyl chloride (Crio Spray, Karl Sanremo, IM, Italy). The file was operated for 60 s with vertical movements of 7–8 mm to the WL to activate NaOCl and EDTA.

The same amount of irrigants was employed in all groups. Sterile paper points were used to dry all canals, and the roots were then split along their longitudinal axis into two halves with a small chisel and a hammer. Division in thirds (apical, middle, and coronal) was determined by marking the roots at 2, 5, and 11 mm from the apex, respectively (Figure 1B).

2.3. SEM-EDX Evaluation (Quantitative Analysis)

Split roots were mounted on aluminum stubs coated with 8–10 nm of gold and analyzed by SEM-EDX (Quanta 200, Fei Company, Eindhoven, Netherlands and INCA-350, Oxford instruments, Oxford, UK) in backscattered mode (BSE). Micrographs were acquired at various magnification from 60× to 15,000×. EDX microanalysis was applied to assess the chemical composition of the different phases visible in the SEM micrographs. To quantify the residual CH, image analysis was performed using Fiji's software (National Institute of Health, Bethesda, MD, USA). The analysis was performed on 500× magnified SEM backscattered electron (BSD) micrographs, exploiting the gray scale contrast generated by different chemical compositions of dentin and CH in BSE mode. The brightness and contrast of the micrographs were adjusted to highlight the difference between the phases, and a gray scale threshold limit was imposed to obtain a binary black and white image, as shown in Figure 2. From the binary image, the area fraction occupied by the white spots was calculated. This protocol was adapted from Conserva [26] and Deari [27].

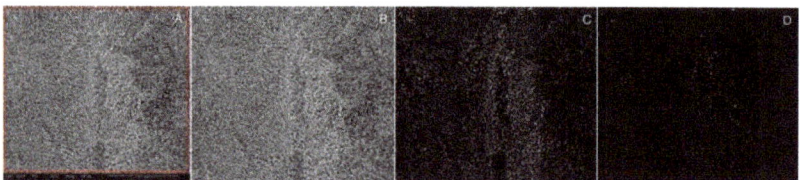

Figure 2. (**A**) Original SEM image where measures were performed; the red square shows where the image is cropped as seen in (**B**). (**C**) Enhancement of contrast highlighting white dots corresponding to CH particles, (**D**) image after binarization.

2.4. Statistical Analysis

STATA 11 (StataCorp LLC, College Station, TX, USA) software was used for statistical analysis. Values in tables are reported as the mean ± standard deviation (SD). Since most data did not follow a normal distribution, the Kruskal–Wallis test followed by the Dunn test were used to compare results among and within groups. A p-value < 0.05 was considered significant.

3. Results

Figure 3 shows a backscattered electron micrograph acquired into a CH-treated tooth canal at 15,000× magnification (Figure 3A) and the relative spot EDX spectra (Figure 3B). Based on the different gray shades of the particles visible in the micrographs and the relative results of the EDX microanalysis, two well-distinguishable phases may be identified. The darker phase, containing high amounts of Ca, P, and O, may be identified as the tooth dentin; the bright globular phase, containing mainly Ca, S, Ba, and O, may be identified as the CH paste remnants. The presence of barium sulfate ($BaSO_4$) in the CH paste, as reported in the safety data sheet of the Calxyl® radiopaque (OCO präparate GmbH, Dirmstein, Germany), added for its X-ray opacity properties, allows clearly distinguishing the CH paste residues in the BSE images, giving to the paste a much brighter contrast compared to the dentin.

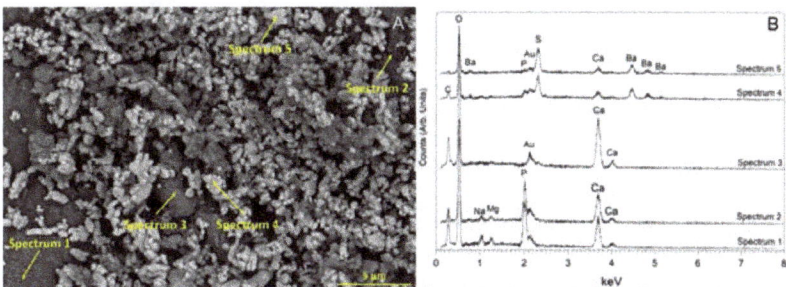

Figure 3. (**A**) SEM image showing the globular aspect of CH residues; arrows indicate the areas analyzed with EDX, (**B**) EDX spectra relative to areas indicated in (**A**).

Table 1 reports the average values of residual calcium hydroxide measured inside the root canal's selected areas according to instrument and level. The Kruskal–Wallis test shows significant differences among groups, both considering the individual levels and the whole root canal. Irrisafe and XP-endo Finisher performed significantly better at the coronal level than the conventional endodontic needle irrigation. Moreover, XP-endo Finisher performed better than Endovac at this level. All instruments removed a significantly higher amount of CH than conventional endodontic needle irrigation at the middle level; moreover, Irrisafe and XP-endo Finisher performed significantly better than Endovac. At the apical level, the amount of CH removed was significantly higher in the Irrisafe and XP-endo Finisher groups than conventional endodontic needle irrigation and Endovac irrigation.

Table 1. Calcium hydroxide residues % (mean ± SD) inside the root canal measured on SEM images.

	Groups				
	CENI	IS	EV	XPF	K-W p-Value
Coronal	4.83 ± 6.0 °	0.88 ± 0.7	2.56 ± 2.7 §	0.66 ± 0.7	0.002
Middle	4.91 ± 5.6 #	0.53 ± 0.9	1.40 ± 1.7 *	0.68 ± 1.1	<0.001
Apical	11.52 ± 8.8 °,+	0.35 ± 0.4	6.39 ± 11.0 *	2.30 ± 5.0	<0.001
Total	7.09 ± 5.9 #	0.59 ± 0.5	3.45 ± 4.6 *	1.21 ± 2.0	<0.001

* versus Irrisafe and XP-endo Finisher $p < 0.05$; § versus XP-endo Finisher $p < 0.05$; # versus Irrisafe, Endovac, and XP-endo Finisher $p < 0.05$; ° versus Irrisafe and XP-endo Finisher $p < 0.05$; + versus coronal and middle levels $p < 0.05$.

When the whole canal is considered, all instruments showed better performance than conventional endodontic needle irrigation in removing CH. Among the three techniques, Irrisafe and XP-endo Finisher were able to remove a significantly higher amount of CH than Endovac.

When results were compared within groups to measure the performance among the three levels of the root canal, the Kruskal–Wallis test highlighted significant differences only respecting the conventional endodontic needle irrigation. Compared to the middle and coronal root canal walls, more CH was detected at the apical level. Figure 4 shows an overview of representative SEM images from the experimental groups at 2, 5, and 11 mm levels.

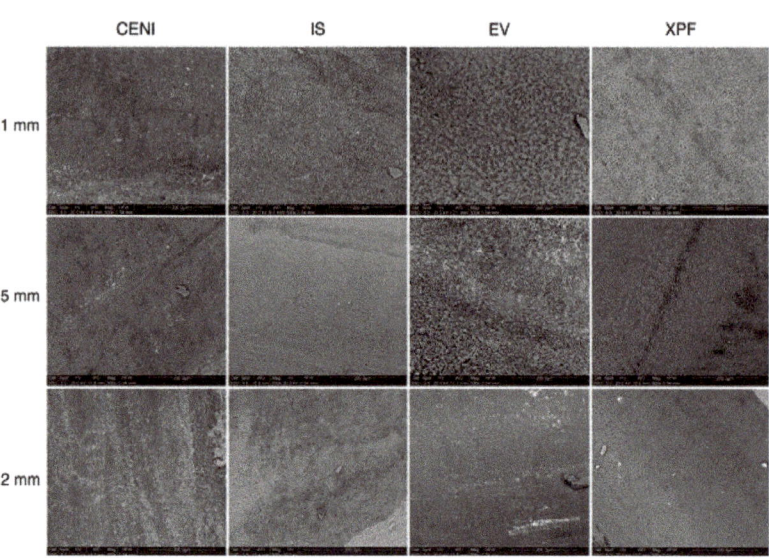

Figure 4. Representative SEM images of areas used for CH residues evaluation for each kind of treatment and root level from the apex.

4. Discussion

This study was designed to assess the ability of four irrigation systems to remove $Ca(OH)_2$ from root canals through a quantitative evaluation. CH paste is a widely used intracanal dressing during root canal therapy due to its alkalinity (pH 12.5) to reduce residual bacteria [4], but the presence of residues on dentin walls can prevent sealer penetration into dentinal tubules, thus compromising the endodontic seal and increasing apical leakage [8]. For the previously mentioned reasons, the intracanal dressings should be completely removed before permanent obturation of the root canal [24]. Many studies have been published regarding the removal of CH or other medicaments from the root canal system using other supplementary systems to the conventional irrigation [15,16,28–30]. The aim of this study was to compare Irrisafe, Endovac, and XP-endo Finisher efficacy with the conventional endodontic needle irrigation. One of the major strengths of the present investigation is represented by the quantitative evaluation performed through SEM images. Different methods have been used to measure residual material inside root canals, spanning from direct visualization to micro-CT, from digital microscopy to scanning electron microscopy [9,13,31]. In most of the cases, studies conducted by SEM analysis achieved a semi-quantitative evaluation. Other studies performed using the grooves model had several advantages with respect to studies investigating smooth root canals wall, because the scoring of the groove's cleanness is presumably more reproducible than the percentage assessment of the whole canal [30]. In this study, standardized grooves were not performed in the canals because a quantitative method was used that allowed measuring the total amount of CH left without visual evaluations by different examiners. In particular, a rectangular area of images was selected. Brightness and contrast were adapted to accentuate CH remnants. The threshold function was used to select the contrasted spots to obtain a binary black and white image, permitting accurately measuring the area of the white spots inside the area selected [26]. Moreover, one of the significant criticisms of the SEM investigation to evaluate the CH removal is the difficulty of discriminating between $Ca(OH)_2$ residues and the smear layer or dentin debris, since EDX spectroscopy analysis reveals Ca^{++} in both cases [9]. In the present study, this problem was overcome by using a Barium sulfate-doped paste of $Ca(OH)_2$. Barium sulfate, probably added by the manufacturer for its X-ray opacity properties, permitted the EDX analysis to perfectly distinguish CH remnants from the dentin debris. According to Silva [31], in the present study, it was decided to preserve the tooth crown as an irrigant reservoir during the endodontic procedures, preventing the same irrigants coronal leak during ultrasonic activation.

The main finding of this investigation was that Irrisafe, Endovac, and XP-endo finisher showed significantly better performance than the conventional endodontic needle irrigation when the whole canal was considered, regardless of the coronal, middle, and apical level. Among the three techniques, XP-endo Finisher and Irrisafe were able to remove a significantly higher amount of CH than Endovac. Altogether, the results suggest that the null hypothesis has to be rejected. In a recent study, XP-endo Finisher was less efficient than ultrasonic activation in the removal of CH from apical grooves [30]. These results are in contrast with the present findings probably because, in this study, the CH removal procedures were executed at 37 °C, and at this temperature, XP-endo Finisher inside the root canal changes shape becoming curved due to the transition from the martensitic state to austenitic state [21,30].

In a comparative study between Passive Ultrasonic Irrigation (PUI) and XP-endo Finisher, the specimens were placed in a controlled-temperature water bath at 37 °C, and the whole canals were analyzed. The XP-endo Finisher was significantly more effective in removing the CH medication in the apical third than PUI [29]. Contrary to the present study, the samples were decoronated, probably causing leakage of the irrigant during ultrasonic activation.

5. Conclusions

The systems investigated in this study were unable to completely remove CH from root canals. However, Irrisafe and XP-endo Finisher were significantly more efficient than EndoVac in the elimination of calcium hydroxide. Conventional endodontic needle irrigation (CENI) was considerably less efficient than the other three systems, especially at the apical level.

Author Contributions: Conceptualization, L.G. (Luigi Generali), F.C.; Data curation, F.I., D.A. and V.C.; methodology, L.G. (Luigi Generali), F.F., F.C. and L.G. (Luciano Giardino); software, P.S.; validation, E.P., L.G. (Luciano Giardino) and L.G. (Luigi Generali); formal analysis, L.G. (Luigi Generali), P.S., F.F. and V.C.; investigation, L.G. (Luigi Generali), C.P., D.A. and C.B., writing—original draft preparation, L.G. (Luigi Generali), F.C., F.I., V.C. and E.P.; writing—review and editing, E.P., F.I., C.P., C.B. All authors have read and agreed to the published version of the manuscript.

Funding: The research was funded from the FAR project (University of Modena and Reggio Emilia Funds for Research) entitled Microstructural and Mechanical investigation of Nickel-Titanium Endodontic instruments—MMiNTEndo.

Informed Consent Statement: Written informed consent has been obtained from the patients to collect teeth for scientific purposes.

Acknowledgments: The SEM microscope is available at the imaging facility (Centro Interdipartimentale Grandi Strumenti (CIGS) of the University of Modena and Reggio Emilia. We thank Mauro Zapparoli from CIGS for technical support.

Conflicts of Interest: The authors declare no conflict of interest.

References

1. Mohammadi, Z.; Dummer, P.M. Properties and applications of calcium hydroxide in endodontics and dental traumatology. *Int. Endod. J.* **2011**, *44*, 697–730. [CrossRef] [PubMed]
2. Lima, R.K.; Guerreiro-Tanomaru, J.M.; Faria-Júnior, N.B.; Tanomaru-Filho, M. Effectiveness of calcium hydroxide-based intracanal medicaments against Enterococcus faecalis. *Int. Endod. J.* **2012**, *45*, 311–316. [CrossRef]
3. Chockattu, S.J.; Deepak, B.S.; Goud, K.M. Comparison of anti-bacterial efficiency of ibuprofen, diclofenac, and calcium hydroxide against Enterococcus faecalis in an endodontic model: An in vitro study. *J. Conserv. Dent.* **2018**, *21*, 80–84. [CrossRef]
4. Govindaraju, L.; Jenarthanan, S.; Subramanyam, D.; Ajitha, P. Antibacterial activity of various intracanal medicament against enterococcus faecalis, streptococcus mutans and staphylococcus aureus: An in vitro study. *J. Pharm. Bioallied Sci.* **2021**, *13*, S157–S161. [CrossRef] [PubMed]

5. Türker, S.A.; Koçak, M.M.; Koçak, S.; Saglam, B.C. Comparison of calcium hydroxide removal by self—Adjusting file, EndoVac, and CanalBrush agitation techniques: An in vitro study. *J. Conserv. Dent.* **2013**, *16*, 439–443. [CrossRef] [PubMed]
6. Margi, P.; Karkala, V.K.; Nidhi, P.S.; Maitry, P.; Krushn, S.; Vinukonda, H.B.; Das, T.D. Efficacy of removal of calcium hydroxide medicament from root canals by endoactivator and endovac irrigation techniques: A systematic review of in vitro studies. *Contemp. Clin. Dent.* **2019**, *10*, 135–142. [CrossRef]
7. Ozyurek, E.U.; Erdogan, O.; Turker, S.A. Effect of calcium hydroxide dressing on the dentinal tubule ppenetration of 2 different root canal sealers: A confocal laser scanning microscopy study. *J. Endod.* **2018**, *44*, 1018–1023. [CrossRef] [PubMed]
8. Kim, S.K.; Kim, Y.O. Influence of calcium hydroxide intracanal medication on apical seal. *Int. Endod. J.* **2002**, *35*, 623–628. [CrossRef] [PubMed]
9. Yaylali, I.E.; Kececi, A.D.; Ureyen Kaya, B. Ultrasonically activated irrigation to remove calcium hydroxide from apical third of human root canal system: A systematic review of in vitro studies. *J. Endod.* **2015**, *41*, 1589–1599. [CrossRef]
10. Yu, D.C.; Schilder, H. Cleaning and shaping the apical third of a root canal system. *Gen. Dent.* **2001**, *49*, 266–270.
11. da Silva, J.M.; Andrade Junior, C.V.; Zaia, A.A.; Pessoa, O.F. Microscopic cleanliness evaluation of the apical root canal after using calcium hydroxide mixed with chlorhexidine, propylene glicol, or antibiotic paste. *Oral Surg. Oral Med. Oral Pathol. Oral Radiol. Endodontol.* **2011**, *111*, 260–264. [CrossRef]
12. Faria, G.; Kuga, M.C.; Ruy, A.C.; Aranda-Garcia, A.J.; Bonetti-Filho, I.; Guerreiro-Tanomaru, J.M.; Toledo Leonardo, R. The efficacy of the self-adjusting file and protaper for removal of calcium hydroxide from root canals. *J. Appl. Oral Sci.* **2013**, *21*, 346–350. [CrossRef]
13. Kenee, D.M.; Allemang, J.D.; Johnson, J.D.; Hellstein, J.; Nichol, B.K. A quantitative assessment of efficacy of various calcium hydroxide removal techniques. *J. Endod.* **2006**, *32*, 563–565. [CrossRef] [PubMed]
14. Rodig, T.; Vogel, S.; Zapf, A.; Hülsmann, M. Efficacy of different irrigants in the removal of calcium hydroxide from root canals. *Int. Endod. J.* **2010**, *43*, 519–527. [CrossRef] [PubMed]
15. Capar, I.; Ozcan, E.; Arslan, H.; Ertas, H.; Aydinbelge, H. Effect of different final irrigation methods on the removal of calcium hydroxide from an artificial standardized groove in the apical third of root canals. *J. Endod.* **2014**, *40*, 451–454. [CrossRef]
16. Arslan, H.; Akcay, M.; Capar, I.; Saygili, G.; Gok, T.; Ertas, H. An in vitro comparison of irrigation using photon-initiated photoacoustic streaming, ultrasonic, sonic and needle techniques in removing calcium hydroxide. *Int. Endod. J.* **2015**, *48*, 246–251. [CrossRef]
17. Haapasalo, M.; Shen, Y.; Qian, W.; Gao, Y. Irrigation in endodontics. *Dent. Clin. N. Am.* **2010**, *54*, 291–312. [CrossRef]
18. Paqué, F.; Balmer, M.; Attin, T.; Peters, O.A. Preparation of oval-shaped root canals in mandibular molars using nickel-titanium rotary instruments: A micro-computed tomography study. *J. Endod.* **2010**, *36*, 703–707. [CrossRef] [PubMed]
19. Lambrianidis, T.; Kosti, E.; Boutsioukis, C.; Mazinis, M. Removal efficacy of various calcium hydroxide/chlorhexidine medicaments from the root canal. *Int. Endod. J.* **2006**, *39*, 55–61. [CrossRef] [PubMed]
20. Kourti, E.; Pantelidou, O. Comparison of different agitation methods for the removal of calcium hydroxide from the root canal: Scanning electron microscopy study. *J. Conserv. Dent.* **2017**, *20*, 439–444. [CrossRef]
21. Zupanc, J.; Vahdat-Pajouh, N.; Schäfer, E. New thermomechanically treated NiTi alloy—A review. *Int. Endod. J.* **2018**, *51*, 1088–1103. [CrossRef] [PubMed]
22. Wigler, R.; Dvir, R.; Weisman, A.; Matalon, S.; Kfir, A. Efficacy of XP-endo finisher files in the removal of calcium hydroxide paste from artificial standardized grooves in the apical third of oval root canals. *Int. Endod. J.* **2017**, *50*, 700–705. [CrossRef]
23. Uygun, A.D.; Gündoğdu, E.C.; Arslan, H.; Ersoy, İ. Efficacy of XP-endo finisher and TRU Shape 3D conforming file compared to conventional and ultrasonic irrigation in removing calcium hydroxide. *Aust. Endod. J.* **2017**, *43*, 89–93. [CrossRef]
24. Keskin, C.; Sariyilmaz, E.; Sariyilmaz, Ö. Efficacy of XP-endo finisher file in removing calcium hydroxide from simulated internal resorption cavity. *J. Endod.* **2017**, *43*, 126–130. [CrossRef] [PubMed]
25. Giardino, L.; Cavani, F.; Generali, L. Sodium hypochlorite solution penetration into human dentin: A histochemical evaluation. *Int. Endod. J.* **2017**, *50*, 492–498. [CrossRef]
26. Conserva, E.; Generali, L.; Bandieri, A.; Cavani, F.; Borghi, F.; Consolo, U. Plaque accumulation on titanium disks with different surface treatments: An in vivo investigation. *Odontology* **2018**, *106*, 145–153. [CrossRef]
27. Deari, S.; Mohn, D.; Zehnder, M. Dentine decalcification and smear layer removal by different ethylenediaminetetraacetic acid and 1-hydroxyethane-1,1-diphosphonic acid species. *Int. Endod. J.* **2019**, *52*, 237–243. [CrossRef]
28. van der Sluis, L.W.; Wu, M.K.; Wesselink, P.R. The evaluation of removal of calcium hy- droxide paste from an artificial standardized groove in the apical root canal using different irrigation methods. *Int. Endod. J.* **2007**, *40*, 52–57. [CrossRef]
29. Hamdan, R.; Michetti, J.; Pinchon, D.; Diemer, F.; Georgelin-Gurgel, M. The XP-endo finisher for the removal of calcium hydroxide paste from root canals and from the apical third. *J. Clin. Exp. Dent.* **2017**, *9*, e855–e860. [CrossRef] [PubMed]

30. Donnermeyer, D.; Wyrsch, H.; Bürklein, S.; Schäfer, E. Removal of calcium hydroxide from artificial grooves in straight root canals: Sonic activation using EDDY versus passive ultrasonic irrigation and XPendo finisher. *J. Endod.* **2019**, *45*, 322–326. [CrossRef]
31. Silva, L.J.M.; Pessoa, O.F.; Teixeira, M.B.G.; Gouveia, C.H.; Braga, R.R. Micro-CT evaluation of calcium hydroxide removal through passive ultrasonic irrigation associated with or without an additional instrument. *Int. Endod. J.* **2015**, *48*, 768–773. [CrossRef] [PubMed]

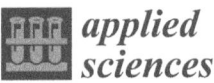

Review

A Brief Review on Micro-Implants and Their Use in Orthodontics and Dentofacial Orthopaedics

Sorana-Maria Bucur [1], Luminița Ligia Vaida [2,*], Cristian Doru Olteanu [3,*] and Vittorio Checchi [4]

1. Faculty of Medicine, Dimitrie Cantemir University of Târgu Mureș, 3-5 Bodoni Sandor Str., 540545 Târgu-Mureș, Romania; bucursoranamaria@gmail.com
2. Department of Dentistry, Faculty of Medicine and Pharmacy, University of Oradea, 1 Universității Str., 410087 Oradea, Romania
3. Faculty of Dental Medicine, Iuliu Hațieganu University of Medicine and Pharmacy, 8 Babeș Str., 400012 Cluj-Napoca, Romania
4. Department of Surgery, Medicine, Dentistry and Morphological Sciences Related to Transplant, Oncology and Regenerative Medicine, University of Modena and Reggio Emilia, 41125 Modena, Italy; vittorio.checchi@unimore.it
* Correspondence: ligia_vaida@yahoo.com (L.L.V.); cristidolteanu@yahoo.com (C.D.O.)

Abstract: The aim of this study was to review the literature and evaluate the failure rates and factors that affect the stability and success of temporary anchorage devices (TADs) used as orthodontic anchorage. Data was collected from electronic databases: MEDLINE database and Google Scholar. Four combinations of term were used as keywords: "micro-implant", "mini-implant", "mini-screw", and "orthodontics". The following selection criteria were used to select appropriate articles: articles on implants and screws used as orthodontic anchorage, published in English, with both prospective and retrospective clinical and experimental investigations. The search provided 209 abstracts about TADs used as anchorage. After reading and applying the selection criteria, 66 articles were included in the study. The data obtained were divided into two topics: which factors affected TAD success rate and to what degree and in how many articles they were quoted. Clinical factors were divided into three main groups: patient-related, implant related, and management-related factors. Although all articles included in this meta-analysis reported success rates of greater than 80 percent, the factors determining success rates were inconsistent between the studies analyzed and this made conclusions difficult.

Keywords: micro-implants; orthodontics; success rate; insertion; loading; biocompatibility; compliance

1. Introduction

Anchorage is one of the most important elements for successful orthodontic treatment. Traditionally, orthodontics employed teeth and extraoral or intraoral appliances for anchorage, often relying on the patient compliance for its effectiveness. Micro-implants (OMIs), also known in orthodontics as temporary anchorage devices (TAD) or mini-implants or mini-screws have been used to realize difficult orthodontic movements. Orthodontic mini-implants can be a powerful aid in resolving challenging malocclusions that require increased anchorage potential. Their use is versatile, minimally invasive, and proves a good ratio between costs and benefits of orthodontic treatments. They can help orthopedic dentofacial treatments by supporting distraction procedures, maxillary protractions, cleft segment expansion, stabilization, and tooth movements into narrow alveolar sites. Anchorage control is essential for an orthodontic treatment's success. The anchorage on micro-implants prevents undesirable movements of tooth elements that were used in classic orthodontic procedures, offers an alternative to orthognathic surgery. As temporary anchorage devices, the use of micro-implants solves difficult problems such as guiding osteo-distractions, fixing maxillary cants after the vertical distraction of a ramus, stabilizing an edentulous premaxilla, moving teeth into atrophic alveolar sites [1]. The skeletal anchorage on micro-implants is a solution to treat adult orthodontic patients with a lack of quantity or quality of dental elements when conventional dental or mobile anchorage is not possible or cases with poor patients' compliance where the wear of mobile devices or elastics is compromised [2]. Their use is the ideal solution in cases where dental anchorage may result in undesirable side effects such as vertical dimension changes produced by the use of conventional inter-maxillary forces [1]. Micro-implants as skeletal anchorage lead to a more effective orthopedic growth modification, and their use helps camouflage orthodontic treatment for those patients who were not eligible for orthognathic surgery [3,4].

Surgical atraumatic techniques, regeneration and osseointegration, an environment favorable for the primary healing, and biocompatible materials are necessary for micro-implants success. Other important issues in using micro-implants as anchorage elements are patients' cooperation and the perception of the pain and trauma produced by surgical insertion and retraction procedures [4].

Many orthodontists avoid using micro-implants as anchorage elements because they are unfamiliar with the surgical procedures required for their insertion or because of fear of failure. Another cause could be a lack of interest in approaching new techniques compared to treatments that are already routine. These limitations should disappear, and orthodontists should also acquire the surgical skills necessary to use micro-implants, The present paper is intended to be a small guide in the practical activity of orthodontists and not only, which can help them in terms of the use of micro-implants by showing the existing types, how to apply them, the clinical situations in which they can be used, and the difficulties that may occur during treatments that use this type of anchorage.

The aim of this study was to review the literature and evaluate the failure rates and factors that affect the stability and success of temporary anchorage devices used as orthodontic anchorage.

2. Materials and Methods

2.1. Eligibility Criteria

Inclusion criteria:

- Scientific articles published from January 2006 to June 2021 (the last 15 years);
- Scientific articles published in the English language;
- Case series, original research, review;
- Mention of the following words in each possible combination: mini-implant; mini-screw; micro-implant; orthodontics.

Exclusion criteria:

- Papers with no clear report of clinical cases;
- Articles published before January 2006;
- Case reports;
- Book chapters, thesis;
- Mini-plates articles.

2.2. Literature Search Strategy

A systematic search of the literature was performed using PubMed and Google Scholar databases. Search strategies are highlighted in Table 1.

Table 1. Literature search strategy.

PubMed	mini-implant; mini-screw; micro-implant; orthodontics
Google Scholar	mini-implant; mini-screw; micro-implant; orthodontics

Titles and abstracts of retrieved studies were screened and all the studies that included one or more of the exclusion criteria were excluded from the study. The articles selected for full text reading were examined by two authors and those that were lacking relevant informations for the purpose of this review were excluded. Any controversy was resolved with the aid of a third reviewer, selected among the authors.

2.3. Risk of Bias

In order to evaluate the methodological quality of included studies, reviewers used the JBI Critical Appraisal Checklist for Case Reports Studies (Table 2) [5].

Table 2. JBI Critical Appraisal Checklist for Case Reports Studies.

JBI Critical Appraisal Checklist for Case Reports
1. Were patient's demographic characteristics clearly described?
2. Was the patient's history clearly described and presented as a timeline?
3. Was the current clinical condition of the patient on presentation clearly described?
4. Were diagnostic tests or assessment methods and the results clearly described?
5. Was the intervention(s) or treatment procedure(s) clearly described?
6. Was the post-intervention clinical condition clearly described?
7. Were adverse events (harms) or unanticipated events identified and described?
8. Does the case report provide takeaway lessons?

An initial search of PubMed and Google Scholar databases identified a total of 209 documents. Of these 114 records were found on PubMed database and 95 on Google Scholar database. The full-texts of 209 articles were then screened and 8 articles were excluded cause the main topic was not relevant for the purpose of this review and 1 record was excluded because the full-text was not in English language. After applying the inclusion criteria when reading titles and abstracts due to type of publication (book or thesis), main topic, language and incapability to retrieve the abstract and/or the full-text we found 50 manuscripts that were not relevant to the purpose of the manuscript.

Furthermore, a manual search of the reference lists of all selected studies was performed and three studies were additionally included after full-text reading. Ultimately, 66 studies were included in the systematic review and processed for data extraction (Figure 1).

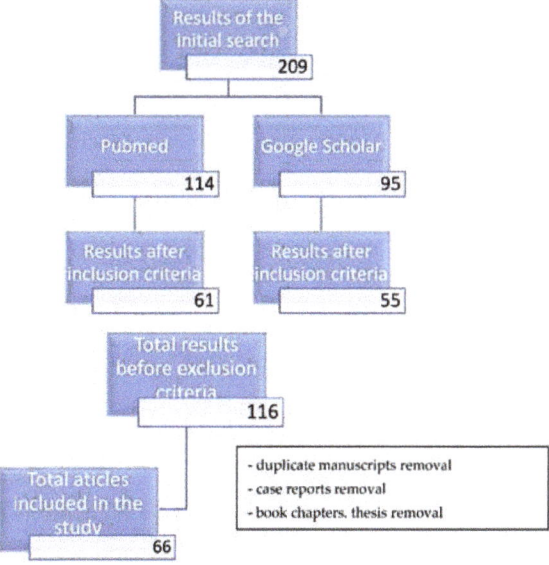

Figure 1. Results of the study selection.

3. Results

3.1. The Success Rate of Micro-Implants

The overall success rate of skeletal anchorage using micro-implants was ranged from 79% to 98.2% [4], described by other studies as being 85.0% [6]. A systematic review published in 2010 [7] included fourteen clinical trials and described the mean overall success rate of 83.8 ± 7.4%, with no significant differences regarding the patient's sex. Little diameters of the mini-screws from 1 to 1.1 mm had lower success rates than the greater ones from 1.5 to 2.3 mm; screws less than 8 mm in length and 1.2 mm in diameter should be avoided [7]. One study reported significantly lower success rates for 6-mm vs. 8-mm long mini-screws (72% vs. 90%) [7]. The recommended diameter and length for a micro-implant placed in the alveolar bone were 1.2 to 1.6 mm respectively 6–7 mm in another study [8]. Other authors [9] concluded that the success rate did not depend on sex, age, and side of placement but significantly increased as total bone density and cancellous bone density increased. The OMIs' success rate was not significantly correlated with the cortical bone density.

3.2. Design

The researchers tried to improve the design of the orthodontic micro-implants to increase torsional strength, stability and reduce bone damage during insertion. An objective function stability quotient (SQ) was built and solved by Korean researchers [10] started from the thread height and pitch of AbsoAnchor SH1312-7 micro-implant (Dentos Inc., Daegu, Korea) as parameters. 3D finite element simulation, torque test, and clinical test led to the creation of four models with optimized thread design and better performance, which indicated that their optimization methodology could be used when designing OMI threads.

The peak insertion torque value is another parameter that influences the OMI's stability. This depends on the manufacturer [11]; the study showed no correlation between the diameter of six different types of self-drilling micro-implants and torque values. Insertion speed did not affect significantly the peak torque values, but the 6 mm OMIs proved to have significantly higher torque values than the 8 and 10 mm ones. Using a screwdriver for limiting the torque or pre-drilling the cortical bone to reduce insertion torque could be a good choice.

3.3. Anatomical and Surgical Details

Over time, several methods have been devised and developed to avoid accidents using micro-implants, the most important being damage to the roots of the neighboring teeth. A precise surgical plan before OMIs' insertion is crucial. Some researchers described the use of radiographic templates and film holders to make a surgical template for guiding OMIs' insertion [12]. The success rate of OMIs was tested by using panoramic radiographs that showed the position and angulation of the screws [6]. The overall success rate was higher for people more than 20 years old and screws on the left side, for the women than for the men, for extraction than for non-extraction group, for OMIs placed on the interradicular midline. OMI success rate significantly increased with an increase in the OMI length and placement height, and with a lesser angulation [6].

Other authors claimed that compared with panoramic radiographs, cone beam computed tomography (CBCT) images can provide more accurate information regarding tooth position, root resorption, and various pathologies; the radiation exposure is less and the cost is lower using panoramic radiographs, which provides acceptable reliability [9].

The efficacy of optical coherence tomography (OCT) was tested comparatively with that of micro-computed tomography (μCT) [13] to detect and analyze cortical bone microdamage immediately after insertion. The visualization of individual microcracks was highly correlated. Even if the depth penetration of OCT was more limited, it has been able to give high-resolution images of the bone microdamage occurring around the micro-implant. Image quality at the surface of the cortical bone is better when compared with μCT imaging, because of the high contrast and the high-resolution quality of OCT systems [13].

The surgical insertion procedure showed contradictory results between flap or without flap techniques on mandibular mini-implants. Loading and healing periods were not significant in the mini-screws success rates [7].

When using micro-implants is important to evaluate the cortical bone thickness and the interradicular spaces to create enough stability for the application of orthodontic forces. Park and Cho [8] found using cone-beam 3D images that in the posterior dentition area the buccal cortical bone is 1 mm or thicker, 1.12 to 1.33 mm for maxilla, and 1.25 to 2.98 mm for mandibula. The cortical bone becomes thicker progressively from the cement-enamel junction to the apical zone. The interradicular distances varied from 1.6 to 3.46 mm in the maxilla with a maximum between the second premolar and the first molar. In mandibula, the interradicular distances were greater than in maxilla and ranged between 1.99 and 4.25 mm. The retromolar zones showed cortical bone from 1.96 to 2.06 mm thicker. The widths of alveolar processes were 3.74–5.78 mm for the maxilla and 3.11–7.84 mm for the mandibula. The mid-palatal area at 20–25 mm posterior than foramen incisivum ranged from 7.04 to 6.99 mm. They concluded that a better location for placing micro-implants was buccal between the second premolar and the first molar for maxilla, buccal from the first premolar to the second molar for mandibula, palatal between molars for maxilla, the mid-palatal and retromolar areas [8].

The cortical bone thickness of the inter-dental area of maxilla and mandible for orthodontic micro-implants placement was investigated by cone-beam computerized tomography [14] by a study that was performed on 32 non-orthodontic adults with normal occlusion. Buccal cortical bone was thicker in the mandible. In the maxilla, the cortical bone was thicker buccal than palatal. In the mandible, the buccal cortical bone vas thickest distal to the first molar, and in the maxilla, it was thickest mesial to the first molar; in the palatal side of maxilla, the cortical bone was thickest mesial to the second premolar. The thinnest cortical bone was found in the buccal side of the maxilla at 4 mm from the alveolar crest and the thickest was at 10 mm, except for the site mesial to the first premolar. The buccal cortical bone thickness mesial or distal to the first inferior molar and palatal cortical bone tended to increase with increasing distance from the alveolar bone [14].

These buccal ideal locations for placing micro-implants were also used in another study that comparatively investigates the anchorage loss in canine retraction with conventional molar anchorage versus titanium micro-implants [15]. In adult patients with a mean age of 19.6 years, the first premolars were extracted to create space for canine retraction. Titanium micro-implants of 1.3 mm in diameter and 9 mm in length were placed between the second premolars and the first molars. The orthodontic mechanics were performed by using closed-coil springs which performed the canine retraction by having on one quadrant a molar anchorage and on the other an anchorage on micro-implants. The results showed no anchorage loss on the micro-implant side and 1.60–1.70 anchorage loss on the molar anchorage side. Other similar studies have aimed to investigate the effectiveness of using mini-implants in canine retraction [16]. The authors used mini-implants of 1.3 mm in diameter and 8 mm in length and their placement was also between the second premolars and the first molars, for each patient in the same quadrants (on the right side), placed at an angle of 30–40° in the maxilla and of 10–20° in the mandible to the long axis of the teeth to increase the contact between the implant and the bone. On the left quadrants, the retraction of the canines was done by using the first molars as anchorage. Orthodontic forces of 100 g were immediately applied; coil springs were used for canine retraction. Results showed that the rates of canine retraction were higher on the implant sides, 0.95 and 0.81 mm/month in maxilla respectively in the mandible and lower on the molar sides, 0.82 and 0.76 mm/month in the maxilla respectively in mandible. The loss of anchorage was less on the implant sides, 0.1 in the maxilla and 0.06 in the mandible and greater on the molar sides, 1.3 mm on the molar side of the maxilla and mandible. There were statistically significant differences between changes in anchorage inclination on the implant side and molar side in both maxilla and mandible: 0.3° on the implant side and 2.45° on the molar side in the maxilla and 0.19° on the implant side and 2.69° on the molar side in mandible. Studies [15,16] demonstrated that micro-implant anchorage is a better alternative to molar anchorage.

Many other studies investigated the ideal insertion angle of orthodontic micro-implants for biomechanical control and cortical anchorage. A study on finite models of maxilla and mandible [17] which used D2 and D3 types of bone and micro-implants of 1.3 mm diameter and 7–8 mm length inserted in different angles on bone's surface shows that the maximum von Mises stress in the implants and the cortical bone decreases as the insertion angle increases. The stress generated at the application of horizontal orthodontic forces was distributed mainly to the cortical bone and less to the cancellous bone. The stress was higher in type D3 bone quality than in type D2. The study demonstrated that the 90° insertion angle is ideal for orthodontic micro-implants' stabilization [17]. The shortcoming of the investigation's method was that the ideal angle for insertion of the screw was not determined in all three spatial planes but only in the horizontal one because the direction of application of the orthodontic force was horizontal. Other studies that investigate only micro-implants placed in the upper jaw demonstrated the opposite, namely that the insertion angle of micro-implants, the cortical bone thickness is not important for the success rate of using orthodontic micro-implants [18,19]. The authors measured horizontal and vertical placement angles using cone-beam computed tomography images. The micro-implants' success rates significantly increased with the distance to the root surface. Cortical bone thickness was affected by placement angles but root proximity was not affected by insertion angles. Other interesting results were that success rates were higher for screws put on the left side, for adult patients than for teenagers, in women than in men. The success rate increased by increasing the horizontal placement angle but the difference was not statistically significant [18].

Contact between orthodontic mini-implants and dental roots during the insertion process is a common problem because inter-radicular spaces are narrow [20]. Such contacts have been associated with root damage and increased implant failure rates. An accurate test to diagnose implant–root contact is therefore indicated. Using specific insertion torque values (the index test) as a diagnostic test of OMIs with root contact could be more accurate less adverse compared with radiographic images. Torque levels of OMIs inserted with root contact were higher than those without. The highest torque differences were identified in the self-drilling compared with the pre-drilling. It is important to record constantly the torque values during the insertion process.

The stress in the cortical bone during and after insertion of self-tapping orthodontic micro-implants using predrilled holes was simulated with a 3-dimensional finite element method [21]. Results showed stresses during insertion that could fracture the cortical bone; hoop stresses of the ultimate tensile strength and radial stresses of the ultimate compressive strength of cortical bone were developed. After insertion, residual radial stresses that could cause bone resorptions were observed. The high insertion-related stresses showed that the bone's response and the micro-implant prognosis depend on the insertion conditions not on the orthodontic force or the timing of its application.

The primary stability of OMIs is influenced by various insertion angles and the direction of the applied orthodontic force. An opinion is that the highest primary stability values were get at an insertion angle of 45° when the mini-implants were loaded by shear force and at 90° when pullout forces were used [22].

Different OMIs proved a wide range of torque at fracture that depended on the manufacturer and the correlation between the diameter of the screw and fracture resistance was poor. The torque is to be considered at the insertion phase to minimize the risk of screw fracture and much care should be for the areas with high-density bone without predrilling [23].

By sequential fluorochrome staining combined with laser confocal microscopy were visualized the damage of cortical bone at insertion and removal of orthodontic micro-implants (OMI) [24]. The presence of a pilot hole demonstrated a minimal effect on microdamage bone characteristics and a minimal effect on maximum insertion torque.

The micro-damages increased with the bone thickness; there was a positive correlation between the bone thickness and the increase in maximum insertion torque. The maximum insertion torque was correlated with the total and diffused bone damaged area. The study concluded that the choice of making pilot holes for orthodontic micro-implants' insertion should depend on the thickness of cortical bone. The bone damages evaluated with two different types of OMI, non-drilling, and self-drilling and pilot holes showed that fractional damaged area, fractional microcracked area, and fractional diffuse damaged area were greater with the self-drilling ones and as the thickness of cortical bone increased [25].

The self-drilling micro-implants create better anchorage than self-tapping ones [26]. Self-drilling micro-implants had higher peak insertion torque and peak removal torque than self-tapping ones. Self-drilling screws demonstrate a higher fracture tendency and better contact between the implant and bone [24,25]; their use is indicated in the maxilla and thin cortical mandibular areas. Negative correlations between Periotest values were mostly demonstrated by the self-drilling micro-implants [27]. The differences between insertion torque values and corresponding assessments of stability scores were higher self-drilling screws.

3.4. Immediate Loading

In the literature, there has been much discussion about the possibility of immediate loading of mini-implants and how it affects the stability of the screw and bone structure.

Immediate loading doesn't affect the osseointegration of OMIs but the anchorage is not always absolutely stationary, extrusion and tipping were observed in areas with thin cortical bone [28]. Immediately loading with orthodontic forces of 200 g does not influence significantly the stability [7] and seemed to accelerate the shaping of periosteal bone after the surgical intervention; there were no statistically significant differences in bone and implant contact values between the loaded OMIs and the unloaded ones [28].

Another study [29] found by histological analysis good osseointegration, bone apposition, and new bone formation in loaded and unloaded OMIs. The contact between bone and micro-implant was higher in the loaded ones. The study concluded that small diameters (1.2–1.3) OMIs made from Titanium alloy are strong enough for immediate loading even in thin cortical bone areas; in this situation drilling a pilot hole reduces the possibility of micro-implants' breakage.

Comparing immediate loading with one-week post-insertion loading of orthodontic micro-implants showed a statistically higher torque loss in delayed insertion; a significant stability loss was seen in both situations in the first week of investigation [30].

Investigating the biomechanical properties of bone around OMIs under immediate loading using nanoindentation testing [31] showed that the trabecular area on the compression site near the implant was significantly harder than in other bone locations.

Another study based on histological, histological-morphometric, and cone beam computed tomography (CBCT) analysis were performed on autoclave-sterilized OMIs and proved that an immediate, light orthodontic load did not influence the bone healing around mini-screws [32]. The osseointegration and the cortical bone thickness increased with the time passed from the insertion of the implants. The absence of infections during the healing showed that OMIs can be autoclaved in the dental practice before insertion time, with no effect on subsequent osseointegration. The predrilling of thick cortical bone reduced the microfractures. The displacement of the periosteum stimulated the healing of the cortical bone [32].

A review article showed the efficiency of using mini-implants as anchorage and concluded that their success depends on proper initial stability and the quality and quantity of loading [16]. Other factors that could compromise the success of using OMIs are the patient's oral hygiene, coexisting pathologies, smoking, the condition of the mucosa, the timing, quantity, and direction of the loading force direction [2,7]. Thus, the micro-implants' success involves factors related to the patient, the orthodontist, and the OMI's design [2,7].

3.5. Microbial Aggregation around Micro-Implants, Biocompatibility

The possibility of microbial aggregation and biofilm formation on micro-implants has been intensively investigated; surface roughness and chemical composition play an important role in this issue. An in-vitro study [33] which uses X-ray photoelectron spectroscopy detected high-carbon contamination and other inorganic elements like Pb, Zn, P, Cu, Cr, Ca on the oxide surfaces of five different types of micro-implants. Those chemical impurities disappeared after Ar(+) ion sputtering. The surface roughness was greater for titanium micro-implants (182 nm) than for the stainless-steel ones. Through scanning electron microscopy, structural defects were observed [34]. These retention sites favored the biofilm's formation when the micro-implants were immersed in human saliva; the microbial flora of the biofilm was reduced when the micro-implants were pretreated with chlorhexidine and fluoride mouth rinses.

Various other methods have been tried to decrease microbial aggregation around micro-implants to prevent their loss. By using silver nanoparticles (AgNPs) were manufactured AgNP-modified titanium micro-implants (Ti-nAg) by coating OMIs with AgNPs or with a AgNP-coated biopolymer (Ti-BP-AgNP) [35]. Comparative data showed that OMIs coated with BP-AgNP had remarkable antibacterial properties by creating inhibition zones for Aggregatibacter actinomycetemcomitans, Streptococcus mutans, and Streptococcus sanguinis, whereas no antibacterial effects were seen on those coated with AgNPs. Scanning electron microscopy showed a silver atomic percent of 1.05 in the group of OMIs coated with regular AgNPs and much greater, 21.2%, in the group coated with BP-AgNP. Ti-BP-AgNP proved to be an excellent implantable biomaterial, with very good antibacterial properties [34].

The heat treatment (APH treatment) increases the hydrophilicity and the roughness of Ti6Al4V micro-implants subjected to anodization and cyclic calcification. APH treatment created a surface of the nanotubular TiO_2 layer which was covered with a compact apatite-like film. APH-treated micro-implants showed better bioactivity and biocompatibility, better bone regenerative characteristics, higher removable torque, and greater contact with bone, compared with untreated (UT) and anodized and heat-treated (AH) ones [36].

Self-drilling orthodontic micro-implants were surface-treated with acid (etched), resorbable blasting media (RBM), partially resorbable blasting media (hybrid) to increase, study and compare the bone-cutting capacity and osseointegration [37]. The hybrid type gave the most stable self-drilling OMIs, without reduction of bone-cutting capacity.

Chitosan modification of the surface of micro-implants might be an approach to enhance the bioactive- and antibacterial properties of orthodontic micro-implants. Chitosan-modified titanium alloy micro-implants showed better biocompatibility with pre-osteoblastic cells which was confirmed by their improved adhesion, proliferation, and cell viability analysis [38]. Biofilm formation of Streptococcus mutans and Streptococcus sobrinus was reduced by 53% and 31%, respectively, on the surface of OMIs.

Nanotechnology is the study, production, and controlled manipulation of materials with a grain size less than 100 nm. As grain size decreases, the interaction between OMIs and the surrounding cellular environment increases. Treating the micro-implants surface with nanophase materials improved their osteo-integration due to a more closely match with the architecture of native trabecular bone [39].

Zirconia micro-implants proved excellent biocompatibility; they were tested and showed initial stability and clinical applicability for orthodontic treatments comparable to that of titanium micro-implants under various compressive and tensile forces [40]. Compressive and tensile forces were recorded at 0.01, 0.02, and 0.03 mm displacement of the implants of zirconia and titanium at various angles of 0°, 10°, 20°, 30°, and 40°; there were no statistically significant differences between the two types of implants made of different materials regarding the maximum insertion torque, maximum removal torque or the amount of movement at displacement test.

3.6. Use in Orthodontic Clinical Practice and Dento-Facial Orthopedics

Micro-implants could help orthopedic and skeletal modifications. Micro-implant-assisted rapid palatal expanders variable as design and using protocols were used for the treatments of Class III [3]. By fixing with micro-implants transversal screws to the hard palate the rapid palatal expansion prevents the tipping of the anchorage teeth, tooth mobility, and resorption of roots and bone which are accidents in using conventional rapid palatal expenders (RPE) [41–43].

Computer tomography and Mimics modeling software, ANSYS simulation software showed that compression and tension forces are directed to the palate bone and produced less rotation or tipping of the maxillary complex in case of using micro-implant-assisted rapid palatal expansion (MARPE) compared to use of conventional rapid palatal expander (RPE) [44]. MARPE made the maxilla bend laterally and prevented unwanted rotation of the maxillary complex, the vertical maxillary dropping [44].

The MARPE was described as efficient in adolescents and an adult-case patient (19 years old) where the palatal anchorage was performed by using four micro-implants. The palatal bones were expanded by 5.41 ± 2.18 mm and 10 mm, respectively [45]. The cross-sectional CT showed the expansion of maxillofacial structures, zygoma, and nasal floor, and the widening of circum-maxillary sutures; the alveolar bone maintained its integrity even the teeth tipped in vestibular direction. The dentoalveolar side effects were minimum: the first molars exhibited buccal tipping of $2.56 \pm 2.64°$ [46].

Another study [47] contradicted these results by finding 41% skeletal enlargement, 12% alveolar bone bending, and 48% dental tipping after MARPE. The mid-palatal suture opening was parallel in both axial and coronal planes. The dental tipping was 4.17° to 4.96° and the buccal bone thickness was reduced by an average of 39% measured at the molars and the premolars [46]. MARPE appears to be an alternative to surgical treatment in the correction of moderate transverse deficiencies in skeletally mature adult patients [43–47].

Micro-implant-supported midfacial skeletal expanders that had been used as anchorage four OMIs (1.8 mm in diameter, 11 mm or 13 mm in length) inserted through the palatal bone, bi-cortically, produced almost pure skeletal rotational movement of the mid cranial structures [48]. Alveolar bone bending and dental tipping were not statistically significant. The localization of the rotational fulcrum of the zygomaticomaxillary complex should be the first step to differentiate the expansion pattern, than angular measurements should be performed. The angular measurements for fulcrums gave very different results than the conventional linear measurement system that can falsely exaggerate the alveolar and dental components of midfacial skeletal expansion [48].

Micro-implant-assisted expanders have proved significant effects on the mid-face, with a degree of asymmetry [49]. On non-growing patients, CBCT images showed a statistically significant difference between the average magnitude of the total expansion of 4.98 mm at the anterior nasal spine and the average of 4.77 mm at the posterior nasal spine. Among the asymmetric patients, one-half of the anterior nasal spine moved more than the contralateral one by 2.22 mm. The expansion achieved was 96% parallel in the antero-posterior direction.

The palatal bone and soft tissue thicknesses were investigated by cone-beam computerized tomography, using a micro-implant-supported maxillary skeletal expander in Class III malocclusion on 58 patients [50]. The antero-posterior reference that has been used was the line connecting the central fossae of the first molars (Level 0). The anterior palatal bone was significantly thicker in males than females in the anterior palate, whilst in the posterior palate there was no significant sex-related difference. The thickness tended to decrease in the posterior direction, except in women at 2 mm lateral from the reference line. In all investigated areas the palatal soft tissue was significantly thicker in males than females. The bone thickness decreased and the soft tissue thickness increased as the lateral distance from the reference line increased. Another similar study [51] showed that the palatal bone was thinner in cases with class III malocclusion than in those with class I malocclusion, with significant differences in some areas. Palatal bone was thicker in the middle region of the midline area. The palatal bone was significantly thinner in area 9.0 mm before the transverse palatine suture in the midline area, 9.0 mm before and after the transverse palatine suture in the middle area, and 9.0 mm after the transverse palatine suture in the lateral area. The study concluded that anterior and middle palatal areas are safer for putting micro-implants, while the thinness of the posterior palatal bone increases the risk of failure and perforations.

Micro-implants can be used as orthodontic anchorage in infra-zygomatic areas. A research study was performed to investigate the insertion torque and pull-out strength of three brands of infra-zygomatic mini-implants. Their mechanical strength proved to depend on their design [52].

Cleft lip and palate is the most common craniofacial malformation clinical characterized by underdeveloped maxilla in transverse and sagittal dimension; it can be corrected by surgical repair of the cleft followed by orthodontic treatment [53]. Bone-anchored rapid palatal expanders had the advantage of directly anchoring the expansion appliance to the palatal bone with less dental secondary effects. The greatest stress caused by the bone expander which used OMIs as anchor system was observed in the mid-palatal suture area at the implant insertion site on the cleft side along the palatal slopes and was equally distributed superiorly to the alveolar and basal bone [53]. In conventional expanders the greatest stress was observed at tooth level both on the cleft side and on the opposite side. The zygomaticomaxillary suture experienced maximum stress, followed by the zygomaticotemporal and nasomaxillary sutures. Displacement in the transverse plane was highest on the cleft side, and in the antero-posterior plane was highest in the posterior region [53].

The OMIs can be used as direct or indirect anchorage elements for molar up-righting in all three spatial planes [54]. The direct method is simpler because it requires one OMI and a single bracket or button, reducing the patient's discomfort and chair time compared to the indirect anchorage. It eliminates the unwanted movement of the anchorage unit. Direct anchorage has limitations in cases of rotated or lingually tipped molars because they need more than a single force to upright their position. OMIs are a reliable solution in the treatment of tipped or impacted molars.

Micro-implant assisted molar intrusion in maxillary helped the prosthetic rehabilitation in mandible [55]. The maxillary molars extruded in time after opposite molar extractions in mandible could be easily intruded by using OMIs placed palatal or both buccal and palatal and placing on them intrusive forces. These procedures created a minimum of 5–8 mm for rehabilitation on implants of the posterior sector of the mandible, in adult patients [55].

The distalization with micro-implant-aided sliding mechanics proved less distal tipping of the posterior teeth and the method seemed efficient for patients with mild arch length discrepancies even without making therapeutic extractions, except the third molars [56]. In the maxilla, the posterior teeth were distalized with 1.4 to 2.0 mm, a media of 3.5° of distal tipping, and 1 mm intrusion; in the mandible, the posterior teeth were distalized with 1.6 to 2.5 mm and 6.6° to 8.3° of distal tipping. The maxillary posterior teeth showed intrusion by 1 mm. There were increases in arch widths at the premolars and molars. The micro-implants' success rate was 89.7% and the mean treatment time was 20 ± 4.9 months. Inter-premolar and intermolar distances have increased. In the adult group, the Frankfort horizontal to mandibular plane angle has decreased. Profile changes were determined by distal repositioning of the upper and lower lips [57].

In cases with maxillary dentoalveolar protrusion, the anchorage on micro-implants was more efficient in retracting the anterior group than the traditional anchorage [57]. The use of micro-implants produced less anchorage loss, and had a better effect for the high-angle patients than had traditional anchorage. Both systems proved their efficiency in reducing dental and alveolar protrusion.

In skeletal Class III, orthognathic surgery the maxillary intervention could be avoided by using OMIs placed in the palatal bone between the upper first and second molars to intrude the posterior teeth. The maxillary occlusal plane rotated clockwise and increased the surgical mandibular setback; the vertical dimension was reduced. The distal movement of the chin was greater than the alternative surgical prediction with no change in the occlusal plane. The intrusion of the maxillary posterior teeth with OMIs prevented the need for upper jaw surgery in adult skeletal Class III patients [58].

The micro-implants as anchorage can be successfully used for the treatment of Class II malocclusions [59]. OMIs were included in a novel en masse distalization concept used for patients with canine sagittal distalizations of half of a cusp or more. One palatal micro-implant on each maxillary side was introduced in the interradicular region. The objective of the study was to get a complete en-masse distalization of the whole upper arch in one step. By maxillary tooth movements and dentoalveolar compensations, the canine neutral relationship and the overjet correction were achieved [59].

OMIs can be used in lingual straight wire appliances for retraction of the frontal maxillary group [60]. The study used 3D finite element models and analysis software ANSYSnsys Workbench 15 (ANSYS, USA). The OMIs were positioned at 8 mm from the alveolar crest. On the OMIs positioned between the two central incisors was applied a vertical traction force for the simulation of the intrusion anterior from the bonded threads. The retraction hooks were positioned between the lateral incisor and the canine at a height of 6 mm. A retraction force of 1.5 N from the retraction hooks to OMIs was applied; the additional intrusive force of 50 g from the two incisors was combined to simulate the effect on labial crown torque. The double wire was more efficient in torque control compared with the single round or rectangular wire or in lingual orthodontics [60]. En-masse bodily movement of anterior teeth seemed to be difficult although the vertical intrusion force increases by using OMIs increased.

En-masse distalization in the maxilla requires antibiotics or a placebo before the micro-implant's placement. However, a study on 38 participants [61] proved that antibiotics provided no benefit in terms of OMIs stability, inflammation of soft tissues, and postinterventional pain. Measurements of inflammatory markers in serum were inefficient in demonstrating soft tissue inflammations. Antibiotic prophylaxis slightly decreased the levels of the biomarkers.

Regardless of the severity of obstructive sleep apnea (OSA), the use of oral appliances is preferred when nasal continuous positive airway pressure (CPAP) is not efficient [62]. Micro-implant assisted rapid maxillary expansion is effective in treating children with OSA and maxillary constriction. The maxillary expansion enlarges the nasal cavity and increases the air quantity that passes through the nasal pathway. In adult patients, the side effects are unwanted teeth movements. Micro-implant assisted rapid maxillary expansion (MARME) could reduce even eliminate the dental side effects. MARME produces skeletal effects that enable a larger mid-palatal suture separation and a larger increase of the nasal cavity volume. The maxillary skeletal expander (MSE) is a special MARME appliance of four mini-screws inserted in the posterior palate with bi-cortical engagements in the palatal and nasal cortical bone. MSE expands the superior and posterior areas of the nasal cavity [62].

The pterygopalatine suture can be split without surgery, by using midfacial skeletal expanders [63]. The device used had a jackscrew unit with four parallel holes for the micro-implant insertion, with two soft supporting arms on each side which are soldered to the molar bands for increasing stability. The jackscrew was seated on the hard palate between the zygomatic buttress bones. After the treatment, the mean palatal suture opening angle was 0.57°. There was no significant difference between males and females regarding the palatal suture opening pattern and 84% of cases had openings between the medial and lateral pterygoid plates on both right and left sides.

Micro-implants are indicated as anchorage elements in cases of periodontal patients who need orthodontic treatment [64]. For the advantages like a simple surgical procedure, low cost, immediate loading, the placement's possibilities the OMIs are indicated for molar intrusion, molar up-righting, and other minor tooth movements [54].

Rupture of the intermaxillary suture with a micro-implant-supported screw was experimentally achieved with an expansion force of 86 N. A high tensile stress concentration was exerted and opened the fused intermaxillary suture [65].

Experimentally on dogs, the bi-cortical micro-implants with two anchorage units demonstrated their efficiency for the difficult movement that is the posterior teeth protraction, in the mandible [66].

3.7. Patients' and Practitioners' Compliance

Another important issue besides investigating the efficiency of the use of micro-implants was the determination of patients' compliance with their use and the perception of pain while performing the insertion procedures. An article from 2008 [67] showed by using a visual analog scale (VAS) that the patients who underwent micro-implant surgery were expected to experience significantly greater pain than they endured. The postinterventional pain decreased continuously from the first to day seven after the surgical procedure. Pain experienced in the initial tooth alignment phase was significantly greater than in extraction procedures, micro-implants' insertion, or tooth or the insertion of separators. Patients' expectations of pain were greater in the case of micro-implants' insertion than in insertion of separators and tooth alignment but not statistically different than in extractions. Patients' pain significantly decreased seven days after the insertion of the micro-implants. Most patients reported little or no pain during micro-implant's insertion and overestimated first overestimated before the intervention the pain and trauma that would have been endured. The only problems caused by micro-implants were the accumulation of food waste around the screws (86%) and minor speech disturbances (37%). A large percentage of patients were satisfied with the implant surgery (76%) and said they would recommend it to others (78%).

Another similar article that investigated pain perception on maxillary OMIs insertion found that VAS score 1 day after placement was significantly less than that 1 day after first premolar extraction for orthodontic purpose or that one day after the fixed appliance was bonded. The results indicated that interdental micro-implants did not produce greater pain than other orthodontic interventions [68].

A questionnaire-based study from 2010 [69] evaluated the pain experienced by orthodontic patients during tooth extractions, maxillary OMIs insertions, and gingival tissue removal before placing the maxillary implants. The pain felt during extractions was significantly greater than during tissue removal or micro-implant placement. The micro-implant placement caused no pain in 30% of patients and was the least painful procedure; the transgingival placement was significantly preferred.

Orthodontic mini implants (OMIs) provide anchorage without depending on the collaboration of patients, they are effective and can be used for various treatment objectives; still, surveys have shown that many orthodontists never or rarely use them [70]. The barriers to implement OMIs in clinical practice are: the need to perform surgical procedures for their placement and risk factors associated, implant failure, costs, numerous implementation issues. Conducting surgical interventions in orthodontic offices is still very uncommon and can be conditioned by variables such as the lack of knowledge and skills of clinicians; the lack of knowledge-management skills of pertinent stakeholders, lack of organization, lack of time and resources, attitudes towards new knowledge, and resistance from the patient. Limitations depend more on the medical staff than on patients [70].

Retrieved OMIs exhibited different degrees of chemical changes on surface characteristics and mechanical behavior. The thread edges and tips were worn out and thin deposits were seen on their surfaces. Traces of foreign elements like iron, sulfur, and calcium, were detected on their surfaces. The maximum insertion torque and the insertion time of retrieved OMIs were increased compared to the initial use. The maximum insertion torque was increased in all OMIs put with the insertion angle of 45° compared with 90°. The reuse for immediate relocation in the same patient may be acceptable; postponed relocation and allogeneic reuse of OMIs are not recommended in clinical practice [71].

For future practice, we can try the mini-implant anchorage in the mechanics of reducing the displacements of the temporomandibular discs [72], in the reposition of the mandible [73], in solving complicated problems such as cranial asymmetries with dentofacial and occlusal effects [74], in orofaciodigital syndrome treatments [75], and as a non-surgical alternative in progressive ankylosis of the temporomandibular joint when patients do not accept the surgical treatment [76].

A great advantage of using micro-implants is the possibility of maintaining better oral hygiene than with the use of conventional anchoring systems, due to the smaller size and lower ability to retain food debris [77]. In the last decade, oral hygiene has been greatly improved by using web media as a means of investigation and education for patients and their parents in cases of pediatric patients [78,79]. The possible side effects of mini-implants as oral mucosa trauma, inflammation, and eventually chronic lesions can be easily treated by photodynamic therapy that is minimally invasive and showed promising results [80].

4. Conclusions

Considering the results of our study we can conclude that the micro-implants' success involves factors related to the patient, the orthodontist, the design and material of these devices and due to the multiple advantages that micro-implants have, they would have been indicated to be commonly used in orthodontic practices.

Author Contributions: Conceptualization, S.-M.B., C.D.O.; methodology, L.L.V., S.-M.B.; supervision, V.C.; writing—original draft, S.-M.B.; writing—review and editing, L.L.V., C.D.O., V.C. All authors have read and agreed to the published version of the manuscript.

Funding: This research received no external funding.

Institutional Review Board Statement: Not applicable.

Informed Consent Statement: Not applicable.

Data Availability Statement: Not applicable.

Conflicts of Interest: The authors declare that they have no conflict of interest regarding this manuscript and did not receive any financial support from any organizations or a research grant.

References

1. Vachiramon, A.; Urata, M.; Kyung, H.M.; Yamashita, D.-D.; Yen, S.L.-K. Clinical Applications of Orthodontic Microimplant Anchorage in Craniofacial Patients. *Cleft Palate-Craniofacial J.* **2009**, *46*, 136–146. [CrossRef] [PubMed]
2. Leo, M.; Cerroni, L.; Pasquantonio, G. Temporary anchorage devices (TADs) in orthodontics: Review of the factors that influence the clinical success rate of the mini-implants. *Clin. Ter.* **2016**, *167*, e70–e77. [CrossRef] [PubMed]
3. Ngan, P.; Moon, W. Evolution of Class III treatment in orthodontics. *Am. J. Orthod. Dentofac. Orthop.* **2015**, *148*, 22–36. [CrossRef] [PubMed]
4. Kyung, H.; Ly, N.; Hong, M. Orthodontic skeletal anchorage: Up-to-date review. *Orthod. Waves* **2017**, *76*, 123–132. [CrossRef]
5. The Joanna Briggs Institute Critical Appraisal Tools for Use in JBI Systematic Reviews Checklist for Case Reports. Available online: http://joannabriggs.org/research/critical-appraisal-tools.html (accessed on 6 October 2021).
6. Park, J.H.; Chae, J.-M.; Bay, R.C.; Kim, M.-J.; Lee, K.-Y.; Chang, N.-Y. Evaluation of factors influencing the success rate of orthodontic microimplants using panoramic radiographs. *Korean J. Orthod.* **2018**, *48*, 30–38. [CrossRef]
7. Crismani, A.G.; Bertl, M.; Čelar, A.G.; Bantleon, H.-P.; Burstone, C.J. Miniscrews in orthodontic treatment: Review and analysis of published clinical trials. *Am. J. Orthod. Dentofac. Orthop.* **2010**, *137*, 108–113. [CrossRef]
8. Park, J.; Cho, H.J. Three-dimensional evaluation of interradicular spaces and cortical bone thickness for the placement and initial stability of microimplants in adults. *Am. J. Orthod. Dentofac. Orthop.* **2009**, *136*, 314.e1–314.e12, discussion 314–315. [CrossRef]
9. Lee, M.-Y.; Park, J.H.; Kim, S.-C.; Kang, K.-H.; Cho, J.-H.; Chang, N.-Y.; Chae, J.-M. Bone density effects on the success rate of orthodontic microimplants evaluated with cone-beam computed tomography. *Am. J. Orthod. Dentofac. Orthop.* **2016**, *149*, 217–224. [CrossRef]
10. Kim, K.-D.; Yu, W.-J.; Park, H.-S.; Kyung, H.-M.; Kwon, O.-W. Optimization of orthodontic microimplant thread design. *Korean J. Orthod.* **2011**, *41*, 25–35. [CrossRef]
11. Whang, C.Z.Y.; Bister, D.; Sherriff, M. An in vitro investigation of peak insertion torque values of six commercially available mini-implants. *Eur. J. Orthod.* **2011**, *33*, 660–666. [CrossRef]
12. Wu, J.C.; Huang, J.-N.; Zhao, S.-F.; Xu, X.-J.; Xie, Z.-J. Radiographic and surgical template for placement of orthodontic microimplants in interradicular areas: A technical note. *Int. J. Oral Maxillofac. Implant.* **2006**, *21*, 629–634.

13. Lakshmikantha, H.T.; Ravichandran, N.K.; Jeon, M.; Kim, J.; Park, H.-S. Assessment of cortical bone microdamage following insertion of microimplants using optical coherence tomography: A preliminary study. *J. Zhejiang Univ. Sci. B* **2018**, *19*, 818–828. [CrossRef]
14. Zhao, H.; Gu, X.-M.; Liu, H.-C.; Wang, Z.-W.; Xun, C.-L. Measurement of cortical bone thickness in adults by cone-beam computerized tomography for orthodontic miniscrews placement. *J. Huazhong Univ. Sci. Technolog. Med. Sci.* **2013**, *33*, 303–308. [CrossRef]
15. Thiruvenkatachari, B.; Pavithranand, A.; Rajasigamani, K.; Kyung, H.M. Comparison and measurement of the amount of anchorage loss of the molars with and without the use of implant anchorage during canine retraction. *Am. J. Orthod. Dentofac. Orthop.* **2006**, *129*, 551–554. [CrossRef]
16. Davis, D.; Krishnaraj, R.; Duraisamy, S.; Ravi, K.; Dilip, S.; Charles, A.; Sushil, N. Comparison of Rate of Canine Retraction and Anchorage Potential between Mini-implant and Conventional Molar Anchorage: An In vivo Study. *Contemp. Clin. Dent.* **2018**, *9*, 337–342. [CrossRef] [PubMed]
17. Jasmine, M.I.F.; Yezdani, A.A.; Tajir, F.; Venu, R.M. Analysis of stress in bone and microimplants during en-masse retraction of maxillary and mandibular anterior teeth with different insertion angulations: A 3-dimensional finite element analysis study. *Am. J. Orthod. Dentofac. Orthop.* **2012**, *141*, 71–80. [CrossRef]
18. Chen, Y.; Kyung, H.M.; Zhao, W.T.; Yu, W.J. Critical factors for the success of orthodontic mini-implants: A systematic review. *Am. J. Orthod. Dentofac. Orthop.* **2009**, *135*, 284–291. [CrossRef] [PubMed]
19. Park, H.-S.; Hwangbo, E.-S.; Kwon, T.-G. Proper mesiodistal angles for microimplant placement assessed with 3-dimensional computed tomography images. *Am. J. Orthod. Dentofac. Orthop.* **2010**, *137*, 200–206. [CrossRef] [PubMed]
20. Reynders, R.M.; Ladu, L.; Ronchi, L.; Di Girolamo, N.; De Lange, J.; Roberts, N.; Plüddemann, A. Insertion torque recordings for the diagnosis of contact between orthodontic mini-implants and dental roots: A systematic review. *Syst. Rev.* **2016**, *5*, 50. [CrossRef] [PubMed]
21. Yu, W.; Park, H.-S.; Kyung, H.-M.; Kwon, O.-W. Dynamic simulation of the self-tapping insertion process of orthodontic microimplants into cortical bone with a 3-dimensional finite element method. *Am. J. Orthod. Dentofac. Orthop.* **2012**, *142*, 834–841. [CrossRef]
22. Araghbidikashani, M.; Golshah, A.; Nikkerdar, N.; Rezaei, M. In-vitro impact of insertion angle on primary stability of miniscrews. *Am. J. Orthod. Dentofac. Orthop.* **2016**, *150*, 436–443. [CrossRef] [PubMed]
23. Smith, A.; Hosein, Y.K.; Dunning, C.E.; Tassi, A. Fracture resistance of commonly used self-drilling orthodontic mini-implants. *Angle Orthod.* **2015**, *85*, 26–32. [CrossRef] [PubMed]
24. Jensen, S.; Jensen, E.; Sampson, W.; Dreyer, C. Torque Requirements and the Influence of Pilot Holes on Orthodontic Miniscrew Microdamage. *Appl. Sci.* **2021**, *11*, 3564. [CrossRef]
25. Shank, S.B.; Beck, F.M.; D'Atri, A.M.; Huja, S.S. Bone damage associated with orthodontic placement of miniscrew implants in an animal model. *Am. J. Orthod. Dentofac. Orthop.* **2012**, *141*, 412–418. [CrossRef]
26. Chen, Y.; Shin, H.-I.; Kyung, H.-M. Biomechanical and histological comparison of self-drilling and self-tapping orthodontic microimplants in dogs. *Am. J. Orthod. Dentofac. Orthop.* **2008**, *133*, 44–50. [CrossRef]
27. Çehreli, S.; Özçirpici, A.A. Primary stability and histomorphometric bone-implant contact of self-drilling and self-tapping orthodontic microimplants. *Am. J. Orthod. Dentofac. Orthop.* **2012**, *141*, 187–195. [CrossRef]
28. Chen, Y.; Kang, S.T.; Bae, S.-M.; Kyung, H.-M. Clinical and histologic analysis of the stability of microimplants with immediate orthodontic loading in dogs. *Am. J. Orthod. Dentofac. Orthop.* **2009**, *136*, 260–267. [CrossRef]
29. Chen, Y.; Lee, J.-W.; Cho, W.-H.; Kyung, H.-M. Potential of self-drilling orthodontic microimplants under immediate loading. *Am. J. Orthod. Dentofac. Orthop.* **2010**, *137*, 496–502. [CrossRef]
30. Migliorati, M.; Drago, S.; Gallo, F.; Amorfini, L.; Dalessandri, D.; Calzolari, C.; Benedicenti, S.; Silvestrini-Biavati, A. Immediate versus delayed loading: Comparison of primary stability loss after miniscrew placement in orthodontic patients—a single-centre blinded randomized clinical trial. *Eur. J. Orthod.* **2016**, *38*, 652–659. [CrossRef]
31. Iijima, M.; Nakagaki, S.; Yasuda, Y.; Handa, K.; Koike, T.; Muguruma, T.; Saito, T.; Mizoguchi, I. Effect of immediate loading on the biomechanical properties of bone surrounding the miniscrew implants. *Eur. J. Orthod.* **2013**, *35*, 577–582. [CrossRef]
32. Catharino, P.C.; Dominguez, G.C.; Dos Santos, P., Jr.; Morea, C. Histologic, Histomorphometric, and Radiographic Monitoring of Bone Healing Around In-Office–Sterilized Orthodontic Mini-implants With or Without Immediate Load: Study in Rabbit Tibiae. *Int. J. Oral Maxillofac. Implant.* **2014**, *29*, 321–330. [CrossRef] [PubMed]
33. Chin, M.Y.; Sandham, A.; de Vries, J.; van der Mei, H.C.; Busscher, H.J. Biofilm formation on surface characterized micro-implants for skeletal anchorage in orthodontics. *Biomaterials* **2007**, *28*, 2032–2040. [CrossRef] [PubMed]
34. Vlasa, A.; Biris, C.; Lazar, L.; Bud, A.; Bud, E.; Varlam, C.M.; Maris, M.; Pacurar, M. Scanning Electron Microscope Analysis of Titanium Alloy Orthodontic Implants. *Mater. Plast.* **2017**, *54*, 345–347. [CrossRef]
35. Venugopal, A.; Muthuchamy, N.; Tejani, H.; Gopalan, A.-I.; Lee, K.-P.; Lee, H.-J.; Kyung, H.M. Incorporation of silver nanoparticles on the surface of orthodontic microimplants to achieve antimicrobial properties. *Korean J. Orthod.* **2017**, *47*, 3–10. [CrossRef]
36. Oh, E.-J.; Nguyen, T.-D.T.; Lee, S.-Y.; Jeon, Y.-M.; Bae, T.-S.; Kim, J.-G. Enhanced compatibility and initial stability of Ti6Al4V alloy orthodontic miniscrews subjected to anodization, cyclic precalcification, and heat treatment. *Korean J. Orthod.* **2014**, *44*, 246–253. [CrossRef]

37. Kim, H.-Y.; Kim, S.-C. Bone cutting capacity and osseointegration of surface-treated orthodontic mini-implants. *Korean J. Orthod.* **2016**, *46*, 386–394. [CrossRef]
38. Ly, N.T.K.; Shin, H.; Gupta, K.C.; Kang, I.K.; Yu, W. Bioactive Antibacterial Modification of Orthodontic Microimplants Using Chitosan Biopolymer. *Macromol. Res.* **2019**, *27*, 504–510. [CrossRef]
39. De Stefani, A.; Bruno, G.; Preo, G.; Gracco, A. Application of Nanotechnology in Orthodontic Materials: A State-of-the-Art Review. *Dent. J.* **2020**, *8*, 126. [CrossRef]
40. Choi, H.W.; Park, Y.S.; Chung, S.H.; Jung, M.H.; Moon, W.; Rhee, S.H. Comparison of mechanical and biological properties of zirconia and titanium alloy orthodontic micro-implants. *Korean J. Orthod.* **2017**, *47*, 229–237. [CrossRef]
41. Harzer, W.; Schneider, M.; Gedrange, T. Rapid Maxillary Expansion with Palatal Anchorage of the Hyrax Expansion Screw?Pilot Study with Case Presentation. *J. Orofac. Orthop.* **2004**, *65*, 419–424. [CrossRef]
42. Bud, E.; Bică, C.; Păcurar, M.; Vaida, P.; Vlasa, A.; Martha, K.; Bud, A. Observational Study Regarding Possible Side Effects of Miniscrew-Assisted Rapid Palatal Expander (MARPE) with or without the Use of Corticopuncture Therapy. *Biology* **2021**, *10*, 187. [CrossRef] [PubMed]
43. Tausche, E.; Hansen, L.; Schneider, M.; Harzer, W. Bone-supported rapid maxillary expansion with an implant-borne Hyrax screw: The Dresden Distractor. *L'Orthodontie Française* **2008**, *79*, 127–135. [CrossRef] [PubMed]
44. MacGinnis, M.; Chu, H.; Youssef, G.; Wu, K.W.; Machado, A.W.; Moon, W. The effects of micro-implant assisted rapid palatal expansion (MARPE) on the nasomaxillary complex—A finite element method (FEM) analysis. *Prog. Orthod.* **2014**, *15*, 52. [CrossRef] [PubMed]
45. Carlson, C.; Sung, J.; McComb, R.W.; Machado, A.W.; Moon, W. Microimplant-assisted rapid palatal expansion appliance to orthopedically correct transverse maxillary deficiency in an adult. *Am. J. Orthod. Dentofac. Orthop.* **2016**, *149*, 716–728. [CrossRef]
46. Zong, C.; Tang, B.; Hua, F.; He, H.; Ngan, P. Skeletal and dentoalveolar changes in the transverse dimension using microimplant-assisted rapid palatal expansion (MARPE) appliances. *Semin. Orthod.* **2019**, *25*, 46–59. [CrossRef]
47. Ngan, P.; Nguyen, U.K.; Nguyen, T.; Tremont, T.; Martin, C. Skeletal, Dentoalveolar, and Periodontal Changes of Skeletally Matured Patients with Maxillary Deficiency Treated with Microimplant-assisted Rapid Palatal Expansion Appliances: A Pilot Study. *APOS Trends Orthod.* **2018**, *8*, 71. [CrossRef]
48. Paredes, N.; Colak, O.; Sfogliano, L.; Elkenawy, I.; Fijany, L.; Fraser, A.; Zhang, B.; Moon, W. Differential assessment of skeletal, alveolar, and dental components induced by microimplant-supported midfacial skeletal expander (MSE), utilizing novel angular measurements from the fulcrum. *Prog. Orthod.* **2020**, *21*, 18. [CrossRef]
49. Elkenawy, I.; Fijany, L.; Colak, O.; Paredes, N.A.; Gargoum, A.; Abedini, S.; Cantarella, D.; Dominguez-Mompell, R.; Sfogliano, L.; Moon, W. An assessment of the magnitude, parallelism, and asymmetry of micro-implant-assisted rapid maxillary expansion in non-growing patients. *Prog. Orthod.* **2020**, *21*, 42. [CrossRef]
50. Yu, S.-K.; Cho, Y.; Seo, Y.-S.; Kim, J.-S.; Kim, D.K.; Kim, H.-J. Radiological evaluation of the bone and soft tissue thicknesses of the palate for using a miniscrew-supported maxillary skeletal expander. *Surg. Radiol. Anat.* **2021**, *43*, 1001–1008. [CrossRef]
51. Chen, W.; Zhang, K.; Liu, D. Palatal bone thickness at the implantation area of maxillary skeletal expander in adult patients with skeletal Class III malocclusion: A cone-beam computed tomography study. *BMC Oral Health* **2021**, *21*, 144. [CrossRef]
52. Wang, C.-H.; Wu, J.-H.; Lee, K.-T.; Hsu, K.-R.; Wang, H.C.; Chen, C.-M. Mechanical strength of orthodontic infrazygomatic mini-implants. *Odontology* **2011**, *99*, 98–100. [CrossRef] [PubMed]
53. Mathew, A.; Nagachandran, K.S.; Vijayalakshmi, D. Stress and displacement pattern evaluation using two different palatal expanders in unilateral cleft lip and palate: A three-dimensional finite element analysis. *Prog. Orthod.* **2016**, *17*, 38. [CrossRef] [PubMed]
54. Magkavali-Trikka, P.; Emmanouilidis, G.; Papadopoulos, M.A. Mandibular molar uprighting using orthodontic miniscrew implants: A systematic review. *Prog. Orthod.* **2018**, *19*, 1. [CrossRef] [PubMed]
55. Rai, D.; Bhasin, S.S.; Rai, S. Orthodontic Microimplants Assisted Intrusion of Supra-erupted Maxillary Molar Enabling Osseointegrated Implant Supported Mandibular Prosthesis: Case Reports. *J. Indian Prosthodont. Soc.* **2014**, *14* (Suppl. 1), 238–242. [CrossRef]
56. Oh, Y.-H.; Park, H.-S.; Kwon, T.-G. Treatment effects of microimplant-aided sliding mechanics on distal retraction of posterior teeth. *Am. J. Orthod. Dentofac. Orthop.* **2011**, *139*, 470–481. [CrossRef]
57. Xu, Y.; Xie, J. Comparison of the effects of mini-implant and traditional anchorage on patients with maxillary dentoalveolar protrusion. *Angle Orthod.* **2017**, *87*, 320–327. [CrossRef]
58. Park, H.-S.; Kim, J.-Y.; Kwon, T.-G. Occlusal plane change after intrusion of maxillary posterior teeth by microimplants to avoid maxillary surgery with skeletal Class III orthognathic surgery. *Am. J. Orthod. Dentofac. Orthop.* **2010**, *138*, 631–640. [CrossRef] [PubMed]
59. Beyling, F.; Klang, E.; Niehoff, E.; Schwestka-Polly, R.; Helms, H.-J.; Wiechmann, D. Class II correction by maxillary en masse distalization using a completely customized lingual appliance and a novel mini-screw anchorage concept—Preliminary results. *Head Face Med.* **2021**, *17*, 23. [CrossRef]
60. Long, H.-Q.; Xuan, J.; Kyung, H.-M.; Bing, L.; Wu, X.-P. Biomechanical Analysis of Micro-implants Lingual Straight Wire Appliance during Retracting Maxillary Anterior Teeth. *Int. J. Morphol.* **2018**, *36*, 1386–1393. [CrossRef]
61. Łyczek, J.; Kawala, B.; Antoszewska-Smith, J. Influence of antibiotic prophylaxis on the stability of orthodontic microimplants: A pilot randomized controlled trial. *Am. J. Orthod. Dentofac. Orthop.* **2018**, *153*, 621–631. [CrossRef] [PubMed]

62. Chang, H.; Chen, Y.; Du, J. Obstructive sleep apnea treatment in adults. *Med. Sci.* **2020**, *36*, 7–12. [CrossRef]
63. Colak, O.; Paredes, N.A.; Elkenawy, I.; Torres, M.; Bui, J.; Jahangiri, S.; Moon, W. Tomographic assessment of palatal suture opening pattern and pterygopalatine suture disarticulation in the axial plane after midfacial skeletal expansion. *Prog. Orthod.* **2020**, *21*, 21. [CrossRef] [PubMed]
64. Zasčiurinskienė, E.; Lund, H.; Lindsten, R.; Jansson, H.; Bjerklin, K. Outcome of periodontal–orthodontic treatment in subjects with periodontal disease. Part II: A CBCT study of alveolar bone level changes. *Eur. J. Orthod.* **2019**, *41*, 565–574. [CrossRef] [PubMed]
65. Boryor, A.; Hohmann, A.; Wunderlich, A.; Geiger, M.; Kilic, F.; Kim, K.B.; Sander, M.; Böckers, T.; Sander, C. Use of a modified expander during rapid maxillary expansion in adults: An in vitro and finite element study. *Int. J. Oral Maxillofac. Implant.* **2013**, *28*, e11–e16. [CrossRef]
66. Wu, J.-C.; Huang, J.-N.; Zhao, S.-F. Bicortical microimplant with 2 anchorage heads for mesial movement of posterior tooth in the beagle dog. *Am. J. Orthod. Dentofac. Orthop.* **2007**, *132*, 353–359. [CrossRef]
67. Lee, T.C.K.; McGrath, C.P.J.; Wong, R.W.K.; Rabie, A.B.M. Patients' Perceptions Regarding Microimplant as Anchorage in Orthodontics. *Angle Orthod.* **2008**, *78*, 228–233. [CrossRef]
68. Chen, C.-M.; Chang, C.-S.; Tseng, Y.-C.; Hsu, K.-R.; Lee, K.-T.; Lee, H.-E. The perception of pain following interdental microimplant treatment for skeletal anchorage: A retrospective study. *Odontology* **2011**, *99*, 88–91. [CrossRef]
69. Baxmann, M.; McDonald, F.; Bourauel, C.; Jäger, A. Expectations, acceptance, and preferences regarding microimplant treatment in orthodontic patients: A randomized controlled trial. *Am. J. Orthod. Dentofac. Orthop.* **2010**, *138*, 250.e1–250.e10, discussion 250–251. [CrossRef]
70. Reynders, R.M.; Ronchi, L.; Ladu, L.; Di Girolamo, N.; De Lange, J.; Roberts, N.; Mickan, S. Barriers and facilitators to the implementation of orthodontic mini-implants in clinical practice: A protocol for a systematic review and meta-analysis. *Syst. Rev.* **2016**, *5*, 22. [CrossRef]
71. Lu, L.; Park, H.-S. Surface characteristics and mechanical behavior of retrieved orthodontic microimplants. *J. Zhejiang Univ. Sci. B* **2018**, *19*, 372–382. [CrossRef] [PubMed]
72. Supplement, D.; Minervini, G.; Nucci, L.; Lanza, A.; Femiano, F.; Contaldo, M.; Grassia, V. Temporomandibular disc displacement with reduction treated with anterior repositioning splint: A 2-year clinical and magnetic resonance imaging (MRI) follow-up. *J. Biol. Regul. Homeost. Agents* **2020**, *34* (Suppl. 1), 151–160, DENTAL SUPPLEMENT.
73. Minervini, G.; Lucchese, A.; Perillo, L.; Serpico, R.; Minervini, G. Unilateral superior condylar neck fracture with dislocation in a child treated with an acrylic splint in the upper arch for functional repositioning of the mandible. *CRANIO®* **2017**, *35*, 337–341. [CrossRef]
74. Deshayes, M.-J. Les déformations crâniennes asymétriques et leur retentissement dento-facial et occlusal [Cranial asymmetries and their dento-facial and occlusal effects]. *L'Orthodontie Française* **2006**, *77*, 87–99. [CrossRef] [PubMed]
75. Minervini, G.; Romano, A.; Petruzzi, M.; Maio, C.; Serpico, R.; Lucchese, A.; Candotto, V.; Di Stasio, D. Telescopic overdenture on natural teeth: Prosthetic rehabilitation on (OFD) syndromic patient and a review on available literature. *J. Boil. Regul. Homeost. Agents* **2018**, *32* (Suppl. 1), 131–134.
76. D'Apuzzo, F.; Minervini, G.; Grassia, V.; Rotolo, R.; Perillo, L.; Nucci, L. Mandibular Coronoid Process Hypertrophy: Diagnosis and 20-Year Follow-Up with CBCT, MRI and EMG Evaluations. *Appl. Sci.* **2021**, *11*, 4504. [CrossRef]
77. Akbulut, Y. The effects of different antiseptic mouthwash on microbiota around orthodontic mini-screw. *Niger. J. Clin. Pract.* **2020**, *23*, 1507–1513. [CrossRef]
78. Di Stasio, D.; Romano, A.N.; Paparella, R.S.; Gentile, C.; Minervini, G.; Serpico, R.; Candotto, V.; Laino, L. How social media meet patients questions: YouTube review for children oral thrush. *J. Biol. Regul. Homeost. Agents* **2018**, *32* (Suppl. 1), 101–106.
79. Di Stasio, D.; Romano, A.; Paparella, R.S.; Gentile, C.; Serpico, R.; Minervini, G.; Candotto, V.; Laino, L. How social media meet patients questions: YouTube review for mouth sores in children. *J. Biol. Regul. Homeost. Agents* **2018**, *32* (Suppl. 1), 117–121. [PubMed]
80. Di Stasio, D.; Romano, A.; Gentile, C.; Maio, C.; Lucchese, A.; Serpico, R.; Paparella, R.; Minervini, G.; Candotto, V.; Laino, L. Systemic and topical photodynamic therapy (PDT) on oral mucosa lesions: An overview. *J. Biol. Regul. Homeost. Agents* **2018**, *32* (Suppl. 1), 123–126. [PubMed]

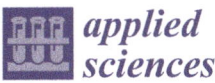

Article

Effect of Digital Technologies on the Marginal Accuracy of Conventional and Cantilever Co–Cr Posterior-Fixed Partial Dentures Frameworks

Celia Tobar, Verónica Rodríguez, Carlos Lopez-Suarez, Jesús Peláez *, Jorge Cortés-Bretón Brinckmann and María J. Suárez

Department of Conservative Dentristy and Bucofacial Prosthesis, Faculty of Odontology, University Complutense of Madrid, 28040 Madrid, Spain; cetobar@ucm.es (C.T.); veranicr@ucm.es (V.R.); carlop04@ucm.es (C.L.-S.); jcortesb@ucm.es (J.C.-B.B.); mjsuarez@ucm.es (M.J.S.)
* Correspondence: jpelaezr@ucm.es

Abstract: The introduction of new digital technologies represents an important advance to fabricate metal–ceramic restorations. However, few studies have evaluated the influence of these technologies on the fit of the restorations. The aim of this study was to evaluate the effect of different manufacturing techniques and pontic design on the vertical marginal fit of cobalt—chromium (Co–Cr) posterior fixed partial dentures (FPDs) frameworks. Methods: Eighty stainless-steel dies were prepared to receive 3-unit FPDs frameworks with intermediate pontic (n = 40) and cantilever pontic (n = 40). Within each design, the specimens were randomly divided into four groups (n = 10 each) depending on the manufacturing technique: casting (CM), direct metal laser sintering (LS), soft metal milling (SM), and hard metal milling (HM). The frameworks were luted, and the vertical marginal discrepancy was assessed. Data analysis was made using Kruskal–Wallis and Mann–Whitney U tests ($\alpha = 0.05$). Results: The vertical marginal discrepancy values of all FPDs were below 50 μm. The HM frameworks obtained the lowest misfit values in both designs. However, no differences were found among intermediate pontic groups or cantilevered groups. Likewise, when differences in a marginal discrepancy between both framework designs were analyzed, no differences were observed. Conclusions: The analyzed digital technologies demonstrated high precision of fit on Co–Cr frameworks and on both pontic designs.

Keywords: marginal adaptation; fixed partial denture; dental technology; cobalt–chromium alloys; scanning electron microscopy

Citation: Tobar, C.; Rodríguez, V.; Lopez-Suarez, C.; Peláez, J.; Brinckmann, J.C.-B.; Suárez, M.J.Effect of Digital Technologies on the Marginal Accuracy of Conventional and Cantilever Co–Cr Posterior-Fixed Partial Dentures Frameworks. *Appl. Sci.* **2021**, *11*, 2988. https://doi.org/10.3390/app11072988

Academic Editor: Vittorio Checchi

Received: 16 February 2021
Accepted: 23 March 2021
Published: 26 March 2021

Publisher's Note: MDPI stays neutral with regard to jurisdictional claims in published maps and institutional affiliations.

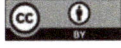

Copyright: © 2021 by the authors. Licensee MDPI, Basel, Switzerland. This article is an open access article distributed under the terms and conditions of the Creative Commons Attribution (CC BY) license (https://creativecommons.org/licenses/by/4.0/).

1. Introduction

Metal–ceramic restorations are still the most widely used for fixed prosthodontics due to their reliability and good long-term prognosis, widely tested, which has led that they are considered to be the gold standard [1–4]. Base metal alloys, especially cobalt–chromium (Co–Cr) alloy, have undergone a higher development in recent decades as an alternative to the costly noble alloys and the lower biocompatibility of nickel-chromium alloys [5,6]. In addition to good biocompatibility, Co–Cr alloys show proper corrosion stability and appropriate mechanical properties, as fracture resistance, hardness and resilience [7–10]. Metal–ceramic restorations have been processed by traditional casting techniques, but currently, new prosthetic technologies have been introduced to fabricate metal-base restorations. Nowadays, Co–Cr frameworks can be processed by computer-aided design and computer-aided manufacturing (CAD-CAM), involving subtractive and additive manufacturing processes. The subtractive or milling method consists of a process controlled by a computer program, which uses power-driven machine tools with a sharp cutting tool to mechanically cut the materials and to achieve specific geometries [11,12]. The main advantages are time-saving, the ability to create fine and precise detail, and the availability of materials [11,13–15]. Nevertheless, it has disadvantages like the high cost and the waste of material [11,16]. Nowadays, metal milling frameworks can be obtained by hard or soft blocks. Soft metal milling is the most recent process within the subtractive method and consists of using metal blanks in a pre-sintered state. These blanks are milled and subsequently sintered in a special furnace until achieving the proper size (volumetric shrinkage of approximately 11%) [13]. This method has the advantages of shorter milling time, fewer machine tools wear (increasing its useful life), and less risk of material contamination due to dry milling [13]. On the other hand, the additive method, especially the direct metal laser sintering (DMLS), produces the metal structures layer by layer by a high-power laser that fuses the alloy powder from a three dimensional (3D) CAD file that contains the framework's design [17–19]. The advantages include no material waste, higher productivity [11], and easy fabrication of complex shapes [18,20]. The main drawbacks are that there may be differences in the final model production and limitations on materials so far [11,12].

A good marginal fit is one of the main criteria to achieve long-term success in fixed prostheses restorations. The lack of an accurate fit can cause severe complications [21–23], and multiple factors, such as tooth preparation, luting procedure, prosthetic design and manufacturing technology, can affect the final adaptation of the restorations [24–28].

Nevertheless, despite its importance, no consensus exists in the literature on what must be considered the optimal fit value [28–32], and most authors continue to refer to the criteria established by McLean and von Fraunhofer [33], which established as clinically acceptable a marginal discrepancy lower than 120 µm. Currently, CAD-CAM restorations have shown high precision in their marginal adaptation, and several authors admit gaps below 100 µm [28,32,34–38]. Different methods have been proposed to measure the marginal adaptation of a restoration. Direct-view microscopic techniques are the most commonly used, although there is no consensus in the methodology and the best technique to follow [26,27,39]. Scanning electron microscopy (SEM) is a conservative method to provide appropriate and realistic marginal fit observations with high magnification, especially with complex margin morphologies [27,28,39]. Nonetheless, this method also has disadvantages as the location of reference points for measurements and the observation angle [26–28,39,40].

There is limited information available regarding the influence of manufacturing techniques on the marginal adaptation of Co–Cr frameworks; thus, it is important to investigate the precision of fit of these restorations. Therefore, the present in vitro study's purpose was to evaluate and compare the vertical marginal discrepancy of posterior Co–Cr fixed partial dentures (FPDs) fabricated with different technologies and with two types of framework design (intermediate or cantilever pontic). The null hypotheses to be tested were that no differences in marginal fit would be found among the Co–Cr frameworks fabricated by the different technologies and framework designs.

2. Materials and Methods

2.1. Experimental Model

Eighty standardized machined stainless-steel master dies, with two abutments and a platform, were fabricated (Mechanical Workshop of Physical Science, University Complutense of Madrid, Spain). The platforms (30 mm in length, 17 mm in width, and 4.5 mm in thickness) [29,39] were designed to receive two designs of posterior 3-unit frameworks: (1) with an intermediate pontic (5 mm between abutments) (n = 40), and (2) cantilever pontic (0.2 mm between abutments) (n = 40). The abutments (n = 160) were designed simulating a first mandibular premolar prepared (5 mm in height, occlusal diameter of 5 mm, a 1 mm-wide chamfer circumferentially finish line, and a 6° angle of convergence of the axial walls) [28,29,32,34,36,39], and randomly screwed on the platform (Figures 1 and 2).

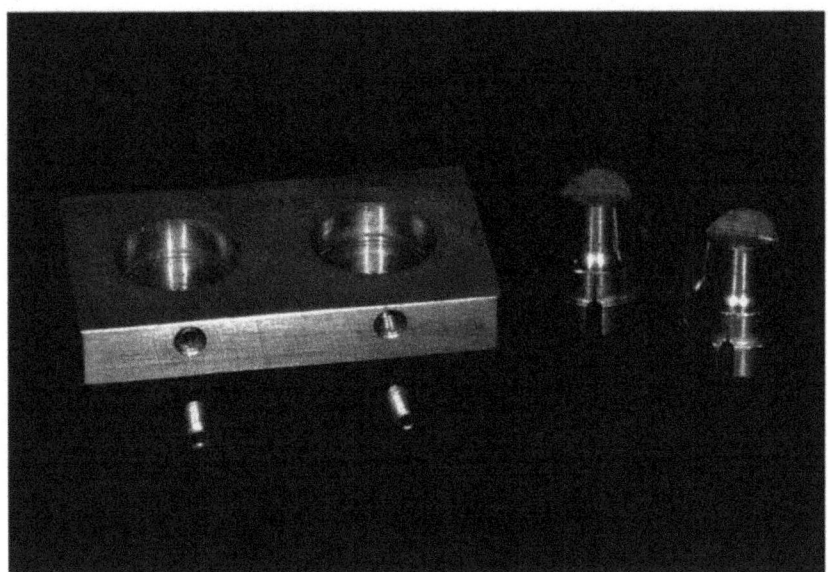

Figure 1. Master die components (platform, screws and abutments) of conventional frameworks.

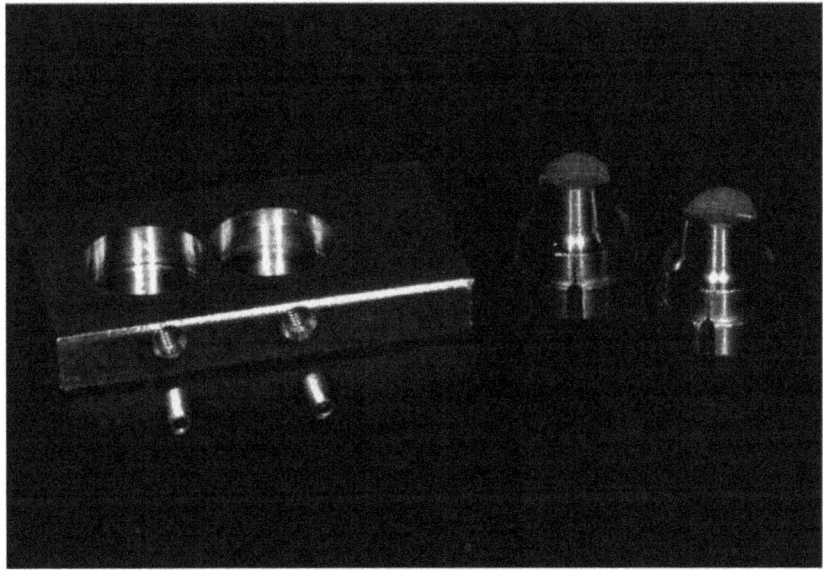

Figure 2. Master die components (platform, screws and abutments) of frameworks with cantilever pontic.

Within each design group, the specimens were randomly divided into four subgroups (n = 10 each, in accordance with the results of power analysis) depending on the manufacturing technique used to fabricate the frameworks: casting (CM), laser sintering (LS), soft metal milling (SM) and hard metal milling (HM). The specimens were used as working dies.

Table 1 displays the group code, coping alloys brands, composition, and manufacturers used in the study.

Table 1. Manufacturing technique, brands, manufacturers and chemical composition of the alloys selected for the study (weight %).

Manufacturing Technique			Dental Alloy Composition (Weight %)									
Group Code		Coping Alloys Brands and Manufacturers										
(1) Intermediate Pontic	(2) Cantilever Pontic		Co	Cr	Mo	W	Si	Fe	C	Mn	Ni	N
CM	CMc	Super 8 (Dental Alloys Products, San Diego, CA, USA)	59.5	31.5	5	-	2	≤1	≤1	≤1	-	-
LS	LSc	ST2724G (Sint-Tech, Clermont-Ferrand, France)	65	28–30	5–6	-	≤1	≤0.5	≤0.02	≤1	≤1	-
SM	SMc	Ceramill® Sintron R 71 L (Amann Girrbach, Koblach, Austria)	66	28	5	-	≤1	≤1	≤0.1	≤1	-	-
HM	HMc	Starbond CoS DISC basic (Scheftner, Mainz, Germany)	59	25	3.5	9.5	1	≤1.5	≤1.5	≤1.5	-	≤1.5

2.2. Fabrication of the Restorations

To fabricate the CM and CMc frameworks, the specimens were scanned and digitized with the Lava Scan ST (3M ESPE, Seefeld, Germany), and the frameworks were designed using CAD software (DWOS version 7.0; Dental Wings, Montreal, QC, Canada). The wax patterns were made with the ProJet 1200 3D printer (3D Systems, Rock Hill, SC, USA) and invested with phosphate graphite-free investment plaster (Vestofix; DFS Diamond GmbH, Riedenburg, Germany). The casting was performed using induction and a centrifugal vacuum-casting machine (MIE-200C/R; Ordenta, Arganda del Rey, Spain) under vacuum pressure of 580 mmHg, at a melting temperature of 1480 °C. After casting, the samples were cleaned with water steam and sandblasted with aluminum-oxide particles (50 µm) under 50 N/cm^2 pressure (EXTRAmatic 9040; Kavo Dental GmbH, Biberach, Germany).

To prepare the LS and LSc frameworks, the scanning and design process was similar to the CM and CMc groups. The CAD design file was transferred to a DMLS unit (PM 100 Dental; Phenix Systems, Clermont-Ferrand, France), and the laser sintering process was performed by building 20 mm layers of alloy powders from the occlusal surface to the margins by applying a Yb-fiber laser at 1650 °C under an argon atmosphere. All the frameworks were cleaned and sandblasted in the same manner as the casted frameworks

To fabricate the SM and SMc frameworks, the specimens were scanned (Ceramill Map400; Amann Girrbach, Koblach, Austria), and the data were entered into specific design software (Ceramill Mind; Amann Girrbach). To compensate for the post-sintering shrinkage, the design was enlarged by 11%. These data were pre-set in the software. The frameworks were manufactured from pre-sintered Co–Cr discs in a milling unit (Ceramill Motion 2; Amann Girrbach). Then, the specimens were placed in a sintering tray (Ceramill Argovent; Amann Girrbach) and introduced into a sintering furnace (Ceramill Algotherm 2; Amann Girrbach) at 1.300 °C under an argon atmosphere to prevent oxidation. All the frameworks were cleaned and sandblasted in the same manner as the casted frameworks.

The manufacturing process for the HM and HMc frameworks also began with scanning the specimens (3Shape D750; 3Shape Dental System, Copenhagen, Denmark) and designing the copings by the specific software (Molder Builder; 3Shape Dental System). Two sintered Co–Cr discs were inserted in the warehouse (PH 2/120 SAUER; DGM Mori, Stipshausen, Germany) of the milling unit (Ultrasonic 10 linear; DMG Mori, Bielefeld, Germany) and machining was carried out.

All the 3D framework designs were done by experienced technicians with the same parameters: 0.5 mm wall-thickness, internal cement space of 50 µm, a premolar shape pontic, and a connector area of 9 mm^2 (3 mm × 3 mm). All the frameworks were cleaned and sandblasted in the same manner as the casted frameworks

The frameworks were luted onto their corresponding specimen using conventional glass–ionomer cement (Ketac-Cem EasyMix; 3 M ESPE), mixed following the manufacturer's instructions, at room temperature (18–24 °C) and relative humidity (50 ± 10%). The cement was placed on the axial walls of the structures, and a constant seating force of 50 N was applied with a torque wrench (Ziacom, Madrid, Spain) fitted to a customized device (Mechanical Workshop of Physical Science, University Complutense of Madrid, Spain) for 10 min.

The marginal accuracy of the restorations was measured under a SEM (JSM-6400; JEOL, Tokyo, Japan) to determinate the vertical marginal discrepancy (or the vertical distance between the restoration margin and the preparation cavosurface angle, measured parallel to the longitudinal axis of the tooth [41]) (Figure 3). The specimens were coated with 24 kt, 19.32 g/m^3 density gold by a Q150RS metallizer (Quorum Technologies, Laughton, United Kingdom) before SEM evaluation and then positioned in a customized clamp perpendicular to the axis of the microscope [32]. To standardize the marginal evaluation, the measuring areas were marked at the same point in the middle of the buccal and lingual surfaces of each abutment in the gap region with an indelible marking pen (Lumocolor permanent; Staedler Mars, Nuremberg, Germany) [28,32,34,39]. The SEM was connected to a computer with the INCA Suite version 4.04 software (Oxford Instruments; Abingdon, Oxfordshire, UK), which was run to capture and calibrate the images at the marked areas, at ×1000 magnification (Figure 4). All the images were captured by the same operator with an acceleration voltage of 20 KV and a 20 mm working distance, achieving a eucentric position, which means that the position at which the primary electron beam hits does not change from one sample to another by following the same coordinates [42]. To increase the number of measurements per specimen, the images were edited by using imaging software (ImageJ version 1.49; U.S. National Institutes of Health, Bethesda, MD, USA), creating lines parallel to the original. Therefore, 60 measurements were recorded for each specimen (30 per abutment) (Figure 5).

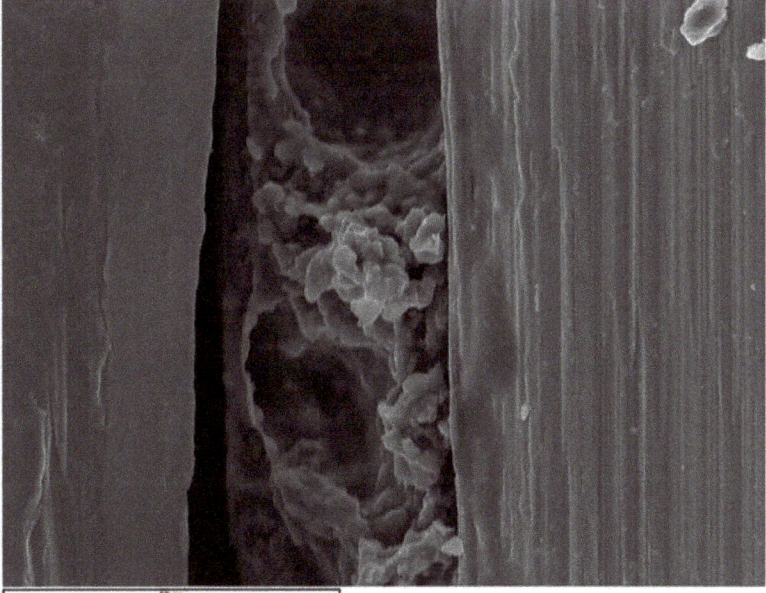

Figure 3. SEM image (1000×) showing the marginal gap in a representative framework of the hard metal milling (HM) group.

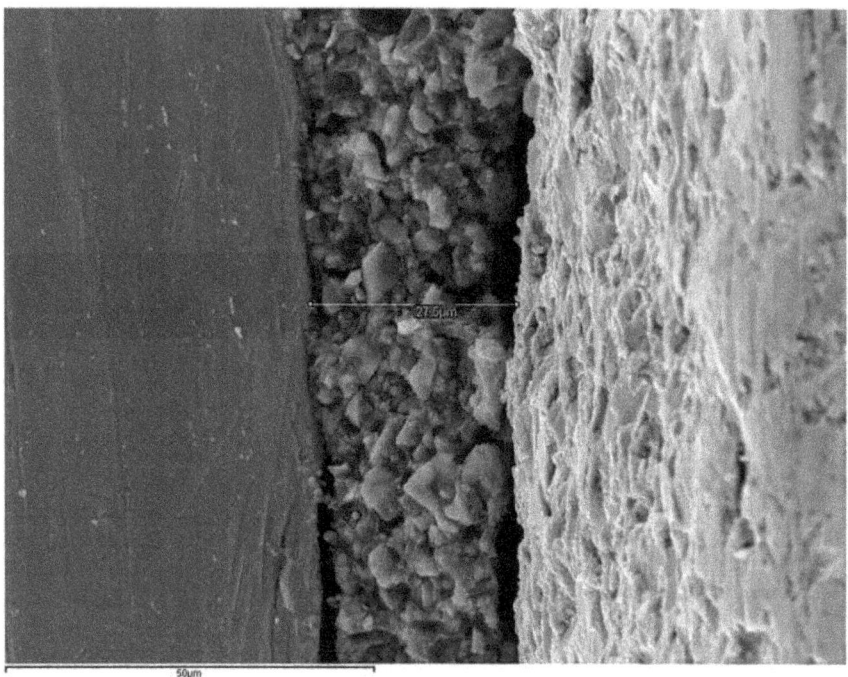

Figure 4. SEM image (1000×) calibrated with INCA software showing a marginal discrepancy of a CMc framework.

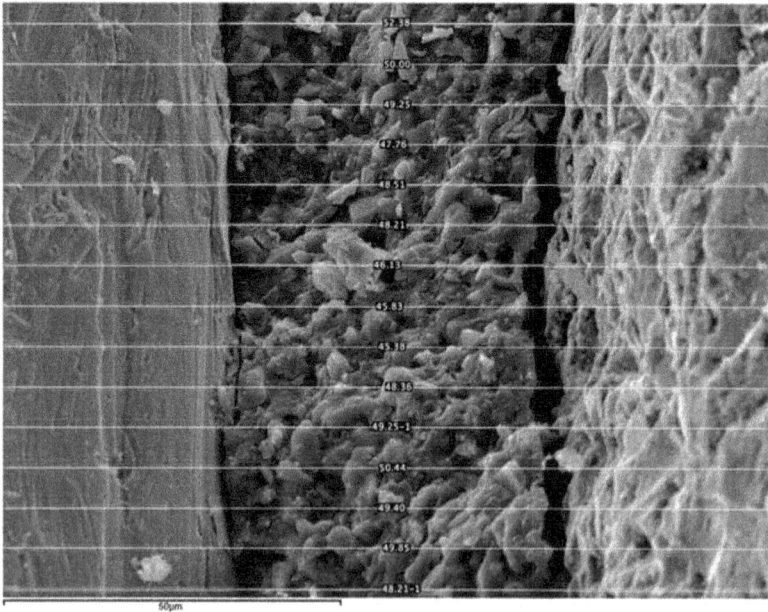

Figure 5. SEM image (1000×) showing the marginal discrepancy measurements with Image software of a direct metal laser sintering (LS) framework.

2.3. Statistical Analysis

SPSS Version 22.0 (SPSS Inc., Chicago, IL, USA) was used for analyzing the data. The mean values and standard deviations (SD) per group were calculated. The Kruskal–Wallis test and post hoc test for multiple comparisons were used for comparisons among the manufacturing techniques. The Mann–Whitney U test was used to compare both framework designs. The level of statistical significance was set to $\alpha = 0.05$.

3. Results

The overall mean and standard deviation marginal discrepancies values of intermediate and cantilever pontic frameworks are listed in Tables 2 and 3, respectively.

Table 2. Mean, standard deviation (SD), minimum and maximum (µm) marginal discrepancies values of in frameworks with intermediate pontic.

Group 1	Mean	SD	Minimum	Maximum
CM	40.11	10.43	26.90	53.90
LS	41.84	10.36	27.16	57.20
SM	39.78	8.77	24.24	53.10
HM	38.67	18.27	22.83	80.01

Table 3. Mean, standard deviation (SD), minimum and maximum (µm) marginal discrepancies values in frameworks with cantilever pontic.

Group 2	Mean	SD	Minimum	Maximum
CMc	34.55	6.93	26.94	50.71
LSc	35.22	10.60	26.17	62.42
SMc	40.81	5.55	32.18	49.21
HMc	34.17	15.85	19.63	71.69

All experimental groups obtained marginal discrepancy values below 50 µm. For the frameworks with an intermediate pontic, the HM group showed the lowest misfit values (38.67 ± 18.27 µm), while the LS subgroup exhibited the highest misfit values (41.84 ± 10.36 µm). The Kruskal–Wallis test revealed no significant differences ($p = 0.677$) in the marginal fit among the different manufacturing techniques. When the cantilever frameworks were analyzed, the HMc group also displayed the lowest marginal discrepancies (34.17 ± 15.85 µm), while the highest misfit values were observed in the SMc group (40.81 ± 5.55 µm). Likewise, no differences ($p = 0.067$) were observed among the manufacturing techniques.

The influence of framework design on the marginal fit was also analyzed, and the Mann–Whitney U test showed no significant differences in any of the tested subgroups: CM and CMc ($p = 0.280$); LS and LSc ($p = 0.123$); SM and SMc ($p = 0.912$); HM and HMc ($p = 0.436$).

4. Discussion

This study evaluated the vertical marginal discrepancy of 3-unit Co–Cr posterior FPDs frameworks with intermediate and cantilever pontic and four different manufacturing techniques. The results of the study showed that all tested groups were able to obtain restorations with an adequate marginal fit within the clinically accepted limits of 120 µm [28,29,33,34,43,44], and support the acceptance of the null hypotheses because no significant differences were found among the manufacturing techniques and between the design of the frameworks.

Up to date, there is no consensus on which metallic framework exhibits the best marginal fit. In the study, the CM group on conventional frameworks with intermediate pontic obtained misfit values similar to other studies [18,39] and lower than other ones [17,20,45,46]. The lower values obtained in the study may be due to the fact that the wax patterns of the frameworks were not made with the conventional manual technique, but they were obtained with the 3D-printing technique, in agreement with the study of

Fathi et al. [47] which obtained better fit in cast crowns with wax patterns fabricated by additive CAD/CAM technique. In the last years, several studies have been published about the marginal fit of restorations made with additive technology. In the study, no differences were shown between CM and LS frameworks. While some authors [48–51] have found better fit values in cast structures compared to sintered ones. Conversely, other authors [15,17,18,45,46,52,53] obtained better fit values in selective laser sintering structures. Therefore, there is no consensus regarding the influence of the LS technique on the marginal fit of the restorations. The HM group obtained the lowest misfit values, although there were no differences with the other groups. Afify et al. [54], in Ni-Cr frameworks, and Tamac et al. [55] obtained the same conclusion in their studies comparing cast, sintered and milled crowns. Neese et al. [16] also reported that the milled structures presented a better fit. However, other authors [56,57] reported a better adaptation of the sintered structures. There are only a few studies that compared the four available techniques for manufacturing metal frameworks, and the differences among studies continue. Recent studies [13,58–60] concluded that milled soft metal structures obtain lower misfit values than the other technologies, while other studies [61] continue to advocate for sintered structures. In the study, no differences could be demonstrated among the four manufacturing techniques. Therefore, it remains unclear nowadays which manufacturing technique offers more advantages regarding the marginal adaptation of the metallic restorations.

In certain situations, the disposition of the abutments may not be ideal for FPDs design, and it is necessary to select cantilevered structures as a treatment option [62]. In the present study, the HMc frameworks also obtained the lowest misfit values, although; no differences were demonstrated with the other cantilevered groups. No previous studies were found comparing different manufacturing techniques on cantilever frameworks regarding the marginal adaptation. Therefore, it was not possible to compare the results of the study with previous studies.

In the study, no differences in marginal adaptation were observed when comparing both frameworks design fabricated with the same technology. Likewise, no previous studies were found to compare the results of the study. Previous studies indicated that cantilevered metal–ceramic FPDs can be used effectively in posterior sectors [62], using non-noble alloys, and to replace a tooth with at least two abutment teeth [63,64]. The evidence on the risk of failure of cantilevered FPDs is controversial when compared with the conventional FPDs with an intermediate pontic. Some authors demonstrated that the survival rates of cantilevered prostheses were lower and with more complications [62,64], while others showed a comparable acceptable survival [65–68], although it may vary according to the variables analyzed. Despite the fact that studies on the behavior of cantilevered FPDs are limited, it is important to evaluate this type of prosthesis because it is a treatment option as an alternative to implants or removable partial dentures in daily clinical practice.

The different results among the studies may be due to the different methodology used and the absence of standardization. Several methods have been proposed for measuring the marginal fit, such as silicone replica [51,69,70], direct-view techniques [28,39], profilometry [71,72], or microcomputed tomography [60,73]. In the study, the marginal fit was evaluated by direct viewing with external measurements on an SEM, based on a previous study that demonstrated that destructive methods are not required to assess the marginal fit [28]. There are other aspects that may also directly influence the marginal fit, such as the finish line, the cementation, and the porcelain veneering [26]. In the study, the finish line design was a chamfer, being the most used finish line in recent studies [16,18,20,28,29,50,53,57]. The marginal fit measurements were performed on cemented frameworks to replicate the clinical practice. Previous studies have found higher misfit values after cementation [30,31,43,50], probably due to the hydraulic pressure or the excess of cement [26]. In the study, glass–ionomer cement was used due to its reduced layer thickness [24], and the predetermined internal space for the luting agent was 50 μm in all the frameworks, allowing an adequate cement flow as previously reported [29]. In addition, the luting procedure was carried out in a standardized way, under a seating force of 50 N, following previous studies that used as reference the 5 Kgf (49 N) [13,24,53,69]. Regarding the veneering porcelain, there is no consensus on whether it affects the marginal fit [18,43,51,74], and in the study, it has not been assessed because the purpose was to analyze only the behavior of the alloy by itself regardless of the veneering ceramic.

Furthermore, the marginal adaptation can also be affected by the manufacturing technique and the Co–Cr alloy selected [60]. Although traditional techniques are handmade processes susceptible to error in any of its phases, and CAD-CAM technologies are automated processes, several factors can affect the marginal fit of the CAD-CAM restorations, such as the accuracy of the scanner, the data scanned transformation to three-dimensional models, and the machine precision [51,75]. In the study, it was analyzed the same Co–Cr alloy with four manufacturing techniques, and it has demonstrated that it provided high precision (below 50 µm) regarding the marginal adaptation, although it may also be due to the precision of the digital technologies employed, including the design and manufacturing of the wax patterns in the casting group.

The study had some limitations. It was performed under standardized conditions, avoiding several variables affecting the clinical practice; however, this allowed testing the marginal adaptation of the frameworks under the same conditions. Another limitation was that only one Co–Cr alloy was analyzed, and it would be interesting to test the technologies analyzed with other alloys. Further research is needed to establish a standardized and reliable method to assess the marginal fit that allows the comparison among the different studies. In addition, more studies are needed on cantilever prostheses since there is a lack of studies to support their clinical behavior. Additional clinical trials are necessary to validate the new technologies in order to achieve greater optimization and standardization. Furthermore, there is a need to review the range of clinical acceptance since digital technologies demonstrate high precision.

5. Conclusions

Within the limitations of this in vitro study, the casting technique with the wax patterns obtained by CAD design and 3D printing, and the CAD/CAM technologies as direct metal laser sintering, hard metal milling and soft metal milling seem to guarantee comparable and clinically acceptable misfit values for fabricating Co–Cr posterior FPDs frameworks with intermediate and cantilever pontic.

Author Contributions: All the authors contributed to the study, writing, review, and editing of the manuscript. Conceptualization and methodology: C.T., V.R., C.L.-S., J.P., J.C.-B.B. and M.J.S.; supervision: M.J.S. and J.P. Data curation, data visualization: C.T., V.R., C.L.-S., J.P. and M.J.S. writing—reviewing and editing: C.T., V.R., C.L.-S., J.P., J.C.-B.B. and M.J.S. All authors have read and agreed to the published version of the manuscript.

Funding: This study was funded by a research grant between the University Complutense of Madrid and Prótesis S.A. (No 381/2015) through the last author.

Institutional Review Board Statement: Not Applicable.

Informed Consent Statement: Not applicable.

Data Availability Statement: The data presented in this study are available on request from the corresponding author.

Acknowledgments: The authors would like to thank dental laboratories Prótesis SA., 3Dental, and Dental Creative for manufacturing the frameworks; and Carmen Bravo, Center of Data Processing, Computing Service for Research Support, University Complutense of Madrid, for her assistance with the statistical analysis.

Conflicts of Interest: The authors reported no conflict of interest related to this study.

References

1. Roberts, H.W.; Berzins, D.W.; Moore, B.K.; Charlton, D.G. Metal-ceramic alloys in dentistry: A review. *J. Prosthodont.* **2009**, *18*, 188–194. [CrossRef]
2. Sailer, I.; Strasding, M.; Valente, N.A.; Zwahlen, M.; Liu, S.; Pjetursson, B.E. A systematic review of the survival and complication rates of zirconia-ceramic and metal-ceramic multiple-unit fixed dental prostheses. *Clin. Oral. Implants. Res.* **2018**, *29*, 184–198. [CrossRef]
3. Ozcan, M. Fracture reasons in ceramic-fused-to-metal restorations. *J. Oral Rehabil.* **2003**, *30*, 265–269. [CrossRef] [PubMed]
4. Limones, A.; Molinero-Mourelle, P.; Azevedo, L.; Romeo-Rubio, M.; Correia, A.; Gomez-Polo, M. Zirconia-ceramic versus metal-ceramic posterior multiunit tooth-supported fixed dental prostheses: A systematic review and meta-analysis of randomized controlled trials. *J. Am. Dent. Assoc.* **2020**, *151*, 230–238e237. [CrossRef]
5. Kelly, J.R.; Rose, T.C. Nonprecious alloys for use in fixed prosthodontics: A literature review. *J. Prosthet. Dent.* **1983**, *49*, 363–370. [CrossRef]
6. Kane, L.M.; Chronaios, D.; Sierraalta, M.; George, F.M. Marginal and internal adaptation of milled cobalt-chromium copings. *J. Prosthet. Dent.* **2015**, *114*, 680–685. [CrossRef]
7. Wataha, J.C. Alloys for prosthodontic restorations. *J. Prosthet. Dent.* **2002**, *87*, 351–363. [CrossRef]
8. Li, K.C.; Prior, D.J.; Waddell, J.N.; Swain, M.V. Comparison of the microstructure and phase stability of as-cast, CAD/CAM and powder metallurgy manufactured Co–Cr dental alloys. *Dent. Mater.* **2015**, *31*, e306–e315. [CrossRef]
9. Lucchetti, M.C.; Fratto, G.; Valeriani, F.; de Vittori, E.; Giampaoli, S.; Papetti, P.; Spica, V.R.; Manzon, L. Cobalt-chromium alloys in dentistry: An evaluation of metal ion release. *J. Prosthet. Dent.* **2015**, *114*, 602–608. [CrossRef] [PubMed]
10. Xin, X.Z.; Chen, J.; Xiang, N.; Gong, Y.; Wei, B. Surface characteristics and corrosion properties of selective laser melted Co–Cr dental alloy after porcelain firing. *Dent. Mater.* **2014**, *30*, 263–270. [CrossRef] [PubMed]
11. van Noort, R. The future of dental devices is digital. *Dent. Mater.* **2012**, *28*, 3–12. [CrossRef] [PubMed]
12. Alghazzawi, T.F. Advancements in CAD/CAM technology: Options for practical implementation. *J. Prosthodont. Res.* **2016**, *60*, 72–84. [CrossRef] [PubMed]
13. Kim, K.B.; Kim, J.H.; Kim, W.C. Three-dimensional evaluation of gaps associated with fixed dental prostheses fabricated with new technologies. *J. Prosthet. Dent.* **2014**, *112*, 1432–1436. [CrossRef] [PubMed]
14. Miyazaki, T.; Hotta, Y. CAD/CAM systems available for the fabrication of crown and bridge restorations. *Aust. Dent. J.* **2011**, *56*, 97–106. [CrossRef] [PubMed]
15. Koutsoukis, T.; Zinelis, S.; Eliades, G.; Al-Wazzan, K.; Rifaiy, M.A.; Al Jabbari, Y.S. Selective Laser Melting Technique of Co–Cr Dental Alloys: A Review of Structure and Properties and Comparative Analysis with Other Available Techniques. *J. Prosthodont.* **2015**, *24*, 303–312. [CrossRef] [PubMed]
16. Nesse, H.; Ulstein, D.M.; Vaage, M.M.; Øilo, M. Internal and marginal fit of cobalt-chromium fixed dental prostheses fabricated with 3 different techniques. *J. Prosthet. Dent.* **2015**, *114*, 686–692. [CrossRef] [PubMed]
17. Castillo-Oyague, R.; Lynch, C.D.; Turrion, A.S.; Lopez-Lozano, J.F.; Torres-Lagares, D.; Suarez-García, M.J. Misfit and microleakage of implant-supported crown copings obtained by laser sintering and casting techniques, luted with glass-ionomer, resin cements and acrylic/urethane-based agents. *J. Dent.* **2013**, *41*, 90–96. [CrossRef]
18. Sundar, M.K.; Chikmagalur, S.B.; Pasha, F. Marginal fit and microleakage of cast and metal laser sintered copings—An in vitro study. *J. Prosthodont. Res.* **2014**, *58*, 252–258. [CrossRef]
19. Traini, T.; Mangano, C.; Sammons, R.L.; Mangano, F.; Macchi, A.; Piattelli, A. Direct laser metal sintering as a new approach to fabrication of an isoelastic functionally graded material for manufacture of porous titanium dental implants. *Dent. Mater.* **2008**, *24*, 1525–1533. [CrossRef]
20. Kim, K.B.; Kim, W.C.; Kim, H.Y.; Kim, J.H. An evaluation of marginal fit of three-unit fixed dental prostheses fabricated by direct metal laser sintering system. *Dent. Mater.* **2013**, *29*, e91–e96. [CrossRef]
21. Ramfjord, S.P. Periodontal aspects of restorative dentistry. *J. Oral Rehabil.* **1974**, *1*, 107–126. [CrossRef] [PubMed]
22. Goldman, M.; Laosonthorn, P.; White, R.R. Microleakage—Full crowns and the dental pulp. *J. Endod.* **1992**, *18*, 43–45. [CrossRef]
23. Felton, D.A.; Kanoy, B.E.; Bayne, S.C.; Wirthman, G.P. Effect of in vivo crown margin discrepancies on periodontal health. *J. Prosthet. Dent.* **1991**, *65*, 357–364. [CrossRef]
24. Piemjai, M. Effect of seating force, margin design, and cement on marginal seal and retention of complete metal crowns. *Int. J. Prosthodont.* **2001**, *14*, 412–416.
25. Beuer, F.; Edelhoff, D.; Gernet, W.; Naumann, M. Effect of preparation angles on the precision of zirconia crown copings fabricated by CAD/CAM system. *Dent. Mater. J.* **2008**, *27*, 814–820. [CrossRef]
26. Contrepois, M.; Soenen, A.; Bartala, M.; Laviole, O. Marginal adaptation of ceramic crowns: A systematic review. *J. Prosthet. Dent.* **2013**, *110*, 447–454.e10. [CrossRef] [PubMed]
27. Nawafleh, N.A.; Mack, F.; Evans, J.; Mackay, J.; Hatamleh, M.M. Accuracy and reliability of methods to measure marginal adaptation of crowns and FDPs: A literature review. *J. Prosthodont.* **2013**, *22*, 419–428. [CrossRef] [PubMed]
28. Ortega, R.; Gonzalo, E.; Gomez-Polo, M.; Lopez-Suarez, C.; Suarez, M.J. SEM evaluation of the precision of fit of CAD/CAM zirconia and metal-ceramic posterior crowns. *Dent. Mater. J.* **2017**, *36*, 387–393. [CrossRef]
29. Gonzalo, E.; Suárez, M.J.; Serrano, B.; Lozano, J.F. A comparison of the marginal vertical discrepancies of zirconium and metal ceramic posterior fixed dental prostheses before and after cementation. *J. Prosthet. Dent.* **2009**, *102*, 378–384. [CrossRef]

30. Wolfart, S.; Wegner, S.M.; Al-Halabi, A.; Kern, M. Clinical evaluation of marginal fit of a new experimental all-ceramic system before and after cementation. *Int. J. Prosthodont.* **2003**, *16*, 587–592.
31. Beschnidt, S.M.; Strub, J.R. Evaluation of the marginal accuracy of different all-ceramic crown systems after simulation in the artificial mouth. *J. Oral Rehabil.* **1999**, *26*, 582–593. [CrossRef] [PubMed]
32. Freire, Y.; Gonzalo, E.; Lopez-Suarez, C.; Suarez, M.J. The Marginal Fit of CAD/CAM Monolithic Ceramic and Metal-Ceramic Crowns. *J. Prosthodont.* **2019**, *28*, 299–304. [CrossRef] [PubMed]
33. McLean, J.W.; von Fraunhofer, J.A. The estimation of cement film thickness by an in vivo technique. *Br. Dent. J.* **1971**, *131*, 107–111. [CrossRef]
34. Ortega, R.; Gonzalo, E.; Gomez-Polo, M.; Suárez, M.J. Marginal and Internal Discrepancies of Posterior Zirconia-Based Crowns Fabricated with Three Different CAD/CAM Systems Versus Metal-Ceramic. *Int. J. Prosthodont.* **2015**, *28*, 509–511. [CrossRef] [PubMed]
35. Att, W.; Komine, F.; Gerds, T.; Strub, J.R. Marginal adaptation of three different zirconium dioxide three-unit fixed dental prostheses. *J. Prosthet. Dent.* **2009**, *101*, 239–247. [CrossRef]
36. Suárez, M.J.; Lozano, J.F.; Salido, M.P.; Martínez, F. Marginal fit of titanium metal-ceramic crowns. *Int. J. Prosthodont.* **2005**, *18*, 390–391.
37. Witkowski, S.; Komine, F.; Gerds, T. Marginal accuracy of titanium copings fabricated by casting and CAD/CAM techniques. *J. Prosthet. Dent.* **2006**, *96*, 47–52. [CrossRef] [PubMed]
38. Boitelle, P.; Mawussi, B.; Tapie, L.; Fromentin, O. A systematic review of CAD/CAM fit restoration evaluations. *J. Oral Rehabil.* **2014**, *41*, 853–874. [CrossRef] [PubMed]
39. Gonzalo, E.; Suárez, M.J.; Serrano, B.; Lozano, J.F. Comparative analysis of two measurement methods for marginal fit in metal-ceramic and zirconia posterior FPDs. *Int. J. Prosthodont.* **2009**, *22*, 374–377.
40. Groten, M.; Axmann, D.; Pröbster, L.; Weber, H. Determination of the minimum number of marginal gap measurements required for practical in vitro testing. *J. Prosthet. Dent.* **2000**, *83*, 40–49. [CrossRef]
41. Holmes, J.R.; Bayne, S.C.; Holland, G.A.; Sulik, W.D. Considerations in measurement of marginal fit. *J. Prosthet. Dent.* **1989**, *62*, 405–408. [CrossRef]
42. Marchionni, S.; Baldissara, P.; Monaco, C.; Scotti, R. A systematic method for predetermined scanning electron microscope analysis in dental science. *Scanning* **2010**, *32*, 97–103. [CrossRef]
43. Quintas, A.F.; Oliveira, F.; Bottino, M.A. Vertical marginal discrepancy of ceramic copings with different ceramic materials, finish lines, and luting agents: An in vitro evaluation. *J. Prosthet. Dent.* **2004**, *92*, 250–257. [CrossRef]
44. Fransson, B.; Oilo, G.; Gjeitanger, R. The fit of metal-ceramic crowns, a clinical study. *Dent. Mater.* **1985**, *1*, 197–199. [CrossRef]
45. Oyague, R.C.; Sanchez-Turrion, A.; Lopez-Lozano, J.F.; Suarez-Garcia, M.J. Vertical discrepancy and microleakage of laser-sintered and vacuum-cast implant-supported structures luted with different cement types. *J. Dent.* **2012**, *40*, 123–130. [CrossRef] [PubMed]
46. Castillo-de-Oyague, R.; Sanchez-Turrion, A.; Lopez-Lozano, J.F.; Albaladejo, A.; Torres-Lagares, D.; Montero, J.; Suarez-Garcia, M. Vertical misfit of laser-sintered and vacuum-cast implant-supported crown copings luted with definitive and temporary luting agents. *Med. Oral Patol. Oral Cir. Bucal* **2012**, e610–e617. [CrossRef]
47. Fathi, H.M.; Al-Masoody, A.H.; El-Ghezawi, N.; Johnson, A. The accuracy of fit of crowns made from wax patterns produced conventionally (hand formed) and via CAD/CAM technology. *Eur. J. Prosthodont. Restor. Dent.* **2016**, *24*, 10–17. [PubMed]
48. Kim, K.B.; Kim, J.H.; Kim, W.C.; Kim, H.Y. Evaluation of the marginal and internal gap of metal-ceramic crown fabricated with a selective laser sintering technology: Two- and three-dimensional replica techniques. *J. Adv. Prosthodont.* **2013**, *5*, 179–186. [CrossRef] [PubMed]
49. Farjood, E.; Vojdani, M.; Torabi, K.; Khaledi, A.A. Marginal and internal fit of metal copings fabricated with rapid prototyping and conventional waxing. *J. Prosthet. Dent.* **2017**, *117*, 164–170. [CrossRef] [PubMed]
50. Karaman, T.; Ulku, S.Z.; Zengingul, A.I.; Guven, S.; Eratilla, V.; Sumer, E. Evaluation and comparison of the marginal adaptation of two different substructure materials. *J. Adv. Prosthodont.* **2015**, *7*, 257–263. [CrossRef]
51. Hong, M.H.; Min, B.K.; Lee, D.H.; Kwon, T.Y. Marginal fit of metal-ceramic crowns fabricated by using a casting and two selective laser melting processes before and after ceramic firing. *J. Prosthet. Dent.* **2019**, *122*, 475–481. [CrossRef] [PubMed]
52. Huang, Z.; Zhang, L.; Zhu, J.; Zhang, X. Clinical marginal and internal fit of metal ceramic crowns fabricated with a selective laser melting technology. *J. Prosthet. Dent.* **2015**, *113*, 623–627. [CrossRef] [PubMed]
53. Xu, D.; Xiang, N.; Wei, B. The marginal fit of selective laser melting-fabricated metal crowns: An in vitro study. *J. Prosthet. Dent.* **2014**, *112*, 1437–1440. [CrossRef]
54. Afify, A.; Haney, S.; Verrett, R.; Mansueto, M.; Cray, J.; Johnson, R. Marginal discrepancy of noble metal-ceramic fixed dental prosthesis frameworks fabricated by conventional and digital technologies. *J. Prosthet. Dent.* **2018**, *119*, 307.e1–307.e7. [CrossRef]
55. Tamac, E.; Toksavul, S.; Toman, M. Clinical marginal and internal adaptation of CAD/CAM milling, laser sintering, and cast metal ceramic crowns. *J. Prosthet. Dent.* **2014**, *112*, 909–913. [CrossRef] [PubMed]
56. Lövgren, N.; Roxner, R.; Klemendz, S.; Larsson, C. Effect of production method on surface roughness, marginal and internal fit, and retention of cobalt-chromium single crowns. *J. Prosthet. Dent.* **2017**, *118*, 95–101. [CrossRef]
57. Ortorp, A.; Jonsson, D.; Mouhsen, A.; von Steyern, P.V. The fit of cobalt-chromium three-unit fixed dental prostheses fabricated with four different techniques: A comparative in vitro study. *Dent. Mater.* **2011**, *27*, 356–363. [CrossRef]

58. Kocaağaoğlu, H.; Kılınç, H.; Albayrak, H.; Kara, M. In vitro evaluation of marginal, axial, and occlusal discrepancies in metal ceramic restorations produced with new technologies. *J. Prosthet. Dent.* **2016**, *116*, 368–374. [CrossRef]
59. Park, J.K.; Kim, H.Y.; Kim, W.C.; Kim, J.H. Evaluation of the fit of metal ceramic restorations fabricated with a pre-sintered soft alloy. *J. Prosthet. Dent.* **2016**, *116*, 909–915. [CrossRef] [PubMed]
60. Kim, E.H.; Lee, D.H.; Kwon, S.M.; Kwon, T.Y. A microcomputed tomography evaluation of the marginal fit of cobalt-chromium alloy copings fabricated by new manufacturing techniques and alloy systems. *J. Prosthet. Dent.* **2017**, *117*, 393–399. [CrossRef] [PubMed]
61. Real-Voltas, F.; Romano-Cardozo, E.; Figueras-Alvarez, O.; Brufau-de Barbera, M.; Cabratosa-Termes, J. Comparison of the Marginal Fit of Cobalt-Chromium Metal-Ceramic Crowns Fabricated by CAD/CAM Techniques and Conventional Methods at Three Production Stages. *Int. J. Prosthodont.* **2017**, *30*, 304–305. [CrossRef]
62. Pjetursson, B.E.; Lang, N.P. Prosthetic treatment planning on the basis of scientific evidence. *J. Oral Rehabil.* **2008**, *35* (Suppl. S1), 72–79. [CrossRef]
63. Henderson, D.; Blevins, W.R.; Wesley, R.C.; Seward, T. The cantilever type of posterior fixed partial dentures: A laboratory study. *J. Prosthet. Dent.* **1970**, *24*, 47–67. [CrossRef]
64. Yang, H.S.; Chung, H.J.; Park, Y.J. Stress analysis of a cantilevered fixed partial denture with normal and reduced bone support. *J. Prosthet. Dent.* **1996**, *76*, 424–430. [CrossRef]
65. Wolfart, S.; Harder, S.; Eschbach, S.; Lehmann, F.; Kern, M. Four-year clinical results of fixed dental prostheses with zirconia substructures (Cercon): End abutments vs. cantilever design. *Eur. J. Oral. Sci.* **2009**, *117*, 741–749. [CrossRef]
66. Rehmann, P.; Podhorsky, A.; Wöstmann, B. Treatment Outcomes of Cantilever Fixed Partial Dentures on Vital Abutment Teeth: A Retrospective Analysis. *Int. J. Prosthodont.* **2015**, *28*, 577–582. [CrossRef]
67. Palmqvist, S.; Swartz, B. Artificial crowns and fixed partial dentures 18 to 23 years after placement. *Int. J. Prosthodont.* **1993**, *6*, 279–285. [PubMed]
68. Zenthöfer, A.; Ohlmann, B.; Rammelsberg, P.; Bömicke, W. Performance of zirconia ceramic cantilever fixed dental prostheses: 3-year results from a prospective, randomized, controlled pilot study. *J. Prosthet. Dent.* **2015**, *114*, 34–39. [CrossRef] [PubMed]
69. Quante, K.; Ludwig, K.; Kern, M. Marginal and internal fit of metal-ceramic crowns fabricated with a new laser melting technology. *Dent. Mater.* **2008**, *24*, 1311–1315. [CrossRef] [PubMed]
70. Laurent, M.; Scheer, P.; Dejou, J.; Laborde, G. Clinical evaluation of the marginal fit of cast crowns—Validation of the silicone replica method. *J. Oral Rehabil.* **2008**, *35*, 116–122. [CrossRef]
71. Mitchell, C.A.; Pintado, M.R.; Douglas, W.H. Nondestructive, in vitro quantification of crown margins. *J. Prosthet. Dent.* **2001**, *85*, 575–584. [CrossRef] [PubMed]
72. Coli, P.; Karlsson, S. Precision of a CAD/CAM technique for the production of zirconium dioxide copings. *Int. J. Prosthodont.* **2004**, *17*, 577–580. [CrossRef] [PubMed]
73. Pimenta, M.A.; Frasca, L.C.; Lopes, R.; Rivaldo, E. Evaluation of marginal and internal fit of ceramic and metallic crown copings using X-ray microtomography (micro-CT) technology. *J. Prosthet. Dent.* **2015**, *114*, 223–228. [CrossRef] [PubMed]
74. Groten, M.; Girthofer, S.; Pröbster, L. Marginal fit consistency of copy-milled all-ceramic crowns during fabrication by light and scanning electron microscopic analysis in vitro. *J. Oral Rehabil.* **1997**, *24*, 871–881. [CrossRef] [PubMed]
75. Persson, A.; Andersson, M.; Oden, A.; Sandborgh-Englund, G. A three-dimensional evaluation of a laser scanner and a touch-probe scanner. *J. Prosthet. Dent.* **2006**, *95*, 194–200. [CrossRef] [PubMed]

Article

Mechanical Properties and Corrosion Resistance of TiAl6V4 Alloy Produced with SLM Technique and Used for Customized Mesh in Bone Augmentations

Nicola De Angelis [1,2,3,*], Luca Solimei [1,2], Claudio Pasquale [1,2], Lorenzo Alvito [4], Alberto Lagazzo [4] and Fabrizio Barberis [4]

[1] Department of Surgical Sciences and Integrated Diagnostics, University of Genova, 16126 Genova, Italy; lucasolimei@hotmail.it (L.S.); clodent@gmail.com (C.P.)
[2] Department of Mechanical and Energetics Engineering, University of Genova, 16126 Genova, Italy
[3] Department of Dentistry, University of Technology MARA Sungai Buloh Malaysia, Shah Alam 40450, Malaysia
[4] Department of Civil, Chemical and Environmental Engineering, University of Genova, 16126 Genova, Italy; l.alvito96@gmail.com (L.A.); alberto.lagazzo@unige.it (A.L.); fabrizio.barberis@unige.it (F.B.)
* Correspondence: nicolaantonio.deangelis@edu.unige.it; Tel.: +39-347-4188-180

Abstract: Bone augmentation procedures represent a real clinical challenge. One option is the use of titanium meshes. Additive manufacturing techniques can provide custom-made devices in titanium alloy. The purpose of this study was to investigate the material used, which can influence the outcomes of the bone augmentation procedure. Specific test samples were obtained from two different manufacturers with two different shapes: surfaces without perforations and with calibrated perforations. Three-point bending tests were run as well as internal friction tests to verify the Young's modulus. Test samples were placed in two different buffered solutions and analyzed with optical microscopy. A further SEM analysis was done to observe any microstructural modification. Three-point flexural tests were conducted on 12 specimens. Initial bending was observed at lower applied stresses for the perforated samples (503 MPa) compared to non-perforated ones (900 MPa); the ultimate flexural strength was registered at 513 MPa and 1145 MPa for perforated and non-perforated samples, respectively. Both microscopic analyses (optical and SEM) showed no significant alterations. Conclusions: A normal masticatory load cannot modify the device. Chemical action in the case of exposure does not create macroscopic and microscopic alterations of the surface.

Keywords: alveolar bone defects; guided bone regeneration; titanium meshes; customized titanium meshes; laser melting process; electron beam melting

1. Introduction

The use of dental implants is a very common procedure [1]. For ideal prosthetic design, implants must be inserted in a correct 3D plan [2]. Patients may present alveolar ridge defects as a consequence of periodontal disease, dental trauma, traumatic extraction, or genetic anomalies, which do not allow the correct implant position [3,4].

Different treatment options have been described to reconstruct these defects, which may include inlay and onlay block bone grafts, crestal splitting, osteogenetic distraction, and guided bone regeneration (GBR) using resorbable and non-resorbable barrier membranes [5]. Of these, GBR seems to be the most reliable and predictable, providing excellent long-term stability [6,7].

The basic principle of GBR involves placing a mechanical barrier to protect the blood clot and to isolate the bony defect from the surrounding connective and epithelial tissue invasion. This space is needed to allow the osteoblasts to access the space intended for bone regeneration. The use of a barrier membrane, especially a resorbable one, has the advantage of facilitating the procedure, but often the shape of the defect itself may create a collapse of the barrier and the loss of the "space maintaining" effect [8].

Titanium meshes, as an alternative to membranes, have been used for a long time as a predictable technique for bone regeneration and, owing to their rigidity, the adaptation onto the defect and maintenance of their shape can be more stable [9]. To overcome the main drawbacks, which are the remaining sharp margins after cutting and the increased surgical time required for their shaping and fitting, pre-shaping of the mesh on a stereolithographic model (STL) of the patient's jaw can be an alternative to significantly shorten the intraoperative time, but with a significant cost increase [10]. More recently, 3D-printed, custom-made titanium devices have been introduced as a modern alternative [11].

Regardless of the production technique for any implantable devices, it is mandatory to control the characteristics to optimize their biological performance [12]. The stiffness of titanium meshes can damage the soft tissue, and the mechanical strength is related to the thickness of the material and pore dimensions. More specifically, the surface properties direct the cellular interactions [13]. These properties, including surface topography and chemical composition, are usually derived by the surface treatments applied [14].

Surface topography and roughness are aspects that can be easily manipulated by post-production surface treatments and that play a strategic role in the determination of cellular interactions, influencing adhesion and differentiation [15,16]. High degrees of roughness represent a major risk for ionic leakage from the material [17] and the bacterial adhesion can be increased, with the consequence of implant failures [18].

Smooth surfaces are able to reduce the biological processes at the interface, keeping the titanium oxidized layer properties unaffected for periods [16]. Thus, the correct micro- and nano-roughness levels can stimulate osteoblast differentiation and maturation, proliferation, and production of both matrices [19]. Although the mesh characteristics should be highly controlled, it is important to note that the biological response depends also on the correct diagnosis and clinical indication. Moreover, if an exposure during the healing phase occurs, it is relevant to demonstrate if, beside the unfavorable outcome, chemical modifications of the exposed surface may affect the bone growth.

The present study investigated two different commercial customized devices, comparing their mechanical properties (flexion test and internal friction) and their macro- and microstructural changes after exposure to different degrees of pH to observe if the modifications of the material were coherent with the clinical findings. Further evaluations were made using SEM with profiles analysis and chemical composition.

2. Materials and Methods

2.1. Samples' Preparation

Specific test samples produced with the laser sintering technique used for customized implantable titanium meshes were obtained from two different manufacturers, BoneEasy (Arada, Ovar, Portugal) and BTK (Vicenza, Italy), and came with two different shapes: surfaces without perforations and with calibrated perforations 1.2 mm in diameter.

The samples were characterized by the following dimensions: 40 mm length, 10 mm width, and 0.5 mm thickness, to conduct the test according to the protocols of ISO5832-3:2014, ASTM F136:2013, ASTM F2934:2014, ASTM F3001:2014, and ASTM B348:2013.

The chemical composition declared by the manufacturer was TiAl6V4 with the following percentages of the different elements: Al 5.5–6.5% and V 3.5–4.5%.

All the tests were conducted on:

- Three BoneEasy specimens (BE) without perforations,
- Three Biotek specimens (BTK) without perforations,
- Three BoneEasy specimens (BE) with perforations, and
- Three Biotek specimens (BTK) with perforations.

2.2. Experiments

In order to simulate the mechanical stress due to the masticatory function over the implanted device, three-point bending tests were run as well as internal friction tests to verify the Young's modulus.

The bending tests were performed using a Zwick/Roell Z0.5 electromechanical testing machine (Standards EN 2562–EN 2746) equipped with a three-point bending device with a span of 40 mm. All the tests were run on rectangular samples 0.5 mm in thickness, 10 mm in width, and 40 mm in length, at a rate of 5 mm/min for the determination of the flexural elastic modulus and a rate of 30 mm/min until break.

The tests for the determination of the internal friction were performed using an experimental setup consisting of a laser vibrometer to measure the displacement of a sample placed on two supporting pins and impulsively hit by a ball and on an oscilloscope to evaluate the resonance frequency. The physics equation that links the geometric parameters of the specimen and its Young's Modulus E' to the material frequency is:

$$f = \frac{\lambda^2 \cdot 10^6}{2\pi L^2} \left(\frac{Eh^2}{12\rho} \right)^{1/2}$$

where E is the Young's Modulus [Gpa], the density is [g/cm^3], h is the specimen thickness [mm], L is the span between the two supports [mm], and λ is the modal coefficient equal to 4.73.

The speed c_o of the elastic longitudinal waves along the bar, expressed in m/s, can be derived as:

$$c_o = \frac{2\pi f L^2}{\lambda^2 r \cdot 10^3}$$

where $= h/(12)^{0.5}$ is the radius of inertia of the sample section [mm]. The Young's Modulus can be calculated through the equation:

$$E = c_o^2 \, 10^{-6}$$

$$Q^{-1} = \frac{1}{\pi f \Delta t} \ln \left(\frac{A_1}{A_2} \right)$$

To reproduce the chemical oral environment with consistent pH variations (food, beverages, and existing pathologies), the test samples were placed into two different buffered solutions at pH 7 and pH 4 and analyzed with optical microscopy (50, 100×) at 7, 14, and 21 days.

2.3. Analysis

A further SEM analysis was done to assess whether different chemical baths could produce external and internal modifications of the alloy structures and also to analyze the composition of the specimens, comparing these with the manufacturer's declarations by means of Specific Energy-dispersive X-ray spectroscopy.

Samples without perforations produced by both companies were cut and incorporated into epoxy resin for inspection of their profiles using SEM and mathematical calculation (Image J and MATLAB software) of the roughness parameters.

3. Results

Three-point flexural tests were conducted on 12 specimens (Figure 1).

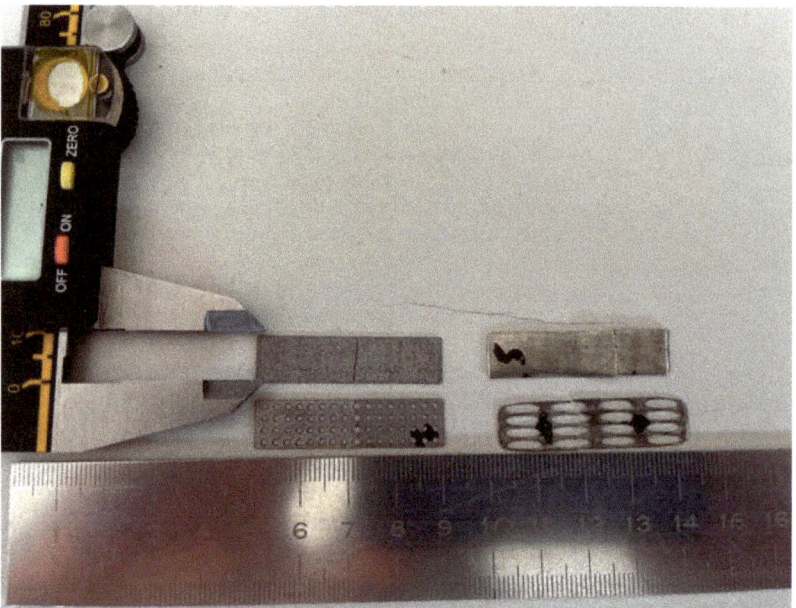

Figure 1. Four of the specimens used for the investigation. Perforated and non-perforated BTK and BoneEasy. The picture was taken after the three-point flexural tests, and it is evident of the fracture of the specimen.

Initial bending was observed at lower applied stresses for perforated samples (503 MPa) compared to non-perforated ones (900 MPa). The ultimate flexural strength was registered at 513 MPa and 1145 MPa for the perforated and non-perforated samples, respectively (Figure 2).

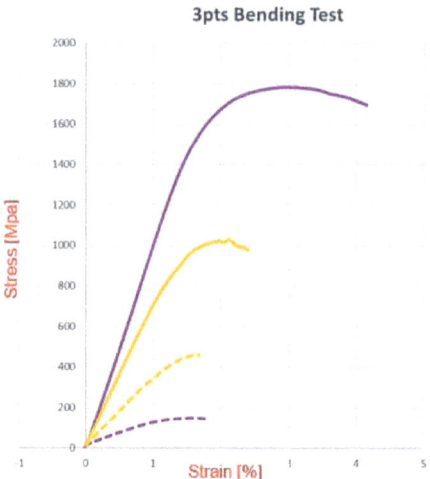

Figure 2. Diagram of three-point flexural strength on four different types of specimens.

Internal friction tests were conducted to determine the Young's modulus, which was reported from 101 to 107 MPa (Figure 3).

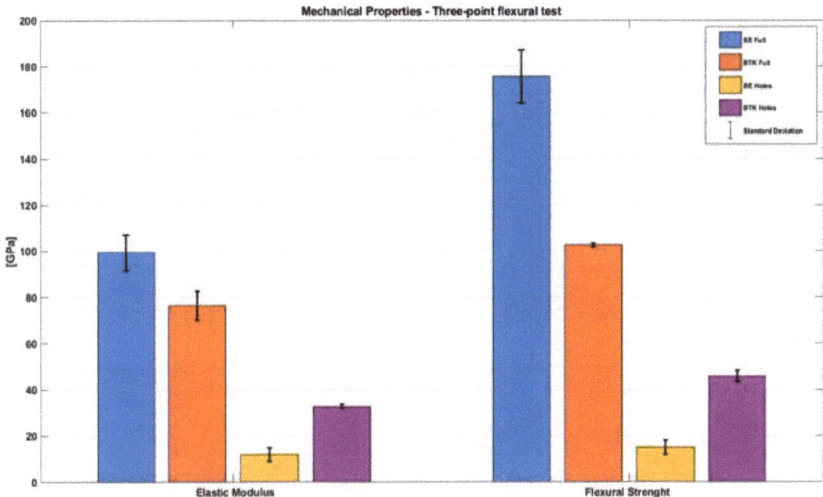

Figure 3. Graphical representation of elastic modulus and flexural strength values on the four types of specimens.

The analysis with an optical microscope at different pH at 7, 14, and 21 days, respectively, did not reveal any macroscopic alteration of the surface (Figure 4).

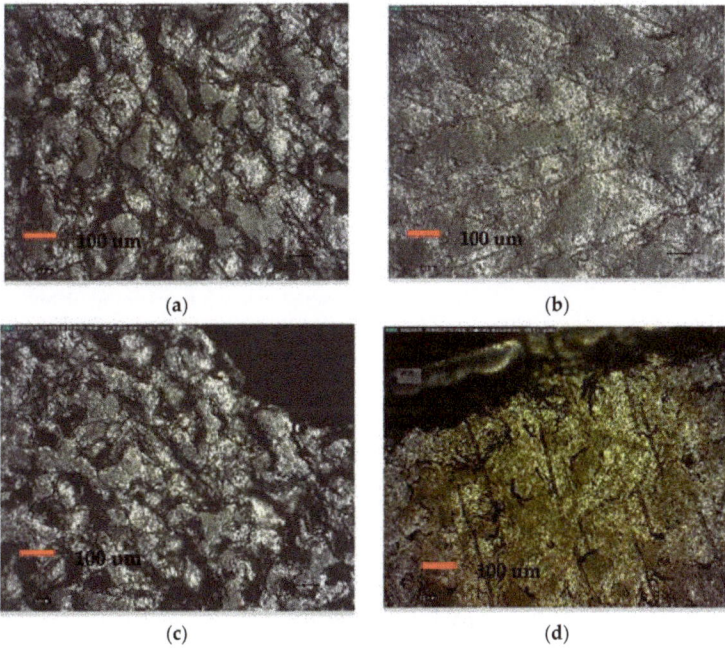

Figure 4. A 200× optical microscopy analysis: (**a**,**b**) on specimens exposed at pH 7 for 21 days, (**c**,**d**) on specimens exposed at pH 4 for 21 days. No macroscopic differences can be seen.

The further SEM analysis done on all the samples showed several microscopic defects of the surface on all the samples exposed at pH 4. Thus, it can be concluded that those imperfections are attributed to a corrosion effect (Figure 5).

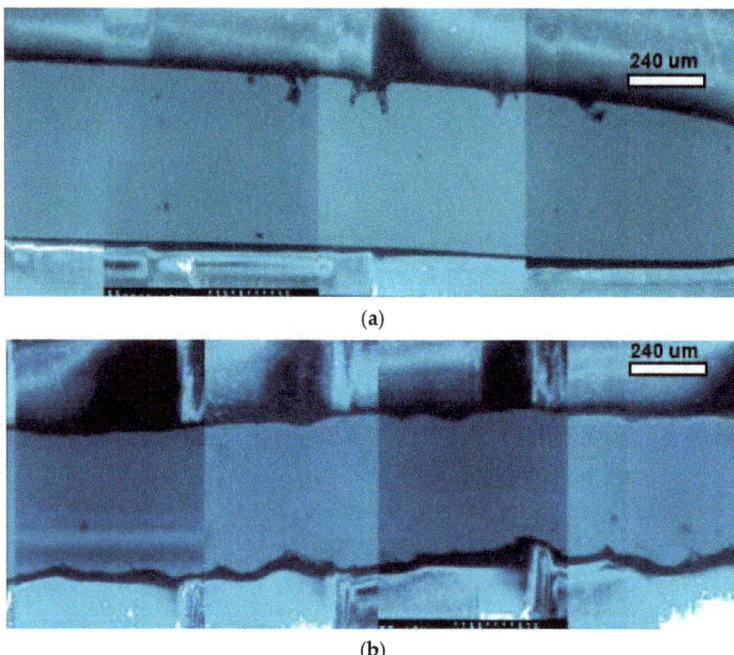

Figure 5. SEM analysis revealed profile and internal defects on both BoneEasy (**a**) and BTK (**b**) samples, probably attributed to the long exposure to a pH 4 buffered solution.

The roughness parameters Ra, Rq, and Sigma of the samples are reported in Tables 1 and 2, where Ra is the roughness average, Rq the root mean square, and Sigma is the standard deviation.

The profile analysis of the lower faces of the BE and BTK specimens at pH 7 showed Sigma values (σ) of 1.165 µm and 21.555 µm, respectively. On the upper face, the same samples showed Sigma values (σ) of 1.697 µm for BE and 13.756 µm for BTK.

After pH 4 immersion, the lower faces of the BE and BTK specimens showed Sigma values (σ) of 0.883 µm and 19.685 µm, respectively. The upper faces of the same samples had Sigma values (σ) of 1.583 µm for BE and 9.073 µm for BTK.

The Sigma values confirmed that the BTK samples were rougher than the BE ones and also that the BTK ones had two different surfaces with different degrees of roughness (Tables 1 and 2, Figure 6).

Table 1. Roughness parameters on lower faces of both samples. The numbers of samples used for the analysis are identified in each column.

Lower Face	BTK 7	BTK 4	BE 7	BE 4
Ra	17.673 µm	15.636 µm	1.466 µm	1.126 µm
Rq	21.553 µm	19.683 µm	1.945 µm	1.474 µm
Sigma	21.555 µm	19.685 µm	1.165 µm	0.883 µm

Table 2. Roughness parameters on upper faces of both samples.

Upper Face	BTK 7	BTK 4	BE 7	BE 4
Ra	12.125 μm	7.601 μm	2.387 μm	2.103 μm
Rq	13.754 μm	9.072 μm	2.833 μm	2.644 μm
Sigma	13.756 μm	9.073 μm	1.697 μm	1.583 μm

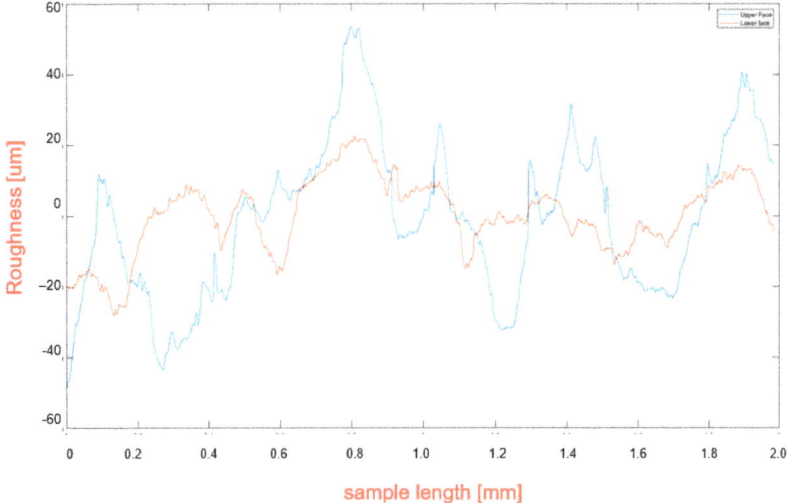

Figure 6. Profile analysis of upper and lower faces.

The profile analysis revealed, also, some internal defects, and the further Energy-dispersive X-ray spectroscopy evidenced the chemical composition of both samples, in which high percentages of carbon were detected (1.25% for BE and 3.65% for BTK) (Figures 7 and 8).

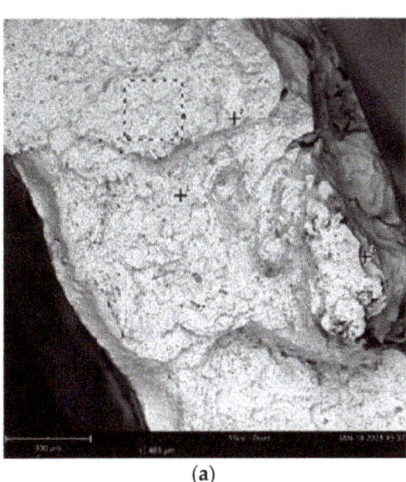

(a)

Figure 7. Cont.

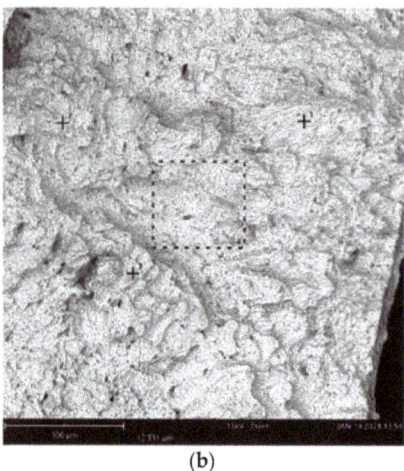

(b)

Figure 7. SEM internal defects on BTK (**a**) and BE (**b**) samples.

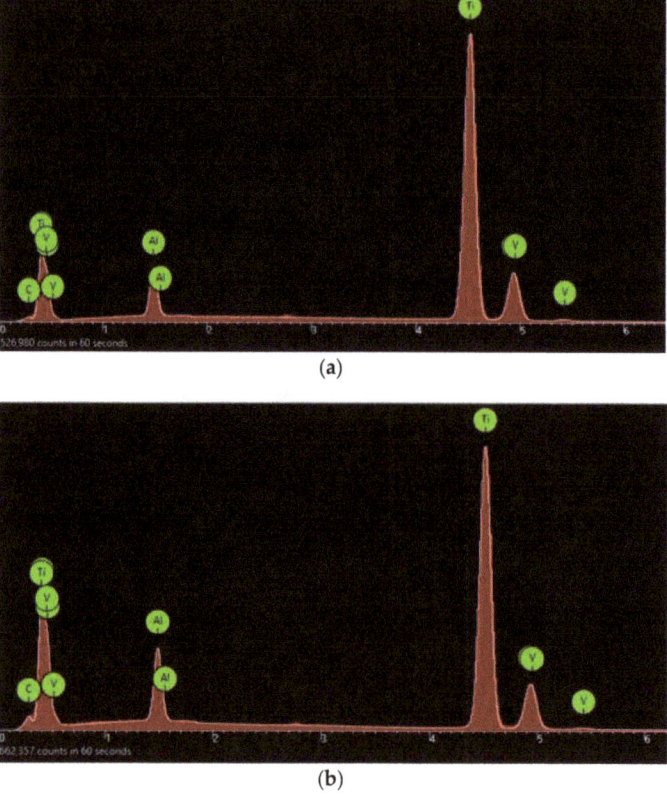

Figure 8. Energy-dispersive X-ray spectroscopy on BE samples (**a**) and BTK samples (**b**). X-axis represents the energy (KeV) and Y-axis represents the number of counts. The highest peak is titanium but an average of 1.25% and 3.65% of carbon can be detected in the BE and BTK samples, respectively.

4. Discussion

Additive manufacturing (AM) is widely applied in the medical field and it is becoming popular in oral surgery. However, only a few studies have analyzed the effect of the laser melting and sintering process (defined as additive manufacturing techniques) on the metal alloys in terms of mechanical and chemical properties [20,21].

Considering that the implant has to be placed in the oral cavity, a variety of factors can influence the final outcome: masticatory function and applied stress on the device, chemical action of the saliva, and, in the case of partial exposure, of foods and beverages, including also any endogenous pathologies, like gastro-esophageal acid reflux.

AM technology offers some advantages compared to conventional techniques [22], such as digital planning and design of the customized mesh, shorter surgical times, and easy adaptation of the device to the bone defect [23–26].

Otawa et al. [27] evaluated the dimensional accuracy of customized AM Ti mesh. The thickness of the polished device was 0.3 mm with perforations of 1.0 mm. The results obtained demonstrated that the x- and y-axes representation showed higher accuracy compared to the z-axis. The mean accuracy error value reported was 139 µm.

Sumida et al. [28] compared the clinical performance of customized AM with conventional Ti meshes for bone augmentation procedures in 26 patients. The customized AM meshes were manufactured with a thickness of 0.5 mm and with 1.0-mm diameter pores. The screw perforations for positioning the AM mesh had a 1.5-mm diameter, and the mesh was manually polished until 0.3-mm thickness was achieved. During implant placement, the Ti meshes were positioned with autogenous bone. The authors reported a higher surgical time for conventional Ti mesh compared to customized AM mesh. Furthermore, conventional meshes were associated with 15.4% of mucosal dehiscence with infection compared to AM procedures.

Inoue et al. [29] evaluated the feasibility of the customized Ti mesh sheets for alveolar bone reconstruction in two patients. A customized SLM Ti mesh sheet was positioned at the same time as placing a commercial implant.

None of the abovementioned studies investigated whether the additive manufacturing process may influence the mechanical properties. From the results of this study, there is a clear difference between perforated and non-perforated samples, with an obvious higher resistance, calculated as ultimate flexural strength, for the samples without any kind of perforation.

An adult human male can produce an occlusal force that averages from 45–68 kg (441.3–666.8 MPa) on molar sites. The values of the ultimate flexural strength for non-perforated samples are much higher, but perforated samples break at 503 MPa and start bending with alteration of the initial shape at 300 MPa. The samples, both perforated and not, from BoneEasy (BE) seem to have a higher resistance than the BTK ones. The elastic modulus of perforated samples is lower than the full samples and more similar to the bone's Young's modulus (10–20 GPa). Although the shape of the customized mesh was different from the samples, with a noticeable difference also of the mechanical properties, this aspect should be considered after the implantation in order to avoid potentially dangerous stresses on the device.

Partial exposure of the mesh is one of the most common complications and it has been demonstrated by several studies that it may average from 0 to 66% [28], regardless of the site and the extension of the bone augmentation.

The existing evidence does not report whether the part exposed to the oral cavity and, thus, to contaminants such as food and beverages but also to sudden and extremely variable chemical conditions, may influence or not the surface of the device, affecting the bone response.

In this study, several conditions were simulated, from the immersion of the sample in saline solution (pH 7) up to the extreme acid buffering with pH 4 for a maximum time of 21 days. The microscopic analysis revealed different Sigma values (standard deviation) for the two examined samples, which was most evident after the immersion in the acid solution. Moreover, the samples from BoneEasy were apparently smoother than the BTK ones and this aspect could imply a lower bacterial adhesion in the case of complications.

The effect of the acid solution, although not reproducible in humans, revealed that both samples were extremely resistant, but the surface showed a moderate corrosion, which was analyzed with SEM and with energy-dispersive X-ray spectroscopy. The presence of high percentages of carbon represents an important and negative aspect, which was found in all samples, with slight differences between the two manufacturers.

Several reasons could be addressed to explain these values, and during the investigations none of the examined bars was touched without gloves, in order to eliminate the superficial contamination of the human epithelial cells. Furthermore, the same values of carbon were detected also from the analysis of the internal margin immediately after the fracture of the sample.

In a recent article, Cruz et al. [29] compared three different types of meshes from BTK, BoneEasy, and Reoss. The result of their profile analysis was coherent with the data retrieved in this investigation. They also found several artifacts embedded into the meshes. Specifically, several deep cracks were found, and it can be assumed that these features existed already after the first production steps of the mesh. The EDS analysis revealed that the embedded residues were aluminum and oxygen. These alterations of the surface were probably induced by the post-production alumina (Al_2O_3) sandblasting process. Apparently, the presence of carbon in both the BTK and BoneEasy samples could not be explained and this undoubtedly represented a certain weakness in the production of these devices. It would be important to understand whether the same findings can be observed also in patients' dedicated meshes, in order to clarify the safety of their use.

5. Conclusions

Within the limitations of this study, it can be assessed that a normal masticatory load cannot modify the device. Mechanical tests revealed that the BE- and BTK-manufactured samples had different responses to the applied stress, and the elastic modulus was significantly lower for perforated samples, with differences between BE and BTK, which showed a value more similar to the Young's modulus of the bone. Chemical action in the case of exposure did not cause macroscopic and microscopic alteration of the surface. Thus, besides the unfavorable clinical outcome, it can be assumed that no structural modifications are expected. It can be concluded that TiAl6V4 is a stable and promising material for customized devices, but more clinical studies are needed to understand the long-term host responses.

Author Contributions: Conceptualization, N.D.A. and L.S.; methodology, N.D.A., F.B. and A.L.; software, L.A. and A.L.; validation, C.P., L.S. and N.D.A.; formal analysis, L.A.; investigation, L.A. and N.D.A.; resources, F.B.; data curation, L.A.; writing—original draft preparation, N.D.A.; writing—review and editing, N.D.A. and A.L.; visualization, L.A.; supervision, F.B.; project administration, F.B. All authors have read and agreed to the published version of the manuscript.

Funding: This research received no external funding.

Institutional Review Board Statement: Not applicable.

Informed Consent Statement: Not applicable.

Data Availability Statement: Not applicable.

Conflicts of Interest: The authors declare no conflict of interest.

References

1. Smeet, R.; Stadlinger, B.; Frank, S. Impact of dental implant surface modifications on osseointegration. *Biomed. Res. Int.* **2016**, *2*, 1–16. [CrossRef]
2. Buser, D.; Martin, W.; Belser, U.C. Optimizing esthetics for implant restorations in the anterior maxilla: Anatomic and surgical considerations. *Int. J. Oral Maxillofac. Implant.* **2004**, *19*, 43–61.

3. Jegham, H.; Masmoudi, R.; Ouertani, H.; Blouza, I.; Turki, S.; Khattech, M. Ridge augmentation with titanium mesh: A case report. *J. Stomatol. Oral Maxillofac. Surg.* **2017**, *118*, 181–186. [CrossRef] [PubMed]
4. Rocchietta, I.; Fontana, F.; Simion, M. Clinical outcomes of vertical bone augmentation to enable dental implant placement: A systematic review. *J. Clin. Periodontol.* **2008**, *35*, 203–215. [CrossRef] [PubMed]
5. Rakhmatia, Y.D.; Ayukawa, Y.; Furuhashi, A.; Koyano, K. Current barrier membranes: Titanium mesh and other membranes for guided bone regeneration in dental applications. *J. Prosthodont. Res.* **2013**, *57*, 3–14. [CrossRef] [PubMed]
6. Li, H.; Zheng, J.; Zhang, S.; Yang, C.; Kwon, Y.-D.; Kim, Y.-J. Experiment of GBR for repair of peri-implant alveolar defects in beagle dogs. *Sci. Rep.* **2018**, *8*, 16532. [CrossRef]
7. Donos, N.; Kostopoulos, L.; Tonetti, M.; Karring, T. Long-term stability of autogenous bone grafts following combined appli-cation with guided bone regeneration. *Clin. Oral Implants Res.* **2005**, *16*, 133–139. [CrossRef]
8. Rakhmatia, Y.D.; Ayukawa, Y.; Furuhashi, A.; Koyano, K. Fibroblast attachment onto novel titanium mesh membranes for guided bone regeneration. *Odontology* **2015**, *103*, 218–226. [CrossRef] [PubMed]
9. Di Stefano, D.A.; Greco, G.B.; Cinci, L.; Pieri, L. Horizontal-guided Bone Regeneration using a Titanium Mesh and an Equine Bone Graft. *J. Contemp. Dent. Pract.* **2015**, *16*, 154–162. [CrossRef] [PubMed]
10. De Moraes, P.H.; Olate, S.; De Albergaria-Barbosa, J.R. Maxillary Reconstruction Using rhBMP-2 and Titanium Mesh: Technical Note About the Use of Stereolithographic Model. *Int. J. Odontostomatol.* **2015**, *9*, 149–152. [CrossRef]
11. Sumida, T.; Otawa, N.; Kamata, Y.; Kamakura, S.; Mtsushita, T.; Kitagaki, H.; Mori, S.; Sasaki, K.; Fujibayashi, S.; Takemoto, M.; et al. Custom-made titanium devices as membranes for bone augmentation in implant treatment: Clinical application and the comparison with conventional titanium mesh. *J. Cranio-Maxillofac. Surg.* **2015**, *43*, 2183–2188. [CrossRef]
12. Saini, M.; Singh, Y.; Arora, P.; Arora, V.; Jain, K. Implant biomaterials: A comprehensive review. *World J. Clin. Cases* **2015**, *3*, 52–57. [CrossRef] [PubMed]
13. Ciocca, L.; Ragazzini, S.; Fantini, M.; Corinaldesi, G.; Scotti, R. Work flow for the prosthetic rehabilitation of atrophic patients with a minimal-intervention CAD/CAM approach. *J. Prosthet. Dent.* **2015**, *114*, 22–26. [CrossRef] [PubMed]
14. Al-Radha, A.S.D.; Dymock, D.; Younes, C.; O'Sullivan, D. Surface properties of titanium and zirconia dental implant materials and their effect on bacterial adhesion. *J. Dent.* **2012**, *40*, 146–153. [CrossRef] [PubMed]
15. Ponsonnet, L.; Reybier, K.; Jaffrezic, N.; Comte, V.; Lagneau, C.; Lissac, M.; Martelet, C. Relationship between surface properties (roughness, wettability) of titanium and titanium alloys and cell behaviour. *Mater. Sci. Eng. C* **2003**, *23*, 551–560. [CrossRef]
16. Elias, C.N.; Oshida, Y.; Lima, J.H.C.; Muller, C.A. Relationship between surface properties (roughness, wettability and morphol-ogy) of titanium and dental implant removal torque. *J. Mech. Behav. Biomed. Mater.* **2008**, *1*, 234–242. [CrossRef] [PubMed]
17. Le Guehennec, L.; Soueidan, A.; Layrolle, P.; Amouriq, Y. Surface treatments of titanium dental implants for rapid osseointe-gration. *Dent. Mater.* **2007**, *23*, 844–854. [CrossRef]
18. Dank, A.; Aartman, I.H.A.; Wismeijer, D.; Tahmaseb, A. Effect of dental implant surface roughness in patients with a history of periodontal disease: A systematic review and meta-analysis. *Int. J. Implant. Dent.* **2019**, *5*, 1–11. [CrossRef] [PubMed]
19. Rosales-Leal, J.I.; Rodríguez-Valverde, M.A.; Mazzaglia, G.; Ramón-Torregrosa, P.J.; Diaz Rodriguez, L.; García-Martínez, O.; Vallecillo-Capilla, M.; Ruiz, C.; Cabrerizo-Vílchez, M.A. Effect of roughness, wettability and morphology of engineered tita-nium surfaces on osteoblast-like cell adhesion. *Colloids Surf. A Physicochem. Eng. Asp.* **2010**, *365*, 222–229. [CrossRef]
20. Revilla-León, M.; Özcan, M. Additive Manufacturing Technologies Used for 3D Metal Printing in Dentistry. *Curr. Oral Health Rep.* **2017**, *4*, 201–208. [CrossRef]
21. Ciocca, L.; Fantini, M.; De Crescenzio, F. Direct metal laser sintering (DMLS) of a customized titanium mesh for pros-thetically guided bone regeneration of atrophic maxillary arches. *Med. Biol. Eng. Comput.* **2011**, *49*, 1347–1352. [CrossRef] [PubMed]
22. Hartmann, A.; Seiler, M. Minimizing risk of customized titanium mesh exposures—A retrospective analysis. *BMC Oral Health* **2020**, *20*, 36. [CrossRef]
23. Otawa, N.; Sumida, T.; Kitagaki, H.; Sasaki, K.; Fujibayashi, S.; Takemoto, M.; Nakamura, T.; Yamada, T.; Mori, Y.; Matsushita, T. Custom-made titanium devices as membranes for bone augmentation in implant treatment: Modeling accuracy of titanium products constructed with selective laser melting. *J. Cranio-Maxillofac. Surg.* **2015**, *43*, 1289–1295. [CrossRef] [PubMed]
24. Trevisan, F.; Calignano, F.; Aversa, A.; Marchese, G.; Lombardi, M.; Biamino, S.; Ugues, D.; Manfredi, D. Additive manufacturing of titanium alloys in the biomedical field: Processes, properties and applications. *J. Appl. Biomater. Funct. Mater.* **2018**, *16*, 57–67. [CrossRef]
25. Inoue, K.; Nakajima, Y.; Omori, M. Reconstruction of the alveolar bone using bone augmentation with selective laser melting titanium mesh sheet: A report of 2 cases. *Implant Dent.* **2018**, *27*, 602–607. [CrossRef]
26. Ortuğ, G. A new device for measuring mastication force (Gnathodynamometer). *Ann. Anat. Anat. Anz.* **2002**, *184*, 393–396. [CrossRef]
27. Shan, X.-F.; Chen, H.-M.; Liang, J.; Huang, J.-W.; Cai, Z.-G. Surgical Reconstruction of Maxillary and Mandibular Defects Using a Printed Titanium Mesh. *J. Oral Maxillofac. Surg.* **2015**, *73*, 1437–e1. [CrossRef] [PubMed]
28. Ciocca, L.; Lizio, G.; Baldissara, P.; Sambuco, A.; Scotti, R.; Corinaldesi, G. Prosthetically CAD-CAM–Guided Bone Augmentation of Atrophic Jaws Using Customized Titanium Mesh: Preliminary Results of an Open Prospective Study. *J. Oral Implant.* **2018**, *44*, 131–137. [CrossRef]
29. Cruz, N.; Martins, M.I.; Santos, J.D.; Gil Mur, J.; Tondela, J.P. Surface Comparison of Three Different Commercial Custom-Made Titanium Meshes Produced by SLM for Dental Applications. *Materials* **2020**, *13*, 2177. [CrossRef]

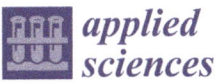

Article

Effect of Photofunctionalization with 6 W or 85 W UVC on the Degree of Wettability of RBM Titanium in Relation to the Irradiation Time

Arturo Sanchez-Perez [1,*], Nuria Cano-Millá [1], María José Moya Villaescusa [1], José María Montoya Carralero [1] and Carlos Navarro Cuellar [2]

[1] Department of Periodontology, Medicine and Dentistry Faculty, Murcia University, 30008 Murcia, Spain; nuria.canom@um.es (N.C.-M.); mjm.villaescusa@um.es (M.J.M.V.); jmmontoya@um.es (J.M.M.C.)
[2] Department of Surgery, Complutense University, 28040 Madrid, Spain; cnavarrocuellar@gmail.com
* Correspondence: arturosa@um.es; Tel.: +34-968-247-946

Citation: Sanchez-Perez, A.; Cano-Millá, N.; Moya Villaescusa, M.J.; Montoya Carralero, J.M.; Navarro Cuellar, C. Effect of Photofunctionalization with 6 W or 85 W UVC on the Degree of Wettability of RBM Titanium in Relation to the Irradiation Time. *Appl. Sci.* **2021**, *11*, 5427. https://doi.org/10.3390/app11125427

Academic Editor: Vittorio Checchi

Received: 18 May 2021
Accepted: 7 June 2021
Published: 11 June 2021

Publisher's Note: MDPI stays neutral with regard to jurisdictional claims in published maps and institutional affiliations.

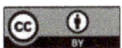

Copyright: © 2021 by the authors. Licensee MDPI, Basel, Switzerland. This article is an open access article distributed under the terms and conditions of the Creative Commons Attribution (CC BY) license (https://creativecommons.org/licenses/by/4.0/).

Featured Application: Due to the inevitable ageing of titanium, the use of a reliable, fast, and inexpensive method to reverse the effects of time on implants is of clinical relevance.

Abstract: Photoactivation with ultraviolet C light can reverse the effects derived from biological ageing by restoring a hydrophilic surface. Ten titanium discs were randomly divided into three groups: a control group, a 6 W group, and an 85 W group. A drop of double-distilled, deionized, and sterile 10 µL water was applied to each of the discs. Each disc was immediately photographed in a standardized and perpendicular manner. Measurements were taken based on the irradiation time (15, 30, 60, and 120 min). UVC irradiation improved the control values in both groups. There was no difference in its effect between the 6 W group and the other groups during the first 30 min. However, after 60 min and up to 120 min, 85 W had a significantly stronger effect. The contact angles with the 85 W ultraviolet light source at 60 and 120 min were 19.43° and 31.41°, respectively, whereas the contact angles for the 6 W UVC source were 73.8° and 61.45°. Power proved to be the most important factor, and the best hydrophilicity result was obtained with a power of 85 W for 60 min at a wavelength of 254 nm.

Keywords: titanium; dental implants; hydrophilic; hydrocarbon; biological ageing; UV photofunctionalization

1. Introduction

Titanium is a material devoid of toxicity and is stable and easy to obtain. Its good physical properties have led to its widespread use in oral implantology.

To improve its clinical characteristics, there have been attempts to increase the bioactivity of titanium implants [1–3]. The focus was on improving osseointegration, which is defined as the direct and functional connection between living, structured bone and the surface of an implant under load.

Among other factors, the physicochemical properties of the implant surface, its topography, and chemical composition have been the focus for improving biocompatibility [4]. Under optimal conditions, this improvement implies an increase in the absorption of ions and molecules, thus stimulating cellular attraction, proliferation, and expansion. The result is a higher degree of contact between the bone and the implant (BIC).

One method to establish surface improvement is through its wettability, which is based on the angle of contact between a droplet of water and the surface of the material being checked (Figure 1).

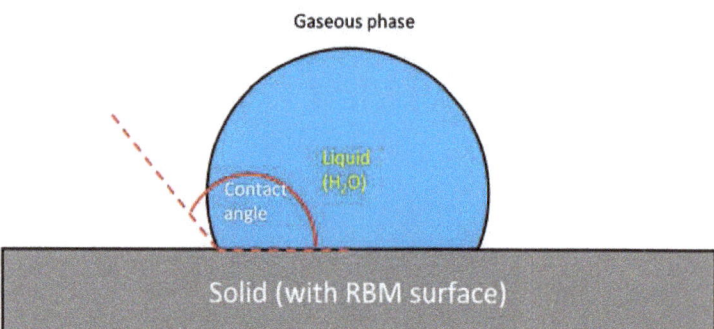

Figure 1. The wettability of a surface depends on the surface energy of the solid, the surface tension of the liquid, and the gaseous phase. Wettability can be established by measuring the contact angle between the liquid and the solid.

Arbitrary degrees of wettability have been established, depending on the angle of contact, and the parameter is classified into four categories: superhydrophobic, hydrophobic, hydrophilic, and superhydrophilic (Figure 2).

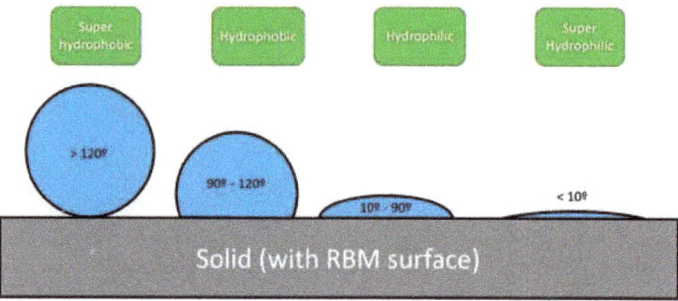

Figure 2. Classification of wettability as a function of contact angle. From superhydrophilic to superhydrophobic.

There are reports that titanium surfaces become contaminated by atmospheric carbon compounds being deposited on their surface, causing them to become progressively more hydrophobic. This process is called biological ageing and has been widely discussed in various works.

Over time, the percentage of carbon deposited on titanium increases from 14% to 63% with important clinical consequences.

Aged titanium surfaces exhibit 50% less absorption of amino acids, proteins, and osteoblast adhesion compared with newly manufactured titanium surfaces. Such alterations are considered unavoidable and depend on the storage time, having been detected as early as four weeks after manufacture.

The physicochemical effect produced by the application of ultraviolet light to the titanium surface is called photofunctionalization, with biological effects. Photofunctionalization is capable of creating a superhydrophilic surface without altering or modifying any other characteristic of the titanium surface. Therefore, it has been proposed as a simple and effective method to reverse the effects of titanium ageing, which can in turn lead to a faster and more complete establishment of bone-titanium integration. Some authors have called this phenomenon superosseointegration.

The purpose of our study was to determine the effect of two UV-C light sources with a wavelength of 254 nm and an energy of 1400 µW/cm^3 to obtain a hydrophilic surface, comparing two UV-C sources with different powers (6 and 85 W) and a control group.

2. Materials and Methods

2.1. Materials

The materials used in this study were as follows:

- Ten titanium discs 6 mm in diameter and 1 mm thick with biological ageing for 4 weeks;
- Ultraviolet light sources:
  - VL-6C (Analyzer, Murcia, Spain),
  - Ultraviolet germicidal sterilizer (Quirumed, Valencia, Spain);
- Ten titanium discs with biological ageing for 4 weeks;
- Nikon D 80 DSLR Camera (Nikon Corp., Tokyo, Japan);
- Sigma macro 110 mm lens (Kabushiki gaisha, Kanagawa, Japan);
- IMAGEJ image analysis program (National Institutes of Health, Bethesda, MD, USA);
- Micropipette Easy 10 KG 578545 (10 µL) (Labbox Labware, S.L., Barcelona, Spain);
- SPSS V23 statistical package IBM (SPSS Inc., Chicago, IL, USA).

2.2. Method

The 10 discs were stored for 4 weeks in darkness and in a temperature- and humidity-controlled environment. Each disc underwent the same process of biological ageing, after which they were randomly distributed into 3 groups using the Internet program random.org:

- Control group;
- 6 W group;
- 85 W group.

All the groups received one 10 µL drop of water from an Easy 10 KG 578545 pipette, which was photographed perpendicularly, and its angulation was measured using ImageJ. Measurements were recorded according to the irradiation time at 15, 30, 60, and 120 min.

In each group, one disc was used as a control, which received no irradiation and was processed according to the same methodology (Figure 3).

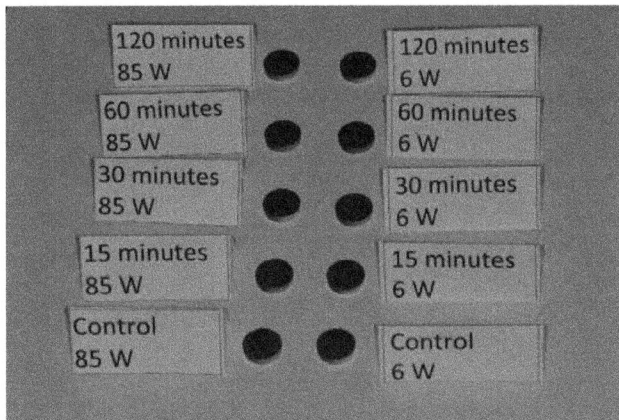

Figure 3. Distribution of discs into groups irradiated with 6 or 85 W according to irradiation time.

Statistical analysis was performed using IBM SPSS ver. 23.0 (IBM Co., Armonk, NY, USA). A normality assumption for the data was tested using the Shapiro–Wilk test.

Descriptive statistics were used to synthesize the collected data. Mean comparisons within the group were computed using analysis of variance, whereas median differences between the groups were analysed using the Mann–Whitney U-test. Statistical significance was considered when $p \leq 0.05$.

All analyses were conducted by an independent statistician who was blind to the procedure performed (http://estadisticamurcia.com/web/#2) (accessed on 7 June 2021).

3. Results

All variables followed a normal distribution except the variable of 6 W and 15 min. The average contact angles for the control discs were 116.19° for the 6 W control group and 117.6° for the 85 W control group. The mean angles obtained at 15, 30, 60, and 120 min with the 6 W ultraviolet (UVC) light source were 69.66°, 74.38°, 73.8°, and 61.45°, respectively. When an ultraviolet (UVC) light bulb of 85 W was used as the source, the average angle obtained at 15 min was 70.25°, 66.28° at 30 min, 19.43° at 60 min, and 31.41° at 120 min. The results obtained are reflected in Tables 1 and 2 and Figures 4–7.

Table 1. Data obtained with the 6 W lamp.

Group	N	Mean	Standard Deviation	95% Confidence Interval for the Mean	
				Lower Limit	Upper Limit
Control	6	116.1983	5.89532	110.0116	122.3851
15 min	6	69.6667	4.86648	64.5596	74.7737
30 min	6	74.3833	3.87475	70.3170	78.4496
60 min	6	73.8000	3.60333	70.0185	77.5815
120 min	6	61.4517	5.85645	55.3057	67.5976
Total	30	79.1000	19.97077	71.6428	86.5572

Table 2. Data obtained with the 85 W lamp.

Group	N	Mean	Standard Deviation	95% Confidence Interval for the Mean	
				Lower Limit	Upper Limit
Control	6	117.6000	5.66533	111.6546	123.5454
15 min	6	70.2583	3.70735	66.3677	74.1490
30 min	6	66.2833	2.94715	63.1905	69.3762
60 min	6	19.4333	1.78176	17.5635	21.3032
120 min	6	31.4167	1.71629	29.6155	33.2178
Total	30	60.9983	35.14705	47.8742	74.1225

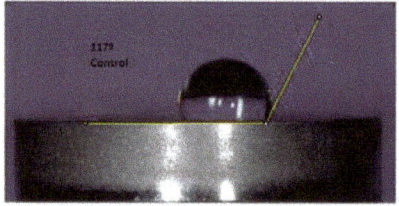
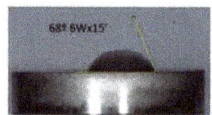
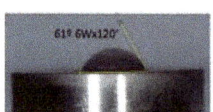
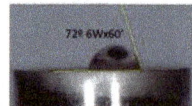
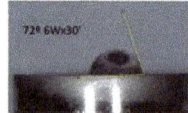

Figure 4. Composition of the different angles obtained with irradiation at 6 W for different time intervals compared with the control.

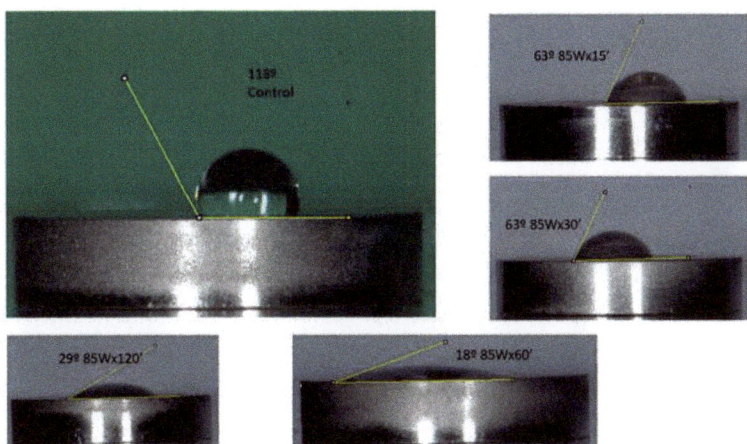

Figure 5. Composition of the different angles obtained with irradiation at 85 W for different time intervals compared with the control.

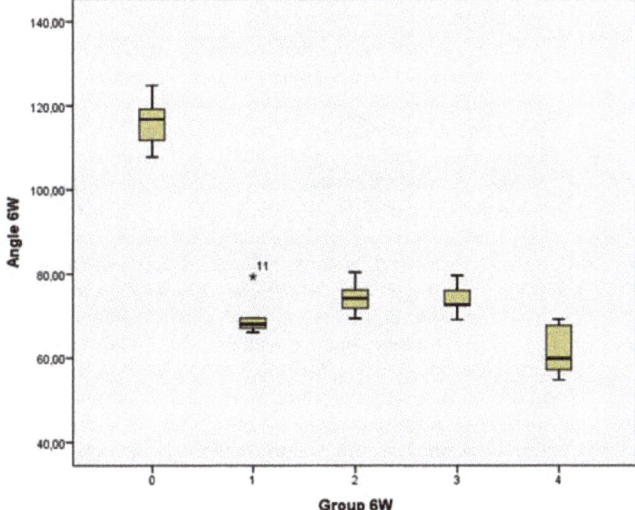

Figure 6. Box plot of angles obtained with a 6 W lamp at different irradiation times, including the control. The graphs show the lower (Q1), mean (Q2), and upper (Q3) quartiles.

The whiskers represent the highest and lowest values. All groups presented statistically significant differences with respect to the control. The 120 min group also showed statistically significant differences from the 30 and 60 min groups.

The whiskers represent the highest and lowest values. All the groups presented statistically significant differences with respect to the control. The 60 and 120 min groups also showed statistically significant differences from the 15 and 30 min groups.

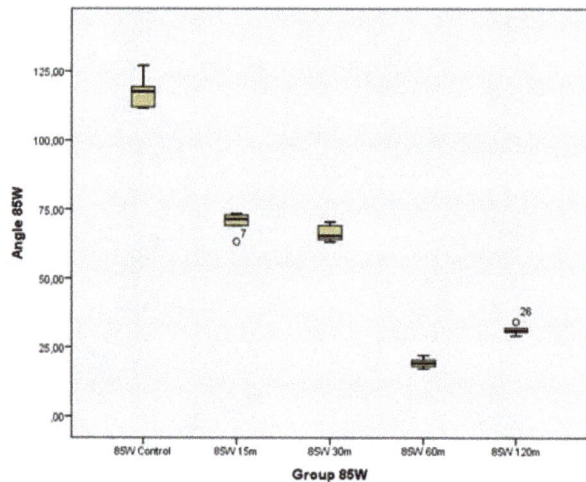

Figure 7. Box plot of angles obtained with an 85 W lamp at different irradiation times, including the control. The graphs show the lower (Q1), mean (Q2), and upper (Q3) quartiles.

4. Discussion

A perfectly clean titanium surface is considered to comprise only titanium and oxygen, which creates a titanium oxide surface. However, such pure surfaces are not available even in the laboratory, as it only a short period of atmospheric exposure is required for the surface to be contaminated with a monolayer of hydrocarbons and inorganic impurities. In a study conducted by Zhao et al. [5], lower carbon pollution was observed on surfaces that had been isolated from the surrounding environment during production compared with those that had not.

It is known that the higher the deposit of hydrocarbon compounds, the lower the hydrophilicity and the greater the angle of contact of the water. Usually, to measure this effect on hydrophilicity, the contact angle of a drop of liquid on the surface being studied is measured, and digital images of the same are analyzed.

The importance of good wettability and a low contact angle is to ensure rapid protein absorption and good cell adhesion to hinder bacterial colonization. Osteoblasts grown on hydrophilic surfaces produce more markers of differentiation by creating an osteogenic microenvironment, potentially contributing to faster and improved osseointegration.

In general, the information provided by implant manufacturers only refers to the maximum sterilization length, which is usually 5 years. However, the need for clinics to have a wide assortment of material available means that they must have an ample supply of stored implants. Due to these circumstances, it is unlikely that dental implants can be used within 4 weeks of manufacturing, implying that most implants will have already undergone a process of ageing prior to insertion.

Different methods have been proposed to preserve the surface of titanium under the best biocompatibility conditions, including packaging in ultravacuum conditions (ultrahigh vacuum), immersion in isotonic solutions, irradiation with ultraviolet C light, the use of cold plasma, and medical ozone. Whereas the first two methods attempt to keep the implant surface intact, the others focus on restoring the surface of titanium oxide, freeing it from impurities.

Perhaps the most viable and economical solution against the inevitable biological ageing of titanium is exposure to UV radiation just before use in a procedure known as photofunctionalization [6].

The underlying mechanism of photofunctionalization appears to be based on the creation of amphiphilic molecules, also called amphipathic molecules. These are molecules that have one hydrophilic (water soluble) end and another hydrophobic end (rejects water). It was stated that modifying the electrostatic properties of the titanium surface plays a decisive role in its bioactivity. The change in surface energy is responsible for this modification. It was also mentioned that this fundamental change is caused by the formation of spaces between the oxygen atoms that allow the adhesion of OH hydroxyl radicals. Other authors attributed this effect to the energy of UVC beam photons, which induces the formation of hydroxyl radicals and hydrogen dissociation. Finally, there are authors who attributed this effect to the rupture of the C=O bonds, removing surface contaminants and regenerating a clean surface that would leave the penta-coordinated titanium (Ti5c) exposed.

Regardless of the exact mechanism, photofunctionalization creates homogeneous conditions for all implants regardless of the date of manufacture, offering the clinician the opportunity to accurately compare individual results. In this way, differences in the osseointegration of products from the same manufacturer can also be eliminated.

This effect has been observed at various UV wavelengths, including ultraviolet A (UVA), ultraviolet B (UVB), and even in combinations of both ultraviolet C light (UVC), which is commonly used due to its higher power. Two previous studies comparing titanium surfaces treated with UVA and UVC showed that despite emerging superhydrophilia on both titanium surfaces, the cellular fixation capacity was significantly greater for the UVC-treated surfaces. Reported findings indicate that photofunctionalization with ultraviolet C light accelerates the process of osseointegration, both in animals and in humans.

This effect may be of help in immediate loading procedures, as well as in short implants and in cases of poor bone quality, low primary stability, or systemic diseases [7–10].

The intention of our work was to determine the effect of both irradiation power and time on the wettability angle of standard surfaces, which does not depend solely on the composition of the material. Surface topography also plays an important role, depending on whether it is a pure titanium surface, acid-etched, or sand-blasted. Rough surfaces lose their hydrophilicity more quickly than smooth surfaces. In addition, an interesting observation is that the hydrophilicity and hydrophobicity of rough surfaces are greater than those of smooth surfaces, while their angles vary widely as a result of biological ageing.

In our study, all surfaces were of the same nature: Grade IV titanium with RBM-TC surface (Ticare, Mozo Grau, Valladolid, Spain), so that the only variables capable of affecting the wettability angle were power and time of exposure.

This study showed that UVC photoactivation modifies titanium surfaces from a hydrophobic (control) to a hydrophilic state at both 6 and 85 W, each showing statistically significant differences from the control group. However, according to the wettability classification based on the contact angle, superhydrophilic surfaces were not achieved, as no angle was less than 10°.

These differences were accentuated by an increase in time. However, the results revealed that the most significant effect depended on the power of the emitter, although the effect was not evident before 30 min. After 60 min, the effect of 85 W was significantly more pronounced (73° versus 19°) and was equally or more effective at 120 min (61° versus 31°). However, in the case of the 85 W group, this improvement did not change to any great extent, changing from a contact angle of 19° at 60 min to 31° at 120°, a paradoxical effect not seen at 6 W. We share the opinion that this is due to the saturation of compounds in the atmosphere, which, once detached from the titanium surface, are re-deposited on the titanium surface with its increased absorption capacity.

This study points to an increase in the hydrophilicity of titanium surfaces treated with UV light, and it would be of particular interest to continue with an in vivo study. Such a study should focus on applying a power of 85 W and a time of 60 min, a combination that yielded the best result in vitro.

Study Limitations

Some authors considered that the effect of the hydrophilicity of a given material and its impact on biological activity may be difficult to interpret [11]. However, the wide diversity of materials and variety of treatments available for implant surfaces complicate generalizing the results.

Our study is based on an in vitro model. We feel that animal studies are needed to check whether the results obtained with a power of 85 watts for 60 min produce an improvement in BIC values.

5. Conclusions

The exposure to UVC ultraviolet light resulted in an increase in the hydrophilicity of titanium surfaces in both groups with respect to the controls, although superhydrophilic surfaces were not obtained. Power, rather than time, was shown to be the most important and significant factor for obtaining hydrophilic surfaces.

Within the limitations of this study, we concluded that the ideal power to improve the wettability of titanium with an RBM-TC surface is 85 watts applied for 60 min at a wavelength of 254 nm. There is no improvement with longer times at this power, as the situation stabilizes and the system becomes saturated.

We consider that these findings can improve the biological process of osseointegration in implant therapy and offer us clues to the use of UVC in dental offices.

Author Contributions: Conceptualization, A.S.-P. and C.N.C.; methodology, N.C.-M.; investigation, N.C.-M.; data curation, M.J.M.V.; writing—original draft preparation, J.M.M.C.; writing—review and editing, A.S.-P.; N.C.-M.; C.N.C.; M.J.M.V., and J.M.M.C.; supervision, A.S.-P. All authors have read and agreed to the published version of the manuscript.

Funding: This research received no external funding.

Institutional Review Board Statement: This study was edited by American Journal Expert.

Informed Consent Statement: Not applicable.

Data Availability Statement: The data obtained in this study are available to those who request them.

Acknowledgments: The authors would like to thank Ticare for their collaboration in manufacturing the titanium discs.

Conflicts of Interest: The authors declare no conflict of interest.

References

1. Ogawa, T.; Nishimura, I. Different bone integration profiles of turned and acid-etched implants associated with modulated expression of extracellular matrix genes. *Int. J. Oral Maxillofac. Implants* **2003**, *18*, 200–210. [PubMed]
2. Albertini, M.; Fernandez-Yague, M.; Lázaro, P.; Herrero-Climent, M.; Rios-Santos, J.-V.; Bullon, P.; Gil, F.-J. Advances in surfaces and osseointegration in implantology. Biomimetic surfaces. *Med. Oral Patol. Oral Cir. Bucal* **2015**, *20*, e316–e325. [CrossRef] [PubMed]
3. Khang, D.; Lu, J.; Yao, C.; Haberstroh, K.M.; Webster, T.J. The role of nanometer and sub-micron surface features on vascular and bone cell adhesion on titanium. *Biomaterials* **2008**, *29*, 970–983. [CrossRef] [PubMed]
4. Sartoretto, S.C.; Alves, A.T.N.N.; Resende, R.F.B.; Calasans-Maia, J.; Granjeiro, J.M.; Calasans-Maia, M.D. Early osseointegration driven by the surface chemistry and wettability of dental implants. *J. Appl. Oral Sci.* **2015**, *23*, 279–287. [CrossRef] [PubMed]
5. Zhao, G.; Schwartz, Z.; Wieland, M.; Rupp, F.; Geis-Gerstorfer, J.; Cochran, D.L.; Boyan, B.D. High surface energy enhances cell response to titanium substrate microstructure. *J. Biomed. Mater. Res. A* **2005**, *74A*, 49–58. [CrossRef] [PubMed]
6. Aita, H.; Att, W.; Ueno, T.; Yamada, M.; Hori, N.; Iwasa, F.; Tsukimura, N.; Ogawa, T. Ultraviolet light-mediated photofunctionalization of titanium to promote human mesenchymal stem cell migration, attachment, proliferation and differentiation. *Acta Biomater.* **2009**, *5*, 3247–3257. [CrossRef] [PubMed]
7. Roy, M.; Pompella, A.; Kubacki, J.; Szade, J.; Roy, R.A.; Hedzelek, W. Photofunctionalization of titanium: An alternative explanation of its chemical-physical mechanism. *PLoS ONE* **2016**, *11*, e0157481. [CrossRef] [PubMed]
8. Sanchez-Perez, A.; Cachazo-Jiménez, C.; Sánchez-Matás, C.; Martín-de-Llano, J.J.; Davis, S.; Carda-Batalla, C. Effects of ultraviolet photoactivation on osseointegration of commercial pure titanium dental implant after 8 weeks in a rabbit model. *J. Oral Implantol.* **2020**, *46*, 101–107. [CrossRef] [PubMed]

9. Ueno, T.; Yamada, M.; Hori, N.; Suzuki, T.; Ogawa, T. Effect of ultraviolet photoactivation of titanium on osseointegration in a rat model. *Int. J. Oral Maxillofac. Implants* **2010**, *25*, 287–294. [PubMed]
10. Suzuki, S.; Kobayashi, H.; Ogawa, T. Implant stability change and osseointegration speed of immediately loaded photofunctionalized implants. *Implant Dent.* **2013**, *22*, 481–490. [CrossRef] [PubMed]
11. Aita, H.; Hori, N.; Takeuchi, M.; Suzuki, T.; Yamada, M.; Anpo, M.; Ogawa, T. The effect of ultraviolet functionalization of titanium on integration with bone. *Biomaterials* **2009**, *30*, 1015–1025. [CrossRef] [PubMed]

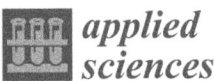

Article

Marginal Adaptation Assessment for Two Composite Layering Techniques Using Dye Penetration, AFM, SEM and FTIR: An In-Vitro Comparative Study

Andrea Maria Chisnoiu [1], Marioara Moldovan [2], Codruta Sarosi [2], Radu Marcel Chisnoiu [3,*], Doina Iulia Rotaru [3], Ada Gabriela Delean [3], Ovidiu Pastrav [3], Alexandrina Muntean [4], Ioan Petean [5], Lucian Barbu Tudoran [6,7] and Mihaela Pastrav [8]

1. Department of Prosthodontics, "Iuliu Hatieganu" University of Medicine and Pharmacy, 32 Clinicilor Street, 400006 Cluj-Napoca, Romania; maria.chisnoiu@umfcluj.ro
2. Department of Polymeric Composites, "Raluca Ripan" Institute of Research in Chemistry, "Babes Bolyai" University, 30 Fantanele Street, 400294 Cluj-Napoca, Romania; marioara.moldovan@ubbcluj.ro (M.M.); codruta.sarosi@ubbcluj.ro (C.S.)
3. Department of Cariology, Endodontics and Oral Pathology, "Iuliu Hatieganu" University of Medicine and Pharmacy, 33 Motilor Street, 400001 Cluj-Napoca, Romania; doina.rotaru@umfcluj.ro (D.I.R.); ada.delean@umfcluj.ro (A.G.D.); ovidiu.pastrav@umfcluj.ro (O.P.)
4. Department of Pedodontics, "Iuliu Hatieganu" University of Medicine and Pharmacy, 31 Avram Iancu Street, 400117 Cluj-Napoca, Romania; alexandrina.muntean@umfcluj.ro
5. Faculty of Chemistry and Chemical Engineering, "Babes Bolyai" University, 11 Arany Janos Street, 400028 Cluj-Napoca, Romania; ioan.petean@ubbcluj.ro
6. Electron Microscopy Centre, "Babes Bolyai" University, 5-7 Clinicilor Street, 400006 Cluj-Napoca, Romania; lucianbarbutudoran@gmail.com
7. Advanced Research and Technology Centre for Alternative Energy, National Institute for Research and Development of Isotopic and Molecular Technologies, 67-103 Donat Street, 400331 Cluj-Napoca, Romania
8. Department of Orthodontics, "Iuliu Hatieganu" University of Medicine and Pharmacy, 31 Avram Iancu Street, 400117 Cluj-Napoca, Romania; mihaela.pastrav@umfcluj.ro
* Correspondence: marcel.chisnoiu@umfcluj.ro; Tel.: +40-721-207-617

Abstract: Do the new, modern dental resin composites improve the sealing in cavities restorations? The present study was designed to compare the effect of two different, but most used layering techniques of the dental composite in reducing the marginal microleakage when a brand-new material is used; Class I black cavities were prepared on 120 human extracted teeth and then restored using oblique and horizontal layering technique. The dye penetration analysis, the atomic force microscopy (AFM), scanning electron microscopy (SEM) together with energy-dispersive X-ray spectroscopy (EDX) and Fourier transform infra-red spectroscopy (FTIR) technique were used to assess the adaptation of the restorative material to the dental structures. Some better results were obtained for oblique layering technique, but the differences to the other method have not been statistically validated. The composite layering technique still remains an open quest and, moreover, in vivo studies should be designed in order to assess microleakage in real conditions of the oral environment.

Keywords: composite restoration; microleakage; oblique layering technique; horizontal layering technique

1. Introduction

One of the most important issues in restorative dentistry is the failure of restorative materials to completely bind to hard dental tissues, both enamel and dentin. The ability of the restoration to perfectly fit to the walls of the cavity and to seal them influences the durability of the treatment. Speaking of perfection, a firm bond between the dental tissues and the restorative material should lead to a snug and concealed marginal adaptation [1]. Despite the technological improvement, for the moment, no material perfectly adheres to the tooth surface. This results in cracks between the restorative material and the margins of the cavity, allowing the microleakage [2].

Microleakage is defined as the passage of bacteria, fluids, molecules or ions, between the restoration and the cavity walls. It has been considered to be involved in the development of recurrent caries, pulpal inflammation or, even the failure of the endodontic treatments [3]. The improper adaptation, the deformation due to load or temperature variations of the restorative material or the contraction during polymerization may result in gaps which will represent a pathway for bacteria and their products to the dentin and, further, to the pulp [4,5].

The composite resin polymerization shrinkage may be the most important factor that leads to microleakage occurrences. Along the factors involved in shrinkage stress, there can be noticed the cavity size and geometry (including the configuration factor—C factor), the application technique (including composite layering and light curing) and the composite characteristics (including modulus of elasticity) [6].

Several procedures were imagined in order to solve or, at least, to improve the sealing problem of the posterior composite resin restorations. One of these procedures is represented by the oblique layering technique which involves the use of 1 to 1.5 mm triangle-shaped increments of resin, so the C factor reduced [7]. The highest value of the C factor is considered to be when the horizontal layering technique is used. This is the most easy-to-use and, probably, the most comfortable technique for the beginner practitioners.

Recent studies indicate that the most important factor in achieving a successful restoration is likely careful and proper placement and light-curing technique, independent of the placement technique [8–10]. Based on these results, the current study has been designed as an innovative and complex research to compare the effect of two different layering techniques of the dental composite in reducing of marginal microleakage, to assess the adaptation of the restorative material to the dental tissue by atomic force microscopy (AFM), to evaluate the efficacy of polymerization in composite resins by Fourier transform infra-red spectroscopy (FTIR) technique and to correlate the observations with the SEM—EDX investigation for these two techniques when using same adhesive system and same restorative material.

2. Materials and Methods

2.1. Preparation of the Sample

One-hundred-twenty teeth were included in this study, maxillary and mandibular molars and premolars, extracted due to orthodontic or periodontal reasons, no more than 4 weeks before the study. Only caries-free teeth were included in the group, without coronary destruction and without pre-existing restorations. In order to meet the hydration conditions, these teeth were preserved in distilled water [11,12].

2.2. Cavities Preparation

A single operator prepared a Class I black cavity on the occlusal surface of each tooth. The depth of the cavity did not exceed 3 mm. These cavities were prepared with 0.12 round turbine burs (MDT, Mc Drill Technology, Parma, Italy) in enamel thickness and 0.14 steel round low-speed handpiece burs (Dendia, Dendia GmbH, Feldkirch, Austria) in dentin thickness, following the ditches and avoiding the cusps. A new bur was used after every 5 cavity preparations. An UNC 15 probe (Hu Friedy Mfg. Co. Inc., Chicago, IL, USA) was used for measuring the depth and the width of the cavity. No additional retentions were prepared, as the cavities were restored with adhesive materials.

2.3. Restoration Technique

The teeth were randomly divided into 2 groups of 60 teeth each based on the restorative layering technique as Group A—oblique layering technique, and Group B—horizontal layering technique. As an adhesive system, a 3 steps system was used, considering that this represents the golden standard in dental adhesion. For both groups (A, B), the enamel was etched for 30 s and dentin for 15 s using 37% Meta Etchant Gel (Meta Biomed Co. Ltd. Osong-eup, Republic of Korea), then washed and gently dried for 5 s. The new G2—BOND Universal (GC Europe) was used, according to the manufacturer instructions—first the Primer, for 10 s, using a microbrush and dried for 5 s, then the Bond, spread evenly using a gentle stream of air and light cured for 10 s, using a LED light-curing lamp (Translux-Wave, Kulzer, Germany). Teeth were then filled by a single operator, with a brand-new composite (G-aenial A'CHORD, GC Europe) using oblique layering technique (Group A) and horizontal layering technique (Group B) with 1 mm thick increments and light-curing for 20 s.

The shade of the composite was different from the tooth in order to facilitate the assessment. In the end, the restorations were finished and polished with red and yellow ring burs, rubber cups, brushes and polishing paste.

2.4. Thermocycling

All specimens were thermocycled for 1000 cycles (5/55 °C, 30 s) in Eppendorf Mastercycler gradient (Eppendorf AG, Hamburg, Germany). Then, the surfaces of the roots were covered with two layers of nail polish and the apices were sealed with orthodontic wax. All samples were immersed in 2% methylene blue dye for 24 h, then the teeth were washed with distilled water and dried. Then they were embedded in acrylic resin (Duracryl Plus, SpofaDental) and, later, sectioned mesio-distally using the microtome (IsoMet TM1000, Buehler, Chicago, IL, USA). There were selected those teeth slices that had no damages after cutting. Each tooth slice was 1 mm thick.

For marginal microleakage assessment, the cut sections were observed under 20× magnification and the area of maximum dye penetration was considered. For the magnification, a stereomicroscope was used (Zeiss CL 1500 ECO) and each sample was photographed using a digital photo camera (Canon EOS 1300D).

Two examiners scored the extent of dye penetration using a scale (0–4) by consensus. Examiners were blind to the technique used.

The scoring criteria [13]:

0—no evidence of dye penetration;
1—dye penetration along the axial cavity walls up to 1/3;
2—dye penetration along the axial cavity walls up to 2/3;
3—dye penetration along the whole axial cavity wall;
4—dye penetration on the pulpal wall.

The AFM analysis was conducted on the composite resin (restorative material) for both groups as well as the correspondent interfaces with enamel and dentine. The AFM images were obtained in tapping mode with a JEOL JSPM 4210 Scanning Probe Microscope, produced by JEOL, Japan, Tokyo. The cantilevers used are NSC 15 type produced by MicroMasch, Estonia, Talinn, having a resonant frequency of about 325 kHz and a force constant of 40 N/m. The images were scanned at area of 5 µm × 5 µm for the restorative material and at 20 µm × 20 µm for the interfaces. At least 3 different macroscopic areas were scanned for each situation. All images were scanned in standard manner using Jeol WIN SPM 2.0 processing soft, the average roughness (Ra) and the root mean squared roughness (Rq) being measured for each image.

The samples for scanning electron microscopy (SEM) were prepared as well as for light microscopy, in order to investigate the enamel-composite and dentin-composite interfaces and the structure of the enamel and dentin. High-resolution scanning electron microscopy (HR-SEM) and energy-dispersive X-ray spectroscopy (EDX) were conducted on a Hitachi SU8230 cold field emission scanning electron microscope. Samples were subsequently sputter-coated with an ~7 nm thick layer of gold and imaged under 30 kV acceleration voltage.

For FTIR analysis, a spectrometer (Jasco 610, Jasco International Co., Ltd., Tokyo, Japan) in an ATR mode was used, with a scanning range from 4000 to 550 cm^{-1} at a speed of 4 cm/s and with an average of 128 measurements in the final spectrum.

2.5. Statistical Analysis

Before statistical analyses, G3*Power calculation (software version 3.1.9.6, Erdfelder, Faul and Buchner, 1996, Heinrich Heine University, Dusseldorf, Germany) was used to identify the adequate number of samples to be included in the study. Considering similar studies, the expected mean values of scores were around 2 and standard deviations around 0.9 [14]. These data indicated an estimated effect size that was used to calculate minimal necessary number of samples for analysis of variance. All data were collected and statistically analyzed using SPSS Statistics (ver. 20.0, IBM, Chicago, IL, USA). The Kruskal–Wallis test followed by the Mann-Whitney U test were used and p values < 0.05 were considered statistically significant.

3. Results

3.1. Microleakage Assesment

The dye penetration varied from Score 0 to Score 4 for both groups, but lower scores were obtained for Group A than Group B (Figures 1 and 2).

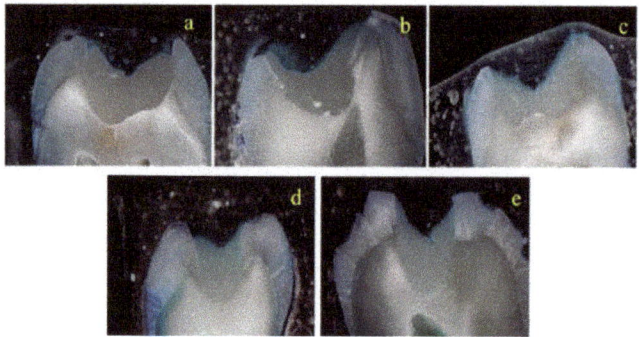

Figure 1. Microleakage scoring: (**a**) Score 0; (**b**) Score 1; (**c**) Score 2; (**d**) Score 3; (**e**) Score 4.

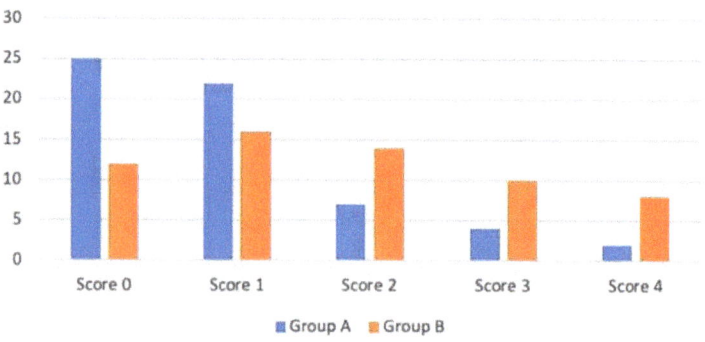

Figure 2. Oblique and horizontal layering technique scoring distribution.

All collected data after scoring were subjected to statistical analysis within the limitations of this study. The mean value in Group A was lower than in Group B. Although there were differences in the results in the two groups, they were not statistically validated ($p > 0.05$) (Table 1).

Table 1. Microleakage in the oblique (Group A) and horizontal (Group B) layering technique.

Microleakage	Mean	Standard Deviation	p-Value
Group A	1	1.1427	0.723
Group B	2	1.3304	

3.2. Atomic Force Microscopy Analysis

For Group A, the fine microstructure of the Composite (C) is presented in Figure 3a. The topographic image reveals a scaly morphology. It is formed up by some submicron boulders (having diameter around 600 nm) very well bonded together with a nanostructured material which is formed by well stacked nanoparticles of about 60 nm. Overall, in Group A, the restorative material proves to be very compact assuring an optimal bulk filling of the cavity. The tri-dimensional image shows a relatively smooth surface having a Ra = 45.6 and Rq = 57.9. Fact deals within the high level of compactness inside of the material.

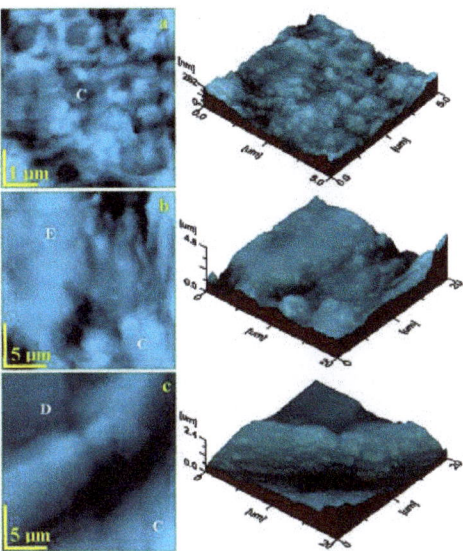

Figure 3. AFM 2D topographic images for Group A samples: (a) composite (restorative material), (b) composite—enamel interface, and (c) composite—dentin interface. Tri-dimensional images are given next to 2D topographic images. C-composite, E-enamel, D-dentin.

The composite—enamel (C–E) interface is presented in Figure 3b. The left side of the topographic image is the enamel featuring a smooth and very compact surface and the right side of the image belongs to composite. Its morphology is similar with the one observed in Figure 3a. The middle vertical of the image in Figure 3b represents the interface. It features a very compact structure with less presence of submicron formation but richest in nanostructured compound which is very well attached to the hydroxyapatite nanoparticles within the enamel. The interface is more visible in the tri-dimensional image as a gap filled with a compact material which assures a strong cohesion between restorative material and enamel. The average thickness of the bonding layer is about of 5 µm. The presence of the bonding interface between composite and enamel leads to a surface roughness increasing of Ra to 315.25 nm and Rq to 412.0 nm (Table 2).

Table 2. Roughness values for the Group A sample.

Roughness		Mean Value	Standard Deviation	p-Value
Ra	C	45.6	13.923	
	C–E	315.25	31.063	0.093
	C–D	240.25	98.63	
Rq	C	57.9	17.583	
	C–E	412.0	35.655	0.184
	C–D	300.75	119.226	

The composite—dentine (C–D) interface is observed by AFM in Figure 3c on the diagonal from left down corner to the right upper corner, the dentine appears on the left upper corner and composite on the right lower corner. The adhesion layer also has a thickness of about 5 µm and is filled up with fine nanostructured bonding material which assures a very good adhesion of the restorative material to the hydroxyapatite nanoparticles from the dentin structure. The tri-dimensional image features the adhesion layer as a well-formed furrow along to the interface proving the strong cohesion between restoration material in Group A sample and dentine. The smoothness of the bonding observed in this case leads to a less increased roughness: Ra to 240.25 nm and Rq to 300.75 nm (Table 2).

Although Ra and Rq values are higher for C–E interface than C–D, the differences are not statistically significant ($p > 0.05$).

For Group B, Composite (C) has a particular morphology as seen in the topographic image in Figure 4a. It is based on a submicron granular material with boulder aspect and diameters varying in a wide range between 200 to 500 nm consolidated in a compact block with a nanostructured material having fine rounded units with diameter of about 80 nm. Such compact area is observed in the upper side of the topographic image in Figure 4a. The lower side of the image features a pore occurred in the restorative material having a diameter of about 1.3 µm and a dendritic–irregular border. The pore is formed in the boulder reach areas, perhaps due to a local lack of nanostructured material. Overall, the composite assures a good in bulk filling of the cavity and features a good cohesion despite the observed pores.

The topographic image in Figure 4b captures the interface between enamel (E) (low side of image) and Composite (C) in the upper side of the image. The enamel area is very smooth and compact corresponding to a perfectly healthy state. The C features two pores with prolonged aspect and irregular borders nearby the interface. The nanostructured material within C perfectly seals those pores and assures an optimal cohesion with the enamel. The bonding layer is difficult to be observed because of the great adhesion to the enamel. The tri-dimensional image allows us to establish the adhesion layer thickness of about 4 µm. The pores presence nearby the interface leads to a surface roughness increasing, presented in Table 3.

The interface C–D is more evident as a gap between dentine to the left and composite to the right in the topographic image, Figure 4c. The gap width is about 3 µm and is completely filled with nanostructured bonding material. A strong cohesion is observed on the both sides, a fact also depicted by the tri-dimensional image. The smoothness observed along the C–D interface leads to a smaller increasing of the roughness. The fact deals with the pore lack nearby dentine.

The Ra and Rq values are higher for C–E interface than C–D, similar to Group A, but the differences are not statistically significant.

Comparing the roughness between the two groups, it results a similar variation for both C–E and C–D interfaces and no statistical difference was validated (Table 4).

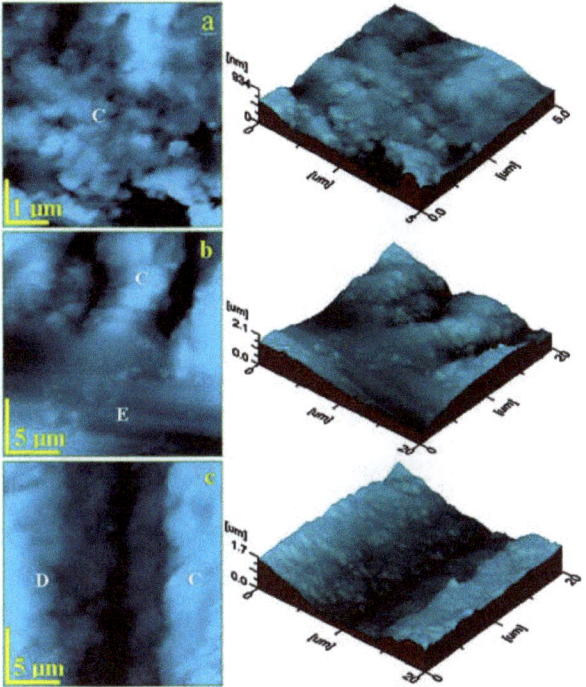

Figure 4. AFM 2D topographic images for Group B samples: (**a**) composite (restorative material), (**b**) C–E interface, and (**c**) C–D interface. Tridimensional images are given next to 2D topographic images.

Table 3. Roughness values for the Group B sample.

	Roughness		Mean Value	Standard Deviation	p-Value
Ra		C	49.83	8.857	
		C–E	318.75	139.047	0.063
		C–D	253.0	88.185	
Rq		C	67.86	11.850	
		C–E	411.75	188.032	0.058
		C–D	309.25	91.729	

Table 4. Roughness values for the Group A and B samples.

	Roughness		Mean Value	Standard Deviation	p-Value
Ra	C–E	Group A	315.25	31.063	0.294
		Group B	318.75	139.047	
	C–D	Group A	240.25	98.63	0.162
		Group B	253.0	88.185	
Rq	C–E	Group A	412.0	35.655	0.091
		Group B	411.75	188.032	
	C–D	Group A	300.75	119.226	0.087
		Group B	309.25	91.729	

3.3. Scanning Electron Microscopy (SEM) and Energy-Dispersive X-ray Spectroscopy (EDX) Analysis

The SEM analysis was performed in order to observe the adhesion between the restoration material and the dental tissues when there was no dye penetration (scores = 0) as well as when the dye penetrated the composite/dental tissue interface (scores > 0).

Analysing the Score 0 samples, adhesive interfaces completely adapted to the restoration material were observed. SEM images show a uniform and efficient polymerization on the entire restored cavity. The hybrid layer has a thin, homogeneous and denser structure in electrons with a relatively uniform thickness (~2 µm), which closely followed the tooth surface and formed a hybrid layer penetrating the thickness of the dental tissue, in some cases on a depth of 10 µm. The high degree of homogeneity of the polymerized adhesive layer was also noticed. It was observed that the resin extensions, which intersect the hybrid layer, have an electronic density similar to the overlying adhesive layer, which demonstrated a continuity of the nanoparticle concentration into depth. Thus, the periphery of the dental tissue was also hybridized and the hybrid layer extends in the entire depth of the demineralized area (Figures 5 and 6).

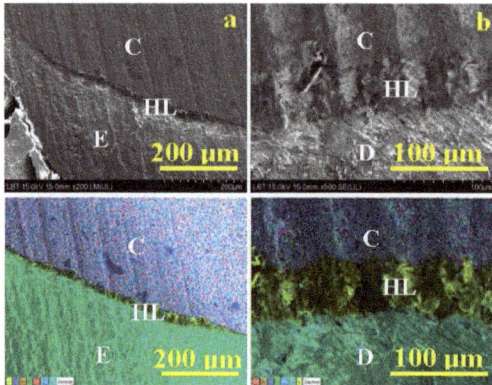

Figure 5. SEM images for Score 0 in Group A: (**a**) Composite (C)—enamel interface (E); (**b**) Composite (C)—dentin (D) interface; HL—hybrid layer. EDX mappings are given below for each SEM electron image.

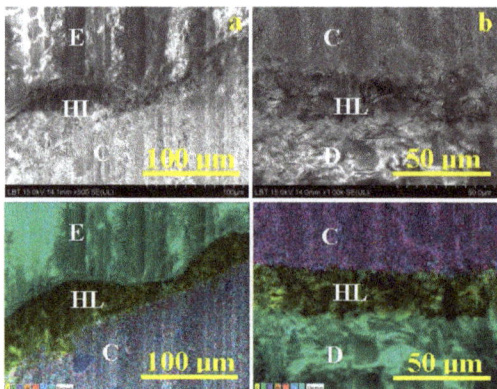

Figure 6. SEM images for Score 0 in Group B: (**a**) Composite (C)—enamel interface (E); (**b**) Composite (C)—dentin (D) interface; HL—hybrid layer. EDX mappings are given below for each SEM electron image.

Regarding the samples with a score higher than 0, there can be noticed cracks at the dental tissue/hybrid layer or composite/hybrid layer interfaces, with a varying length for different samples. Gaps and fissures were observed at the composite/dentin interface more than at the composite/enamel interface, indicating that the adhesion to the dentin is likely to be influenced by several factors than the enamel (Figure 7).

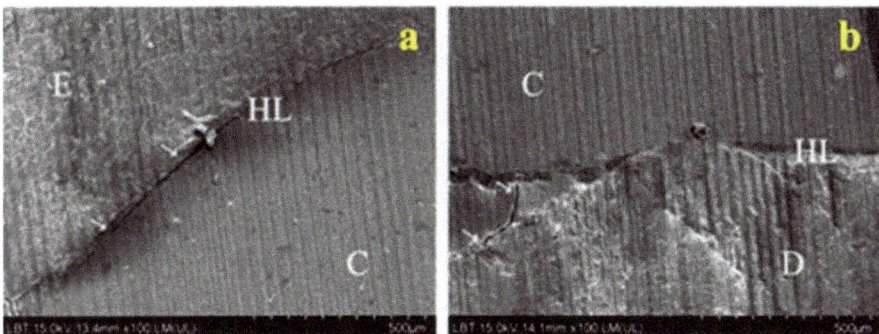

Figure 7. SEM images for Score 3: (**a**) Composite (C)—enamel interface (E); (**b**) Composite (C)—dentin (D) interface; HL—hybrid layer.

The EDX images indicate a high content of atomic oxygen (O), calcium (Ca), silica (Si), carbon (C) and phosphorus (P) and a medium content of barium (Ba). The analysis indicated a high concentration of phosphorus and calcium in dentin which suddenly drops at the dentin/composite interface. Regarding the adhesive layer, an increase in carbon was observed for all samples, suggesting that the monomers contained that element. In addition, the images revealed small concentrations of aluminum and silica in dentin as well as in the adhesive layer.

3.4. Fourier Transform Infra-Red Spectroscopy (FTIR)

The intensity of the peak at 995 cm^{-1} associated with PO from apatite, the majority component of enamel and dentin, is highlighted (Figure 8). The weak bands of 1214 and 1455 cm^{-1} are attributed to the organic components of dentin (dentinal collagen).

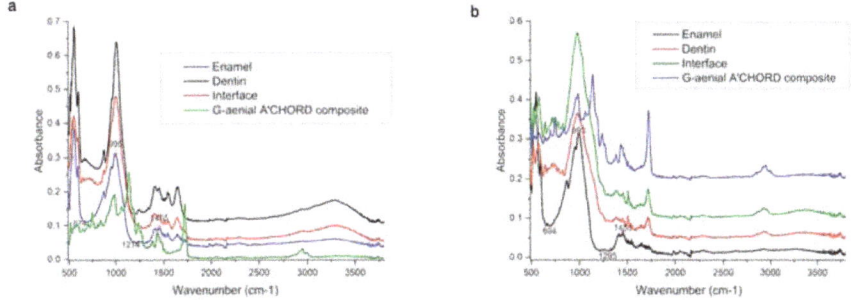

Figure 8. FTIR spectrum based on the restorative layering technique: (**a**)- oblique layering technique; (**b**)- horizontal layering technique.

The IR spectrum corresponding to the adhesive intertubular interface infiltrated in demineralized dentin highlights together with the characteristic bands of apatite ~950 cm^{-1} and dentinal collagen 1637 cm^{-1} (CC), 1455 cm^{-1} (CH$_2$), specific bands of the monomer mixture at 1719 cm^{-1} (specific for urethane carbonyl), 2870–2965 cm^{-1} (CH$_2$ from the structure of the urethane monomer), as well as the 638 cm^{-1} band attributed to the aromatic cycle in Bis-GMA.

The intensity of the bands associated with the Bis-MEPP monomer from composite resin composition suggest that the monomer resin diffuses deeply in the demineralized area of the dentin, meaning the affinity of the monomer to the dental structure.

4. Discussion

It is a continuous quest for the perfect restorative material and restoration technique that ensure the ideal adherence to the tooth surface for eliminating the microleakage. It is, also, very important to maintain the marginal seal in time and to minimize the clinical issues due to microleakage, like marginal discolorations or recurrent caries [15].

The ability of restorative material to reduce the microleakage along the restauration/dental wall interface is crucial in its clinical success. There are several methods that have been proposed in order to assess the correctness of a restoration and the degree of microleakage alongside the margins. One of the most used methods is the dye diffusion. This method involves the use of different dyes like methylene blue, eosin, aniline blue, Indian ink or fluorescein [16].

It is important to mention that the diameter of the dye particles should be smaller than the diameter of dentinal tubules (1–4 µm), otherwise they might be retained by the dental structures or the restorative material, representing a source of errors. According to other dye penetration studies, it is recommended to use a dye with a particle diameter equal to the bacterial size or smaller (~2 µm) [17]. For this reason, in this study methylene blue solution was used as a dye, since its particle size is smaller than bacteria (1.2 nm^2) [18].

Microleakage that occurs along the restorative material/dental tissue interface is the most important issue when composite resins are used for restorations. In order to reduce the shrinkage associated with resins polymerization, different methods of restoration placement were imagined in trying to reduce the bonded to unbonded restoration surface ratio [19]. One of this methods is represented by the oblique layering technique which reduces the contraction forces that occur between opposing walls, and, by that, the cuspal fissures or gap formation [20].

In order to simulate the degradation of composite bond in this study, the aging by thermocycling was used. Different authors suggested different dwell times. These ranged from 4 to 180 s, without any justification. After a careful analysis of more studies, Gale and Darewell [21] noticed wide variations in the thermocycling regimens and concluded that there no rule must be respected when choosing a regimen by the contrary, Rossomando et al. [22] concluded that the dwell time should be of maximum 10 s in order to be clinically relevant.

One more issue that needs to be mentioned in microleakage studies is related to the scoring systems. The evaluation in these studies, usually uses the observer's interpretation, so the leakage scoring can be considered a semi-measurable method [23,24]. In addition, various studies mention that dye leakage in different sections of the restoration may show significant differences [25,26]. For this reason, it is mandatory to assess the leakage on more just one section from a tooth, in order to increase the accuracy of the study.

For the moment, there are no quantitative methods that can be applicate for the microleakage determination. The microleakage was measured through quantification in the present study.

The method within stereomicroscopic studies is based on the interpretation of the dye leakage on the cavity walls and is defined as a semi-quantitative approach where the leakage is calculated solely at the surface where the section is made [27].

The present study showed that the marginal microleakage was present in both groups, but in different proportions. Even if the differences were not statistically validated, the teeth restored by oblique layering technique showed lower scores compared to those restored by horizontal layering technique. Therefore, this difference can be due to the different layering technique that was used.

The results are in agreement with Sarfi et al. [14] and Ghavamnasiri et al. [28] who concluded that, regarding the microleakage, there are not any differences between different layering techniques. In addition, similar results were obtained by Santhosh et al. [29] and Usha et al. [30]. By the contrary, Eakleet et al. [31] found that the oblique layering technique had the most leak-free margins when the proximal box ended on enamel.

Oliveira et al. [32] showed that there are no significant differences between the level of shrinkage stress at the tooth-restoration interface when these two techniques of resin composite placement are used. However, Versluis et al. [33] observed that the highest degree of cusp flexion occurs in the horizontal technique followed by the oblique one. Other studies, like those that belong to Kwon et al. [34] or de Park et al. [35] found that the incremental layering technique leads to a significantly less cuspal deflection when compared to bulk filling technique, however, when comparing the horizontal with oblique layering techniques, there is no significant difference.

AFM seemed to be a useful tool for the assessment of marginal adaptation. The AFM uses a software with great mathematical accuracy for the mapping and characterization of surfaces [36,37] and provides 3D high-resolution offering quantitative data related to the length of marginal gaps. Furthermore, the samples to be investigated by AFM do not require special preparations (such as metallization or fixing) which reduces the occurrence possibility of the artifacts that could affect the analysis [36,38].

According to SEM images analysis of the Score 0 samples, the increased adhesion of the composite to the dental structures can be explained by the existence of a clearly defined hybrid layer on the entire interface in all specimens treated in this study. The granular appearance of the adhesive is due to the SiO_2 filling content of the adhesive. The formation of a homogeneous hybrid layer means the closure of any communication path between the pulp chamber and the outside, meaning a perfect sealing of the dentinal wound.

Regarding the SEM images analysis of the samples with a score higher than zero, the cracks can be due to the low bond strength at the composite/dental structure interface, which could not face the resin polymerization shrinkage and could not provide an adequate interfacial seal for these samples. These issues can, also, be due to the drying of the tooth sections in the air while manipulating or the dehydration under vacuum during SEM analysis. However, because these gaps or cracks were noticed mainly when horizontal layering technique was used and since all samples were treated in the same way, they can be attributed to the low adhesion between the composite and dental structure.

It is not a novelty that the hybrid layer is the most important element in adhesive-dentin bond strength [39,40]. It is formed by resin that covers the collagen fibrils. The bonding agent needs to uniformly penetrate the collagen system and be completely polymerized in order to generate high bond strength.

Considering the EDX analysis, the silica and aluminum in the adhesive layer and dentin is the result of the presence of nanofiller in their composition, and further confirms that resin tags were produced by the adhesive systems. EDX analysis also revealed increased quantities of silica and aluminum in the composite structures, suggesting the presence of an inorganic filler in the material.

The most of the composites contain methacrylate resins and the polymerization process is initiated by light. Almost the whole polymerization process occurs in the first minutes after irradiation [41]. In order to ensure the polymerization for all the restorative material, increments of maximum 2 mm thickness are applied, so the light will penetrate and activate the polymerization in depth [42].

To assess the efficacy of polymerization in composite resins, some laboratory analysis are documented in the literature. Fourier transform infra-red spectroscopy (FTIR) is one of them and it represents a technique that compares the vibration bands of the residual unpolymerized methacrylate C=C stretching mode at 1640 cm^{-1} to the aromatic C=C stretching mode at 1610 cm^{-1} in order to evaluate the degree of conversion. FTIR spectroscopy is based on the absorption of radiation in the infrared frequency range in accordance with the molecular vibrations of the functional groups contained in the polymer chain [43].

In the present study, FTIR was used to observe the polymerization characteristics of a composite resin when is used in two different ways. In both situations, similar spectra curves can be observed, which indicates a similar mechanism is prevailing, based exclusively upon the relative amounts of resin and filler and is, probably, explained by a restricted mobility of the reactants.

The horizontal layering technique, in which each successive layer is in contact with the pulpal wall or the previously placed layer and all axial walls, produces high values of C factor. Thus, this technique shows the highest shrinkage stress during polymerization [29].

When the oblique layering technique is used, successive layers of triangular shape are placed, so the C factor and the distortion of the cavity walls are reduced [44]. Due to the shape of the layers, they cover less of the wall surfaces than in horizontal layering. This leads to less stress at the tooth/restoration interface [32].

This may explain the difference in the degree of dye penetration observed in the two groups. The present study shows that the specimens in the first group perform better than the teeth in the second group.

In this study, each composite layer was light-cured exclusively from the occlusal aspect. The light from the light-curing lamp initially acts on the outer layer of the resin. This leads to the traction of the pulpal wall, thus increasing the level of stress in this area [33].

Our results are consistent with the results of previous studies, like Derhami et al. [45], Hilton et al. [46] and Demarco et al. [47], who established the margins along the occlusal cavities can be less exposed to microleakage due to the thickness of the enamel in that region. Polymerization shrinkage does not cause important problems when restorations are located only in enamel, because enamel is a solid substrate for bonding [48]. Bonding to the dentin has more deficiencies due to the tubular structure and intrinsic wetness [49].

5. Conclusions

A strong and durable bond of the composite to both enamel and dentin is the secret for clinical success when speaking of restorative dentistry. None of the composite layering technique used in this study was able to eliminate marginal microleakage. Even if it seemed that the oblique technique showed a better adaptation of the restorative material to the dental tissue, the statistical analysis did not confirm that. The composite layering technique still remains an open quest and, moreover, in vivo studies should be designed in order to assess microleakage in real conditions of the oral environment.

Author Contributions: Conceptualization, A.M.C. and M.M.; methodology, C.S., O.P.; software, I.P., L.B.T.; validation, R.M.C., A.M., and A.G.D.; formal analysis, M.P.; investigation, A.M.C., M.M., R.M.C.; resources, D.I.R.; data curation, A.M.C., C.S.; writing—original draft preparation, R.M.C., D.I.R., O.P., A.G.D.; writing—review and editing, M.P., A.M.; visualization, D.I.R., I.P., L.B.T.; supervision, A.M.C., M.M.; project administration.; funding acquisition, O.P., M.P., M.M.; A.G.D., A.M., D.I.R. and O.P. have equal contribution to the work reported with A.M.C. All authors have read and agreed to the published version of the manuscript.

Funding: This research received no external funding.

Institutional Review Board Statement: Not applicable.

Informed Consent Statement: Not applicable.

Data Availability Statement: Not applicable.

Acknowledgments: The authors of the present paper acknowledge the Research Center in Physical Chemistry "CECHIF" of Babes Bolyai University for AFM assistance.

Conflicts of Interest: The authors declare no conflict of interest.

References

1. Shih, W.Y. Microleakage in different primary tooth restorations. *J. Chin. Med. Assoc.* **2016**, *79*, 228–234. [CrossRef] [PubMed]
2. Martin, E. Adaptation and micro-leakage of composite resin restorations. *Aust. Dent. J.* **1984**, *29*, 362–370. [CrossRef]
3. Chisnoiu, R.; Pastrav, O.; Delean, A.; Prodan, D.; Boboia, S.; Moldovan, M.; Chisnoiu, A. Push-out Bond Strengths of Three Different Endodontic Sealers A comparative study. *Mater. Plast.* **2015**, *6*, 239–242.
4. Meiers, J.C.; Kresin, J.C. Cavity disinfectants and dentin bonding. *Oper. Dent.* **1996**, *21*, 153–159. [PubMed]
5. Chisnoiu, R.; Moldovan, M.; Păstrav, O.; Delean, A.; Chisnoiu, A.M. The influence of three endodontic sealers on bone healing: An experimental study. *Folia Morphol.* **2016**, *75*, 14–20. [CrossRef]
6. Unterbrink, G.L.; Liebenberg, W.H. Flowable resin composites as "filled adhesives": Literature review and clinical recommendations. *Quint Int.* **1999**, *30*, 249–257.
7. Klaff, D. Blending Incremental and Stratified Layering Techniques to Produce an Aesthetic Posterior Composite Resin Restoration with a Predictable Prognosis. *J. Esthet. Restor. Dent.* **2001**, *13*, 101–113. [CrossRef]
8. Matei, R.I.; Todor, L.; Cuc, E.A.; Popescu, M.R.; Dragomir, L.P.; Rauten, A.M.; Porumb, A. Microscopic aspects of junction between dental hard tissues and composite material depending on composite insertion: Layering versus bulk-fill. *Rom. J. Morphol. Embryol.* **2019**, *60*, 133–138.
9. Ferracane, J.L.; Lawson, N.C. Probing the hierarchy of evidence to identify the best strategy for placing class II dental composite restorations using current materials. *J. Esthet. Restor. Dent.* **2021**, *33*, 39–50. [CrossRef]
10. Pardo Díaz, C.A.; Shimokawa, C.; Sampaio, C.S.; Freitas, A.Z.; Turbino, M.L. Characterization and Comparative Analysis of Voids in Class II Composite Resin Restorations by Optical Coherence Tomography. *Oper. Dent.* **2020**, *45*, 71–79. [CrossRef]
11. Majety, K.K.; Pujar, M. In vitro evaluation of microleakage of class II packable composite resin restorations using flowable composite and resin modified glass ionomers as intermediate layers. *J. Conserv. Dent.* **2011**, *14*, 414–417. [CrossRef]
12. Chisnoiu, R.M.; Moldovan, M.; Prodan, D.; Chisnoiu, A.M.; Hrab, D.; Delean, A.G.; Muntean, A.; Rotaru, D.I.; Pastrav, O.; Pastrav, M. In-Vitro Comparative Adhesion Evaluation of Bioceramic and Dual-Cure Resin Endodontic Sealers Using SEM, AFM, Push-Out and FTIR. *Appl. Sci.* **2021**, *11*, 4454. [CrossRef]
13. Jafari, T.; Alaghehmad, H.; Moodi, E. Evaluation of cavity size, kind and filling technique of composite shrinkage by finite element. *Dent. Res. J.* **2018**, *15*, 33–39.
14. Sarfi, S.; Neerja, S.; Ekta, G.; Dildeep, B. Comparing microleakage inSilorane based composite and nanofilled composite using different layering techniques in class I restorations: An in vitro study. *IAIM* **2017**, *4*, 23–32.
15. Sahu, D.; Somani, R. Comparative evaluation of microleakage of various glass-ionomer cements: An in vitro study. *Int. J. Prev. Clin. Dent. Res.* **2018**, *5*, 17–20.
16. Youssef, M.N.; Youssef, F.A. Effect of enamel preparation method on in vitro marginal microleakage of a flowable composite used as pit and fissure sealant. *Int. J. Paediatr. Dent.* **2006**, *16*, 342–347. [CrossRef]
17. Paromita, M.; Abiskrita, D.; Utpal, K.D. Comparative evaluation of microleakage of three different direct restorative materials (silver amalgam, glass ionomer cement, cention N), in Class II restorations using stereomicroscope: An in vitro study. *Indian J. Dent. Res.* **2019**, *30*, 277–281.
18. Celik, C.; Bayaktar, Y.; Ozdemir, B.E. Effect of Saliva Contamination on Microleakage of Open Sandwich Restorations. *Acta Stomatol. Croat.* **2020**, *54*, 273–282. [CrossRef] [PubMed]
19. Moezyzadeh, M.; Kazemipoor, M. Effect of different placement techniques on microleakage of class V composite restorations. *J. Dent.* **2009**, *6*, 121–129.
20. Tsujimoto, A.; Jurado, C.A.; Barkmeier, W.W.; Sayed, M.E.; Takamizawa, T.; Latta, M.A.; Miyazaki, M.; Garcia-Godoy, F. Effect of Layering Techniques on Polymerization Shrinkage Stress of High- and Low-viscosity Bulk-fill Resins. *Oper. Dent.* **2020**, *45*, 655–663. [CrossRef]
21. Gale, M.S.; Darvell, B.W. Thermal cycling procedures for laboratory testing of dental restorations. *J. Dent.* **1999**, *27*, 89–99. [CrossRef]
22. Rossomando, K.J.; Wendt, S.L., Jr. Thermocycling and dwell times in microleakage evaluation for bonded restorations. *Dent. Mater.* **1995**, *11*, 47–51. [CrossRef]
23. Weinmann, W.; Thalacker, C.; Guggenberger, R. Siloranes in dental composites. *Dent. Mater.* **2005**, *21*, 68–74. [CrossRef]
24. Hilton, T.J.; Schwartz, R.S.; Ferracane, J.L. Microleakage of four Class II resin composite insertion techniques at intra oral temperature. *Quint. Int.* **1997**, *28*, 135–144.
25. Neiva, I.F.; de Andrada, M.A.C.; Baratieri, L.N.; Monteiro, S.; Ritter, A.V. An in vitro study of the Effect of Restorative Technique on Marginal Leakage in Posterior Composites. *Oper. Dent.* **1998**, *23*, 282–289.
26. Yap, A.U.J.; Wang, H.B.; Siow, K.S.; Gan, L.M. Polymerization Shrinkage of Visible-Light-Cured Composites. *Oper. Dent.* **2000**, *25*, 98–103.
27. Albers, H.F. *Tooth-Colored Restoratives. Principles and Techniques*; BC Decker Inc.: London, UK, 2002; pp. 90–93.
28. Bagis, Y.H.; Baltacioglu, I.H.; Kahyaogullari, S. Comparing Microleakage and the Layering Methods of Silorane-based Resin Composite in Wide Class II MOD Cavities. *Oper. Dent.* **2009**, *34*, 578–585. [CrossRef]
29. Santhosh, L.; Bashetty, K.; Nadig, G. The influence of different composite placement techniques on microleakage in preparations with high C- factor: An in vitro study. *J. Conserv. Dent.* **2008**, *11*, 112–116. [CrossRef]

30. Usha, H.; Kumari, A.; Mehta, D.; Kaiwar, A.; Jain, N. Comparing microleakage and layering methods of silorane-based resin composite in class V cavities using confocal microscopy: An in vitro study. *J. Conserv. Dent.* **2011**, *14*, 164–168.
31. Eakle, W.S.; Ito, R.K. Effect of insertion technique on microleakage in mesio-occlus-odistal composite resin restorations. *Quint. Int.* **1990**, *21*, 117–123.
32. Oliveira, K.M.; Lancellotti, A.C.; Ccahuana-Vasquez, R.A.; Consani, S. Influence of filling technique on shrinkage stress in dental composite restorations. *J. Dent. Sci.* **2013**, *8*, 53–60. [CrossRef]
33. Verluis, A.; Douglas, W.H.; Cross, M.; Sakaguchi, R.L. Does an Incremental Filling Technique Reduce Polymerization Shrinkage Stresses? *J. Dent. Res.* **1996**, *75*, 871–878. [CrossRef] [PubMed]
34. Kwon, Y.; Ferracane, J.; Lee, I.B. Effect of layering methods, composite type and flowable liner on the polymerization shrinkage stress of light cured composites. *Dent. Mater.* **2012**, *28*, 801–809. [CrossRef] [PubMed]
35. Park, J.; Chang, J.; Ferracane, J.; Lee, I.B. How should composite be layered to reduce shrinkage stress: Incremental or bulk filling? *Dent. Mater.* **2008**, *24*, 1501–1505. [CrossRef]
36. Batista, L.H.C.; Silva, J.G.; Silva, M.F.A.; Tonholo, J. Atomic force microscopy of removal of dentin smear layers. *Microsc. Microanal.* **2007**, *13*, 245–250. [CrossRef]
37. Kakaboura, A.; Fragouli, M.; Rahiotis, C.; Silikas, N. Evaluation of surface characteristics of dental composites using profilometry, scanning electron, atomic force microscopy and gloss-meter. *J. Mater. Sci. Mater. Med.* **2007**, *18*, 155–163. [CrossRef]
38. Botta, A.C.; Duarte, S.; Paulin Filho, P.I.; Gheno, S.M. Effect of dental finishing instruments on the surface roughness of composite resins as elucidated by atomic force microscopy. *Microsc. Microanal.* **2008**, *14*, 380–386. [CrossRef]
39. Borges, A.; Hasna, A.A.; Matuda, A.G.N.; Lopes, S.R.; Mafetano, A.P.V.P.; Arantes, A.; Duarte, A.F.; Barcellos, D.C.; Torres, C.R.G.; Pucci, C.R. Adhesive systems effect over bond strength of resin-infiltrated and de/remineralized enamel. *F1000Research* **2019**, *11*, 1743. [CrossRef]
40. Yamauchi, K.; Tsujimoto, A.; Jurado, C.A.; Shimatani, Y.; Nagura, Y.; Takamizawa, T.; Barkmeier, W.W.; Latta, M.A.; Miyazaki, M. Etch-and-rinse vs self-etch mode for dentin bonding effectiveness of universal adhesives. *J. Oral Sci.* **2019**, *27*, 549–553. [CrossRef]
41. Stansbury, J.W. Dimethacrylate network formation and polymer property evolution as determined by the selection of monomers and curing conditions. *Dent. Mater.* **2012**, *28*, 13–22. [CrossRef]
42. Pilo, R.; Oelgiesser, D.; Cardash, H.S. A survey of output intensity and potential for depth of cure among light-curing units in clinical use. *J. Dent.* **1999**, *27*, 235–241. [CrossRef]
43. Moraes, L.G.P.; Rocha, R.S.F.; Menegazzo, L.M.; Araújo, E.B.; Yukimito, K.; Moraes, J.C.S. Infrared spectroscopy: A tool for determination of the degree of conversion in dental composites. *J. Appl. Oral Sci.* **2008**, *16*, 145–149. [CrossRef] [PubMed]
44. Chandrasekhar, V.; Rudrapati, L.; Badami, V.; Tummala, M. Incremental techniques in direct composite restoration. *J. Conserv. Dent.* **2017**, *20*, 386–391. [PubMed]
45. Derhami, K.; Colli, P. Microleakage in Class 2 composite restorations. *Oper. Dent.* **1995**, *20*, 100–105. [PubMed]
46. Poggio, C.; Chiesa, M.; Scribante, A.; Mekler, J.; Colombo, M. Microleakage in Class II composite restorations with margins below the CEJ: In vitro evaluation of different restorative techniques. *Med. Oral Patol Oral Cir Bucal.* **2013**, *18*, e793–e798. [CrossRef] [PubMed]
47. Demarco, F.F.; Ramos, O.L. Influence of different restorative techniques on microleakage in class II cavities with gingival wall in cementum. *Oper. Dent.* **2001**, *26*, 253–259. [PubMed]
48. Roberson, T.M.; Heymann, H.O.; Ritter, A.V. *Introduction to Composite Restorations. Sturdevant's Art & Science Operative Dentistry*, 4th ed.; Mosby: St. Louis, MI, USA, 2002; pp. 473–499.
49. Eick, J.D.; Cobb, C.M.; Chappel, R.P.; Spencer, P.; Robinson, S.J. The dentinal structure: Its influence on dentinal adhesion. Part I. *Quint. Int.* **1991**, *22*, 967–977.

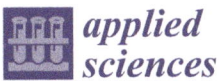

Article

Changes in Crystal Phase, Morphology, and Flexural Strength of As-Sintered Translucent Monolithic Zirconia Ceramic Modified by Femtosecond Laser

Shanshan Liang [1,†], Hongqiang Ye [2,†] and Fusong Yuan [3,*]

1. Second Clinical Division, Peking University Hospital of Stomatology, Beijing 100081, China; dentist_lss@163.com
2. Department of Prosthodontics, Peking University School and Hospital of Stomatology, Beijing 100081, China; yehongqiang@hsc.pku.edu.cn
3. Center of Digital Dentistry, Department of Prosthodontics, Peking University School and Hospital of Stomatology, Beijing 100081, China
* Correspondence: yuanfusong@bjmu.edu.cn; Tel.: +86-010-8219-5892
† These authors contributed to this work equally.

Abstract: Conventional bonding technology suitable for silica-based ceramics is not applicable to zirconia, due to its polycrystalline phase composition, chemical stability, and acid corrosion resistance. The development of an effective treatment to improve its surface roughness and mechanical properties remains an unresolved problem. Therefore, to solve this problem, this in vitro study evaluated the changes in surface morphology and flexural strength of translucent monolithic zirconia surfaces treated with femtosecond laser technology. As-sintered translucent zirconia specimens were subjected to airborne particle abrasion and femtosecond laser treatments, while control group specimens received no treatment. After treatment, the roughness and morphology of the treated zirconia surfaces were examined. The flexural strength and X-ray diffraction of the treated specimens were measured and analyzed. Statistical inferential analysis included one-way analysis of variance at a set significance level of 5%. The surface roughness after femtosecond laser treatment was significantly improved when compared with the control group and the group that received the airborne particle abrasion treatment ($p < 0.05$). In comparison with the airborne particle abrasion group, the flexural strength of the group that received the femtosecond laser treatment was significantly improved ($p < 0.05$). The femtosecond laser approach using appropriate parameters enhanced the roughness of the zirconia without reducing its flexural strength; therefore, this approach offers potential for the treatment of zirconia surfaces.

Keywords: zirconia; airborne particle abrasion; femtosecond laser; flexural strength; surface roughness

Citation: Liang, S.; Ye, H.; Yuan, F. Changes in Crystal Phase, Morphology, and Flexural Strength of As-Sintered Translucent Monolithic Zirconia Ceramic Modified by Femtosecond Laser. *Appl. Sci.* 2021, 11, 6925. https://doi.org/10.3390/app11156925

Academic Editor: Vittorio Checchi

Received: 31 May 2021
Accepted: 22 July 2021
Published: 28 July 2021

Publisher's Note: MDPI stays neutral with regard to jurisdictional claims in published maps and institutional affiliations.

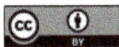

Copyright: © 2021 by the authors. Licensee MDPI, Basel, Switzerland. This article is an open access article distributed under the terms and conditions of the Creative Commons Attribution (CC BY) license (https://creativecommons.org/licenses/by/4.0/).

1. Introduction

Zirconia is highly popular in clinical use for dental restorations, due to its exceptional flexural strength, chemical resistance, and good aesthetics [1]. Depending on whether a glass-matrix phase is present or absent, or whether the material contains an organic matrix highly filled with ceramic particles, all-ceramic materials can be classified into three families: (1) glass-matrix ceramics, (2) polycrystalline ceramics, and (3) resin-matrix ceramics [2]. However, unlike other dental ceramic materials, zirconia has a polycrystalline phase composition without a glass phase composition, as well as good chemical stability and acid corrosion resistance. Owing to this, conventional bonding technology suitable for silica-based ceramics is not effective for zirconia. Thus, an important scientific problem in the use of zirconia materials is the effective treatment of zirconia to improve its surface roughness and mechanical properties [3].

Contemporary surface treatment technologies used for zirconia ceramics include airborne particle abrasion (APA), acid etching, laser etching, silicon coating, pre-treatment agents, and other technologies and combinations thereof. APA with 50 μm Al_2O_3 under 0.2 MPa pressure at a distance of 10 mm from the zirconia surface has been found to be an effective method for improving bond strength [4]. However, this approach may lead to sub-surface damage to the zirconia, resulting in microcracks and debris, which may reduce the mechanical properties of yttria-stabilized tetragonal zirconia polycrystal (Y-TZP), thus affecting its longevity. Studies have shown that APA may cause fractures in zirconia restorations and influence the long-term durability of the bond strength between zirconia ceramics and resin [5–7]. The reduced retention rate after APA may be related to microcracks in the zirconia, and APA may, therefore, have an adverse effect on flexural strength and other long-term mechanical properties of restorations [3].

Other surface modification methods are therefore required to replace aluminum oxide APA and to avoid adverse effects on the mechanical properties and long-term durability of zirconia [4]. Recently, scholars worldwide have trialed advanced technologies, such as thermal acid etching solutions [7,8], plasma technology [6,9], tribochemical silica coating [10,11], ultrashort-pulse lasers [12,13], and fusion sputtering technology [14,15], to treat zirconia surfaces.

Thermal chemical etching solutions have been employed for pre-treating zirconia ceramics. It has been found that this method improves roughness and, therefore, increases the zirconia–resin cement bond strength [7]; however, the configuration of a safe and effective thermal acid etching solution remains unclear, as thermal acid etching may also affect the physical properties of zirconia [8].

The application of plasma technology for the surface modification of zirconia ceramics has also been studied. Fernandes et al. [6] reported that non-thermal plasma modification without significant damage promoted adequate adhesion, but the bond strength was not found to be significantly different from that under aluminum oxide APA. Plasma modification resulted in a significant increase in the surface free energy of the zirconia ceramic, but no significant changes in surface roughness were observed. The application of plasma treatment in zirconia bonding, therefore, cannot replace APA [9].

Tribochemical silica coating is a commonly used silicon coating technology at present, which uses 30 μm alumina particles covered with silica for sandblasting at 0.23 MPa on the zirconia surface [10]. By increasing the silicon content on the surface of the zirconia, the silica layer can react with the cement-containing silane [11]. As a result, through copolymerization between the silane and the resin cement, the bond strength between the zirconia resin can be improved.

In addition, it has been reported that application of the fusion sputtering technique promotes a rough surface and significantly enhances the zirconia–resin microshear bond strength [14,15]. However, the influence of fusion sputtering technology on the crystal phase change and mechanical properties of zirconia, as well as the long-term bond strength remains unclear.

Holthaus et al. [16] found that the application of laser treatment could potentially replace traditional surface treatment by APA, due to the high speed and precise control of the laser. A more regular micro-texture and a reduction in contamination were obtained through the application of a femtosecond laser (FSL), compared with CO2 and Nd-YAG lasers, for zirconia surface micromachining [12]. Ruja et al. [13] evaluated the use of an ultrashort-pulse laser to irradiate the zirconia ceramic surface, so as to improve adhesive properties in the resin–zirconia interface. The results showed that the topography of the zirconia ceramic surface was regularly roughened and wettability was increased, while an improvement in microtensile bond strength was promoted without a significant tetragonal–monoclinic phase transformation [13]. This may be attributed to the fact that the energy of the laser was absorbed by the surface of the zirconia, and the thermal induction process produced shell-like ruptures on the surface [17].

Through the use of FSLs, the surfaces of zirconia ceramics could be effectively modified without inducing thermal or mechanical damage [17,18]. While limited research has been conducted on the surface pre-treatment of zirconia ceramics using laser technology, the ideal effect of zirconia modification by laser, in order to improve the bond strength, has not yet been achieved [19]. Therefore, the changes in surface morphology and flexural strength upon applying the FSL technique require further exploration.

This study aims to evaluate the effect of zirconia surface modification using the FSL method. The null hypothesis was that the application of the FSL would not affect the surface morphology and flexural strength of translucent monolithic zirconia ceramic material.

2. Materials and Methods

2.1. Zirconia Specimen Preparation

A total of 36 disc-shaped fully sintered translucent monolithic zirconia ceramic (UPCERA, ST, Shenzhen, China) specimens (10 mm diameter × 2 mm thickness) and 36 rectangular fully sintered translucent monolithic zirconia specimens (25 mm long × 4 mm wide × 3 mm thick) were prepared from a dental zirconia blank (in which the content of Y_2O_3 was 4.5–6%). A precision cutting machine was used to prepare the specimens, which were sintered using a programmable furnace according to the manufacturer's instructions. The temperature of the furnace was heated from room temperature, at a rate of 8 °C/min, to 1200 °C, then increased at a rate of 2 °C/min from 1200 °C to 1450 °C, maintained at 1450 °C for 2 h, and finally cooled at a rate of 10 °C/min to room temperature. Depending on the employed surface pre-treatment method, the 36 disc-shaped fully sintered zirconia specimens were randomly divided into three groups, with each group containing 12 specimens. Disc-shaped specimens were employed for observation of surface topography and assessment of roughness. Rectangular specimens were used for flexural strength testing. In order to avoid potential failure of specimens due to edge defects, a 45° diagonal angle was introduced on the edges of all the rectangular specimens. Specimen preparation was carried out in accordance with the requirements of the ISO/CD 6872:2015 standard [20]. The calculation of the sample size of this study was carried out with reference to similar studies [21].

2.2. Zirconia Surface Treatment

The 72 sintered translucent zirconia specimens were classified into Groups I, II, and III, with each group containing 12 circular and 12 rectangular specimens. Group I was the control, with no treatment (NT) of the surface of the specimens. Group II underwent APA, whereby the surfaces of the specimens were air abraded (Renfert GmbH, Hilzingen, Germany) with 50 μm aluminum oxide (Al_2O_3) particles at a perpendicular distance of 10 mm from the surface under 0.20 MPa of pressure for 20s. Group III underwent FSL treatment, whereby the surfaces of the specimens were microtextured with FSL (Amplitude Systemes, Tangerine laser head, Bordeaux, France) having a wavelength of 1030 nm, pulse width of 400 fs, repetition frequency of 200 kHz, peak power of 5 W, and single-pulse energy of 25 μJ. The FSL ablation was controlled using a three-axis numerically controlled laser galvanometer scanning system (175 mm lens focal length, ~80 mm spot diameter, 2000 mm/s light spot scanning speed, 0.1 μm minimum step size along the z-axis, and 10 mm maximum step size; see Figure 1).

2.3. Surface Structure and Roughness Assessment

The surface roughness of the specimens was measured using a confocal three-dimensional (3D) laser scanning microscope (VK-X210, Osaka, Japan). For each specimen, the surface roughness of three areas was measured under 200× magnification ($n = 12$/group). The 3D surface roughness parameter R_a was calculated using VK Analyzer software. The acquisition R_a (μm) value was derived from the average of three analyzed areas, using a simple average-type smoothing filter. The disc-shaped specimens of each group were sputter-coated with gold (108AUTO sputter coater, Cressington, Watford,

UK), and the surface topographies of the specimens ($n = 3$/group) were observed using a scanning electron microscope (SEM, SU8010, Tokyo, Japan) under vacuum conditions and secondary electron detector of SE(UL), with 5.0 kV working voltage, at 500× and 10,000× magnifications.

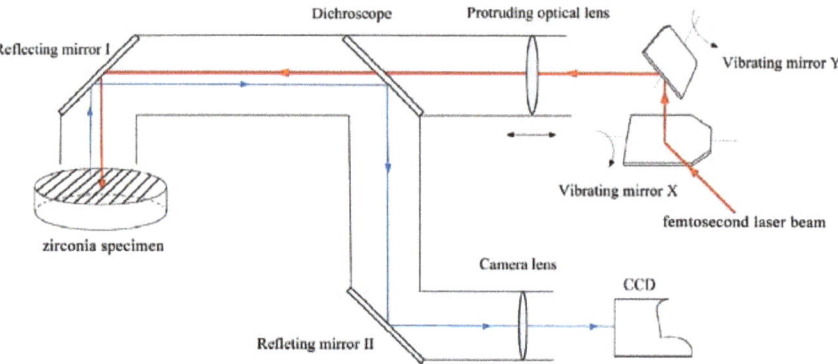

Figure 1. Schematic of the FSL surface treatment system and laser trajectory during surface treatment of the specimen. The red line indicates the propagation path of the FSL in the system, and the blue line indicates the light from the surface treatment result received by the charge-coupled device, which monitored the real-time processing results as the laser processed the specimen surface.

2.4. X-ray Diffraction Analysis (XRD)

The crystalline phases of the specimens were determined using an X-ray powder diffractometer (XRD) system (Bruker D8 ADVANCE, Karlsruhe, Germany), with the following measurement conditions: Cu K-α radiation, tube voltage of 40 kV, tube current of 40 mA, scanning angle range of $2\theta = 25$–$60°$, scanning speed of 17.7 s/step, and step size of $0.02°$.

2.5. Flexural Strength Test (Three-Point Bending Test)

Flexural strength tests were conducted using a universal testing machine (5969R9273, Instron, Norwood, MA, USA) with 1 mm/min crosshead speed and 13 mm span, according to a three-point bending test. During a flexural strength test, the treated surface was placed in contact with the loading stylus (compressive loading zone). The upper limit of the load cell value applied was 2500 N [20]. The fracture loads of the specimens are expressed in Newtons, and their flexural strength was measured in megapascals, using the equation [20] $\sigma = 3Pl/2wb^2$, where P is the fracture load (N), l is the span (mm), w is the specimen width (mm), and b is the specimen height (mm).

2.6. Statistical Analysis

Descriptive statistics and inferential statistic measures were employed to analyze the flexural strength (MPa) and surface roughness (Ra). The mean and standard deviation were calculated, and the normality of the data distribution was confirmed by the Shapiro–Wilk test. A one-way analysis of variance (ANOVA) and Least Significance Difference (LSD) post hoc tests were performed, in order to analyze the results among all groups (NT, APA, and FSL). All calculations were performed using SPSS 20 statistical software (SPSS Inc., Chicago, IL, USA). The significance level was set at $\alpha = 0.05$.

3. Results

3.1. Scanning Electron Microscopy Observations

The SEM images shown in Figure 2 present the surface topographies of the specimens that underwent the different surface treatment methods. Specifically, Figure 2a,b represents the NT group, where Figure 2a shows that the surface was relatively flat, and Figure 2b reveals the unit cell-like microstructure of the zirconia sample after heat treatment. Many grain boundaries can be observed, and the arrangement is dense. There are no voids between the grains. Figure 2c, which represents the APA group, shows that the surface was uniformly rough with sharp edges and corners. A few microcracks can be observed in the image shown in Figure 2d. Finally, the image of the FSL group, depicted in Figure 2e, shows that the surface was uniform and flat without deep grooves. Figure 2f shows an irregular structure with rounded edges and a few pores.

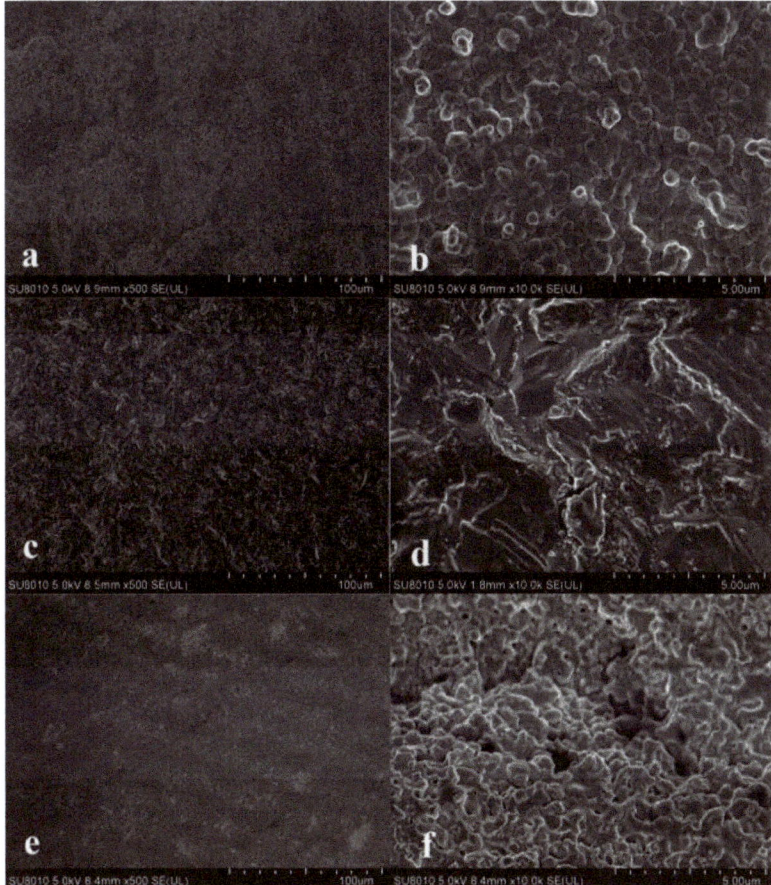

Figure 2. SEM images of zirconia surfaces from different groups at 500× and 10,000× magnifications: (**a,b**) NT; (**c,d**) APA; and (**e,f**) FSL. NT: no treatment group; APA: airborne particle abrasion group; FSL: femtosecond laser group.

3.2. Surface Roughness Evaluation

The surface roughness results (measured by the R_a amplitude value) are recorded in Table 1. One-way ANOVA analysis showed that there were statistical differences between the three groups ($p < 0.05$; Figure 3a). Compared with the NT group ($R_a = 0.98 \pm 0.18$ μm) and the APA group ($R_a = 1.12 \pm 0.28$ μm), it was found that the FSL group achieved significantly superior roughness ($R_a = 1.42 \pm 0.16$ μm; Table 1). Therefore, the highest roughness of the zirconia surface was due to the FSL treatment (Figure 3a).

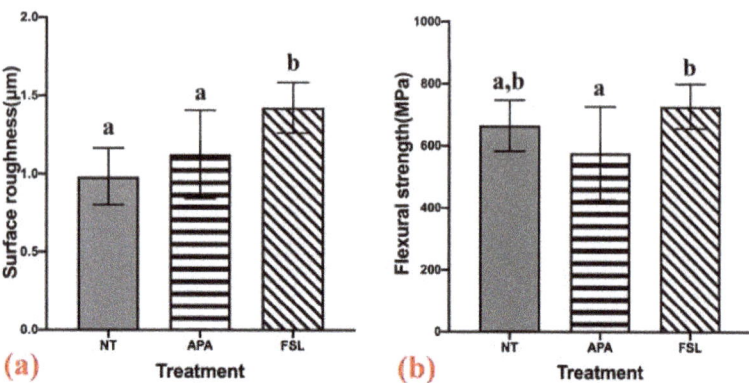

Figure 3. (**a**) The mean surface roughness values (R_a), where the R_a value for the FSL group was significantly the highest ($p < 0.05$); (**b**) the mean flexural strength values ($p < 0.05$), where the result in the FSL group was significantly higher than that in the APA group ($p < 0.05$). NT: no treatment group; APA: airborne particle abrasion group; FSL: femtosecond laser group.

Table 1. Statistical description of surface roughness of the three surface treatment groups (μm).

Group	N	Mean	SD	SE	95% Confidence Interval of the Mean		Minimum	Maximum
					Lower Bound	Upper Bound		
NT	12	0.9820	0.1821	0.0526	0.8663	1.0977	0.71	1.28
APA	12	1.1248	0.2813	0.0812	0.9461	1.3035	0.89	1.81
FSL	12	1.4237	0.1613	0.0466	1.3213	1.5262	1.22	1.69

The mean difference is significant at the 0.05 level. NT: no treatment group; APA: airborne particle abrasion group; FSL: femtosecond laser group.

3.3. Flexural Strength

Table 2 shows the mean flexural strength values (MPa), along with the standard deviation, for the three groups. The one-way ANOVA analysis indicated a statistical difference among the three groups ($p < 0.05$; Figure 3b). No significant difference was found between FSL and NT or between APA and NT, but a significant difference was found between FSL and APA (Figure 3b). The effect of the FSL treatment was, therefore, found to be superior to that of the APA treatment (Figure 3b).

Table 2. Statistical description of the flexural strengths of the three surface treatments (Mpa).

Group	N	Mean	SD	SE	95% Confidence Interval of the Mean		Minimum	Maximum
					Lower Bound	Upper Bound		
NT	12	665.4604	82.2518	23.7441	613.2001	717.7207	563.78	825.14
APA	12	577.0494	150.0842	43.3256	481.6905	672.4083	415.92	927.46
FSL	12	727.7890	71.7360	20.7084	682.2101	773.3678	611.99	887.62

The mean difference is significant at the 0.05 level. NT: no treatment group; APA: airborne particle abrasion group; FSL: femtosecond laser group.

3.4. XRD

Through analysis of the XRD pattern (Figure 4) on zirconia, we found that strong diffraction peaks of the tetragonal phase were identified in both the NT and APA groups. The zirconia surface with no treatment was completely tetragonal-phase (Figure 4a). Compared with the APA group, the diffraction peaks of the tetragonal phase for the NT group were dominant. The tetragonal phase ratio of the surface treated with APA was low, with a small amount of monoclinic phase (about 9.23%) and cubic phase (4.10%), as shown by the small peaks of monoclinic crystal and cubic phases (Figure 4b); however, the XRD of the sample treated with FSL suggested that there may be an amorphous phase, as it was also possible to form salt crystals on the surface of the ceramic treated by FSL (Figure 4c).

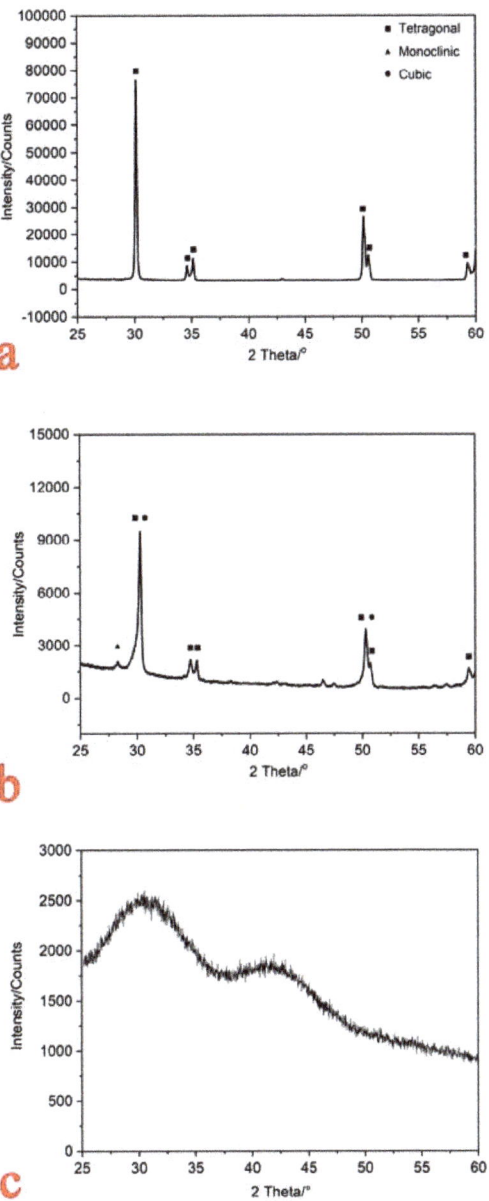

Figure 4. XRD images of zirconia surface from different groups: (**a**) For NT (no treatment group), the zirconia surface for NT was completely tetragonal-phase; (**b**) for APA (airborne particle abrasion group), the tetragonal phase ratio of the surface was low, with a small amount of monoclinic and cubic phases; and (**c**) for FSL (femtosecond laser group), there may be an amorphous phase, as it was also possible to form salt crystals on zirconia surfaces treated with FSL.

4. Discussion

The purpose of this study was to evaluate the effect of femtosecond laser treatment on the surface roughness and flexural strength of translucent zirconia. Compared with the no treatment group, the surface roughness of translucent zirconia was significantly increased in the femtosecond laser group, while the flexural strength measured via three-point bending of zirconia modified by the femtosecond laser was found not to be significantly different from that of samples in the no treatment group. Thus, the null hypothesis of the study was partly rejected.

The bending strength and fatigue resistance of translucent zirconia are higher than those of glass ceramics [22]. Thus, translucent zirconia is a material that offers both mechanical strength and aesthetic performance, and its clinical applications are becoming more and more extensive [22]. However, translucent zirconia may be adversely affected by the use of high-pressure airborne abrasion, as microcracks and defects are generated, and flexural strength is reduced [23]. To date, limited studies have evaluated the effect of FSL modification on Y-TZP surfaces and, to the best of our knowledge, no existing study has evaluated the effect of FSL for treating the surface of translucent zirconia.

Studies have reported that the application of FSL forms groove- or pit-like structures on the surface of zirconia specimens, thereby increasing their surface roughness; however, this was accompanied by a reduction in flexural strength [24]. This approach may lead to sub-surface damage to the zirconia due to 50 µm alumina blasting, which may cause microcracks that limit the life of zirconia restorations [25]. In this study, we explored a specific parameter of FSL in the surface modification of translucent zirconia, in order to improve surface roughness without producing significant grooves or pits. Even though no statistical significance was found, the results in this study revealed that surface roughness was improved. As studies incorporating the FSL method continue to improve, FSL may become more suitable as a surface treatment for zirconia materials.

Although the use of APA with Al_2O_3 particles is popular for the treatment of zirconia surfaces in order to increase the bond strength, studies have shown that the increased roughness imparted by this technique is accompanied by an increased fracture risk, thereby weakening the structure through the introduction of microcracks [26–28]. The results of our study demonstrated that FSL-treated translucent zirconia showed significantly higher mean R_a values than those in the APA and NT groups, and there was no significant difference in the R_a value between the APA and NT groups. These findings are consistent with those of the study of Inokoshi et al. [29], where the surface roughness of highly translucent Y-PSZ modified using Al_2O_3 APA was not significantly enhanced, except for that of specimens comprising KATANA UTML (Kuraray Noritake, Japan). In contrast, FSL ablation of zirconia ceramic significantly enhanced surface roughness and improved the zirconia ceramic–resin bond strength, due to the presence of groove-like structures [30]. In our study, the translucent zirconia surface obtained following the FSL treatment presented uniform irregular structures without groove-like structures or pits, as confirmed in the SEM image shown in Figure 2e. Surface topography can be modified by femtosecond laser surface treatment and surface roughness of the zirconia can be increased; thus, the bond strength can be improved [31].

The main height parameters for evaluating surface roughness are average roughness (R_a), the root mean square of the height of each point of the contour (R_q), and the ten-point height of microscopic unevenness (R_z). The Ra value can represent the arithmetic mean deviation of the surface roughness profile amplitude parameter. Consequently, the R_a value was used in this study to evaluate the surface roughness [32]. Compared with the control group, roughness in the APA group did not increase significantly, which may have been due to the particular cutting texture produced during the processing of the untreated translucent zirconia specimens, which yielded a certain roughness after sintering. The surfaces of the specimens were not polished in this experiment, in order to maintain the original surface morphologies of the final sintered translucent zirconia. On one hand, this allowed for simulation of the surface of a final sintered zirconia crown without polishing;

on the other hand, when the surface of a zirconia specimen is highly polished, FSL irradiates a smooth surface, producing reflections, which may affect the treatment of the zirconia surface. In this study, the surfaces of the zirconia specimens were not polished, allowing the FSL to fully exert its plasma effect at a lower energy density. This may also contribute to the discrepancy in the roughness results between APA and FSL treatments reported in this study when compared with those in other studies. Various surface analysis systems, such as SEM and Atomic Force Microscopy (AFM), are useful for qualitative analysis, but three-dimensional microscopy was used for quantitative evaluation of the surface roughness variation.

The results of XRD showed that the monoclinic content of the APA group was increased, which indicated that aluminum airborne abrasion may lead to t–m phase transformation. At present, there is controversy about the influence of sandblasting on mechanical properties [33]. Some scholars have reported that t–m phase transformation can increase volume and produce protective residual compressive stress, thus preventing the further expansion of microcracks and, consequently, leading to enhanced mechanical strength. This is called the phase transformation toughening mechanism [34]. However, other scholars have indicated that small grain size (within 200 nm) can have a negative impact on the phase transformation and toughening mechanism, consequently reducing the mechanical strength of translucent ZrO_2 [35]. In this experiment, the XRD results indicated that the sintered translucent zirconia specimen appeared to be amorphized after the FSL treatment, which may have been caused by the phenomenon of "avalanche ionization" during interaction of the high-power and high-repetition FSL with the zirconia specimen surface, resulting in high-speed motion [36]. The hypothesis is that the plasma carries a certain element, which is deposited on the surface of the specimen to form a coating, resulting in amorphization [37]. It is also possible to form salt crystals on the surface of the ceramic; however, the interfacial topography between the "amorphized" zirconia layer after FSL and the substrate was not investigated, and further experimental verification is required.

Air particle abrasion may lead to sub-surface damage of the zirconia surface by 50 μm alumina, which may lead to microcracks that limit the life of zirconia restorations [38]. It has been reported that impact-induced defects were observed on zirconia surfaces modified by APA treatment; thus, the longevity of APA-treated zirconia ceramic prostheses may be shortened [39]. Consistent with previous studies, in our study, the surface treated with APA presented a number of microcracks and defects as revealed in Figure 2d, which may lead to a reduction in the flexural strength of the zirconia specimens. In contrast, in a study reported by Wang et al. [40], APA enhanced the flexural strength of zirconia, regardless of the particle size, air pressure, or blasting time. Song et al. [41] reported that flexural strength was significantly higher in the group of air-abraded zirconia specimens than that in the group without any treatment. The content of the monoclinic phase of the lower zirconia surface determines the mechanical behavior of the zirconia specimens, as this is where tensile stress is dispersed. Furthermore, this study indicated that APA of the inner surface of zirconia specimens, in order to improve their bonding performance, might also enhance their fracture strength [40]. In this experiment, we applied 50 μm Al_2O_3 particles to treat the surface of the translucent zirconia specimen, in order to reduce tetragonal–monoclinic phase transformation.

There are two main methods for testing the bending strength of ceramics: uniaxial bending and biaxial bending. In uniaxial bending tests, a cuboid specimen is supported by two points and loaded vertically at one point (i.e., a three-point bending test) or two points (i.e., a four-point bending test). In a biaxial bending test, a thin disk is supported by a ring or three balls close to it, and a load is applied through a ball or a piston in its central area, or a smaller ring in its center. The above methods have been recognized in international standards [20]. Therefore, a three-point bending test was used to evaluate the used methods after surface treatment in this study. New possible methods for the mechanical analysis of materials have been reported as a future perspective for classic dynamometer systems, such as Dynamic Mechanical Analysis (DMA) and Brillouin's micro-spectroscopy [42].

Importantly, the flexural strength results presented herein were consistent with the observed SEM images. However, further investigations are required to evaluate the long-term stability of zirconia treated using different methods. It should also be noted that, in the experimental setup, line-patterning of zirconia surfaces was achieved; thus, tuning the FSL parameters should allow for independent variation of the pattern depth, overall roughness, and surface finish. More specifically, increasing both the fluence and the number of pulses will allow for deeper patterning, with the maximum achievable depth being 1 μm. However, increasing the number of pulses can have a detrimental effect on the quality of the lines produced, and surface damage can occur (e.g., intergranular cracking, open porosity, and nanodroplet formation), depending on the FSL parameters employed [43]. In future experiments, our research team will try to design an integrated processing device featuring a femtosecond laser. After the zirconia restorations are sintered, the dental technician can hold the working end of the device to modify the tissue surface of dental zirconia restorations, in order to achieve a clean, efficient, and damage-free effect.

One limitation of this study is that the long-term effects of FSL modification technology on the flexural strength of zirconia were not investigated. Therefore, an evaluation of resin–zirconia bond strength and durability using different surface modification methods will be reported in a future article.

5. Conclusions

1. Femtosecond laser technology offers potential for zirconia surface treatment.
2. Through the employment of appropriate parameters, femtosecond laser treatment can be used to modify the surface of zirconia, in order to enhance its roughness without decreasing flexural strength.

Author Contributions: Conceptualization, F.Y.; methodology, F.Y. and S.L.; software, H.Y.; validation, F.Y., S.L. and H.Y.; formal analysis, F.Y.; investigation, S.L.; resources, S.L.; data curation, H.Y.; writing—original draft preparation, S.L.; writing—review and editing, F.Y.; visualization, F.Y.; supervision, F.Y.; project administration, F.Y.; funding acquisition, F.Y. All authors have read and agreed to the published version of the manuscript.

Funding: This research was funded by the National Key R&D Program of China [Grant no. 2020YFB1312801], and the State Key Lab of Advance Metals and Materials [Grant no. 2021-Z08].

Institutional Review Board Statement: Not applicable.

Informed Consent Statement: Not applicable.

Data Availability Statement: The data presented in this study are available on request from the corresponding author.

Conflicts of Interest: The authors declare no conflict of interest.

References

1. Denry, I.; Kelly, J.R. State of the art of zirconia for dental applications. *Dent. Mater.* **2008**, *24*, 299–307. [CrossRef]
2. Gracis, S.; Thompson, V.P.; Ferencz, J.L.; Silva, N.R.; Bonfante, E.A. A new classification system for all-ceramic and ceramic-like restorative materials. *Int. J. Prosthodont.* **2015**, *28*, 227–235. [CrossRef]
3. Scaminaci Russo, D.; Cinelli, F.; Sarti, C.; Giachetti, L. Adhesion to Zirconia: A Systematic review of current conditioning methods and bonding materials. *Dent. J.* **2019**, *7*, 74. [CrossRef]
4. Thompson, J.Y.; Stoner, B.R.; Piascik, J.R.; Smith, R. Adhesion/cementation to zirconia and other non-silicate ceramics: Where are we now? *Dent. Mater.* **2011**, *27*, 71–82. [CrossRef] [PubMed]
5. Hallmann, L.; Ulmer, P.; Wille, S.; Polonskyi, O.; Köbel, S.; Trottenberg, T.; Bornholdt, S.; Haase, F.; Kersten, H.; Kern, M. Effect of surface treatments on the properties and morphological change of dental zirconia. *J. Prosthet. Dent.* **2016**, *15*, 341–349. [CrossRef] [PubMed]
6. Fernandes, V.V.B., Jr.; Dantas, D.C.B.; Bresciani, E.; Huhtala, M.F.R.L. Evaluation of the bond strength and characteristics of zirconia after different surface treatments. *J. Prosthet. Dent.* **2018**, *120*, 955–959. [CrossRef]
7. Casucci, A.; Monticelli, F.; Goracci, C.; Mazzitelli, C.; Cantoro, A.; Papacchini, F.; Ferrari, M. Effect of surface pre-treatments on the zirconia ceramic–resin cement microtensile bond strength. *Dent. Mater.* **2011**, *27*, 1024–1030. [CrossRef] [PubMed]

8. Lv, P.; Yang, X.; Jiang, T. Influence of hot-etching surface treatment on Zirconia/Resin shear bond strength. *Materials* **2015**, *8*, 8087–8096. [CrossRef]
9. Lükemann, N.; Eichberger, M.; Stawarczyk, B. Different surface modifications combined with universal adhesives: The impact on the bonding properties of zirconia to composite resin cement. *Clin. Oral. Investig.* **2019**, *23*, 3941–3950. [CrossRef]
10. Wu, X.; Xie, H.; Meng, H.; Yang, L.; Chen, B.; Chen, Y.; Chen, C. Effect of tribochemical silica coating or multipurpose products on bonding performance of a CAD/CAM resin-based material. *J. Mech. Behav. Biomed. Mater.* **2019**, *90*, 417–425. [CrossRef]
11. Chen, B.; Yan, Y.; Xie, H.; Meng, H.; Zhang, H.; Chen, C. Effects of tribochemical silica coating and alumina-particle air abrasion on 3Y-TZP and 5Y-TZP: Evaluation of surface hardness, roughness, bonding, and phase transformation. *J. Adhes. Dent.* **2020**, *22*, 373–382. [CrossRef] [PubMed]
12. Bitencourt, S.B.; Ferreira, L.C.; Mazza, L.C.; Dos Santos, D.M.; Pesqueira, A.A.; Theodoro, L.H. Effect of laser irradiation on bond strength between zirconia and resin cement or veneer ceramic: A systematic review and meta-analysis. *J. Indian. Prosthodont. Soc.* **2021**, *21*, 125–137. [CrossRef] [PubMed]
13. Ruja, M.A.; De Souza, G.M.; Finer, Y. Ultrashort-pulse laser as a surface treatment for bonding between zirconia and resin cement. *Dent. Mater.* **2019**, *35*, 1545–1556. [CrossRef]
14. Aboushelib, M.N. Fusion sputtering for bonding to zirconia-based materials. *J. Adhes. Dent.* **2012**, *14*, 323–328. [CrossRef] [PubMed]
15. Hussein, N.A.; El Kady, A.S.; Aboushelib, M.S. The effect of fusion sputtering surface treatment on microshear bond strength of zirconia and MDP-containing resin cement. *Dent. Mater.* **2019**, *35*, e107–e112. [CrossRef]
16. Holthaus, M.G.; Treccani, T.; Rezwan, K. Comparison of micropatterning methods for ceramic surfaces. *J. Eur. Ceram. Soc.* **2011**, *31*, 2809–2817. [CrossRef]
17. Akpinar, Y.Z.; Kepceoglu, A.; Yavuz, T.; Aslan, M.A.; Demirtag, Z.; Kılıc, H.S.; Usumez, A. Effect of femtosecond laser beam angle on bond strength of zirconia-resin cement. *Lasers. Med. Sci.* **2015**, *30*, 2123–2128. [CrossRef] [PubMed]
18. Aivazi, M.; Hossein Fathi, M.; Nejatidanesh, F.; Mortazavi, V.; HashemiBeni, B.; Matinlinna, J.P.; Savabi, O. The evaluation of prepared microgroove pattern by femtosecond laser on alumina-zirconia nano-composite for endosseous dental implant application. *Lasers Med. Sci.* **2016**, *31*, 1837–1843. [CrossRef]
19. Gomes, A.L.; Ramos, J.C.; Santos-del Riego, S.; Montero, J.; Albaladejo, A. Thermocycling effect on microshear bond strength to zirconia ceramic using Er:YAG and tribochemical silica coating as surface conditioning. *Lasers Med. Sci.* **2015**, *20*, 787–795. [CrossRef] [PubMed]
20. International Organization for Standardization. ISO 6872:2015. Dentistry-Ceramic materials. Geneva: International Organization for Standardization. 2015. Available online: https://www.iso.org/standard/59936.html (accessed on 30 June 2015).
21. Mao, L.; Kaizer, M.R.; Zhao, M.; Guo, B.; Song, Y.F.; Zhang, Y. Graded ultra-translucent Zirconia (5Y-PSZ) for strength and functionalities. *J. Dent. Res.* **2018**, *97*, 1222–1228. [CrossRef] [PubMed]
22. Kwon, S.J.; Lawson, N.C.; McLaren, E.E.; Nejat, A.H.; Burgess, J.O. Comparison of the mechanical properties of translucent zirconia and lithium disilicate. *J. Prosthet. Dent.* **2018**, *120*, 132–137. [CrossRef] [PubMed]
23. Zhang, X.; Liang, W.; Jiang, F.; Wang, Z.; Zhao, J.; Zhou, C.; Wu, J. Effects of air-abrasion pressure on mechanical and bonding properties of translucent zirconia. *Clin. Oral. Investig.* **2021**, *25*, 1979–1988. [CrossRef] [PubMed]
24. Vicente, M.; Gomes, A.L.; Montero, J.; Rosel, E.; Seoane, V.; Albaladejo, A. Influence of cyclic loading on the adhesive effectiveness of resin-zirconia interface after femtosecond laser irradiation and conventional surface treatments. *Lasers. Surg. Med.* **2016**, *48*, 36–44. [CrossRef] [PubMed]
25. Okada, M.; Taketa, H.; Torii, Y.; Irie, M.; Matsumoto, T. Optimal sandblasting conditions for conventional-type yttria-stabilized tetragonal zirconia polycrystals. *Dent. Mater.* **2019**, *35*, 169–175. [CrossRef] [PubMed]
26. Guess, P.C.; Zhang, Y.; Kim, J.-W.; Rekow, E.D.; Thompson, V.P. Damage and reliability of Y-TZP after cementation surface treatment. *J. Dent. Res.* **2010**, *89*, 592–596. [CrossRef]
27. Aung, S.S.M.P.; Takagaki, T.; Lyann, S.K.; Ikeda, M.; Inokoshi, M.; Sadr, A.; Nikaido, T.; Tagami, J. Effects of alumina-blasting pressure on the bonding to super/ultra-translucent zirconia. *Dent. Mater.* **2019**, *35*, 730–739. [CrossRef] [PubMed]
28. Zhao, P.; Yu, P.; Xiong, Y.; Yue, L.; Arola, D.; Gao, S. Does the bond strength of highly translucent zirconia show a different dependence on the airborne-particle abrasion parameters in comparison to conventional zirconia? *J. Prosthodont. Res.* **2020**, *64*, 60–70. [CrossRef] [PubMed]
29. Inokoshi, M.; Shimizu, H.; Nozaki, K.; Takagaki, T.; Yoshihara, K.; Nagaoka, N.; Zhang, F.; Vleugels, J.; Van Meerbeek, B.; Minakuchi, S. Crystallographic and morphological analysis of air abraded highly translucent dental zirconia. *Dent. Mater.* **2018**, *34*, 508–518. [CrossRef]
30. Prieto, M.V.; Gomes, A.L.C.; Martín, J.M.; Lorenzo, A.A.; Mato, V.S.; Martínez, A.A. The effect of femtosecond laser treatment on the effectiveness of resin-zirconia adhesive: An in vitro study. *J. Lasers Med. Sci.* **2016**, *7*, 214–219. [CrossRef]
31. Okutan, Y.; Kandemir, B.; Gundogdu, Y.; Kilic, H.S.; Yucel, M.T. Combined application of femtosecond laser and air-abrasion protocols to monolithic zirconia at different sintering stages: Effects on surface roughness and resin bond strength. *J. Biomed. Mater. Res. B Appl. Biomater.* **2021**, *109*, 596–605. [CrossRef]
32. Tonietto, L.; Gonzaga, L., Jr.; Veronez, M.R.; Kazmierczak, C.S.; Arnold, D.C.M.; Costa, C.A.D. New method for evaluating surface roughness parameters acquired by laser scanning. *Sci. Rep.* **2019**, *9*, 15038. [CrossRef]

33. Botelho, M.G.; Dangay, S.; Shih, K.; Lam, W.Y.H. The effect of surface treatments on dental zirconia: An analysis of biaxial flexural strength, surface roughness and phase transformation. *J. Dent.* **2018**, *75*, 65–73. [CrossRef]
34. Ozer, F.; Naden, A.; Turp, V.; Mante, F.; Sen, D.; Blatz, M.B. Effect of thickness and surface modifications on flexural strength of monolithic zirconia. *J. Prosthet. Dent.* **2018**, *119*, 987–993. [CrossRef]
35. Zhang, F.; Spies, B.C.; Vleugels, J.; Reveron, H.; Wesemann, C.; Müller, W.D.; van Meerbeek, B.; Chevalier, J. High-translucent yttria-stabilized zirconia ceramics are wear-resistant and antagonist-friendly. *Dent. Mater.* **2019**, *35*, 1776–1790. [CrossRef] [PubMed]
36. Joglekar, A.P.; Liu, H.H.; Meyhöfer, E.; Mourou, G.; Hunt, A.J. Optics at critical intensity: Applications to nanomorphing. *Proc. Natl. Acad. Sci. USA* **2004**, *101*, 5856–5861. [CrossRef]
37. Zheng, Q.; Fan, Z.; Jiang, G.; Pan, A.; Yan, Z.; Lin, Q.; Cui, J.; Wang, W.; Mei, X. Mechanism and morphology control of underwater femtosecond laser microgrooving of silicon carbide ceramics. *Opt. Express.* **2019**, *27*, 26264–26280. [CrossRef] [PubMed]
38. Okada, M.; Taketa, H.; Hara, E.S.; Torii, Y.; Irie, M.; Matsumoto, T. Improvement of mechanical properties of Y-TZP by thermal annealing with monoclinic zirconia nanoparticle coating. *Dent. Mater.* **2019**, *35*, 970–978. [CrossRef] [PubMed]
39. Qeblawi, D.M.; Muñoz, C.A.; Brewer, J.D.; Monaco, E.A. The effect of zirconia surface treatment on flexural strength and shear bond strength to a resin cement. *J. Prosthet. Dent.* **2010**, *103*, 210–220. [CrossRef]
40. Wang, H.; Aboushelib, M.N.; Feilzer, A.J. Strength influencing variables on CAD/CAM zirconia frameworks. *Dent. Mater.* **2008**, *24*, 633–638. [CrossRef]
41. Song, J.Y.; Park, S.W.; Lee, K.; Yun, K.D.; Lim, H.P. Fracture strength and microstructure of Y-TZP zirconia after different surface treatments. *J. Prosthet. Dent.* **2013**, *110*, 274–280. [CrossRef]
42. Pagano, S.; Lombardo, G.; Caponi, S.; Costanzi, E.; Di Michele, A.; Bruscoli, S.; Xhimitiku, I.; Coniglio, M.; Valenti, C.; Mattarelli, M.; et al. Bio-mechanical characterization of a CAD/CAM PMMA resin for digital removable prostheses. *Dent. Mater.* **2021**, *37*, 118–130. [CrossRef] [PubMed]
43. Roitero, E.; Lasserre, F.; Anglada, M.; Mücklich, F.; Jiménez-Piqué, E. A parametric study of laser interference surface patterning of dental zirconia: Effects of laser parameters on topography and surface quality. *Dent. Mater.* **2017**, *33*, e28–e38. [CrossRef] [PubMed]

Article

Evaluation of Dental Surface after De-Bonding Orthodontic Bracket Bonded with a Novel Fluorescent Composite: In Vitro Comparative Study

Marco Farronato [1,*], Davide Farronato [2], Francesco Inchingolo [3], Laura Grassi [1], Valentina Lanteri [1,4] and Cinzia Maspero [1,4]

1. Department of Biomedical, Surgical and Dental Sciences, School of Dentistry, University of Milan, 20100 Milan, Italy; laura.grassi@unimi.it (L.G.); valentina.lanteri@unimi.it (V.L.); cinzia.maspero@unimi.it (C.M.)
2. Department of Medicine and Surgery, Insubria University, 21100 Varese, Italy; davide.farronato@uninsubria.it
3. Medicine Interdisciplinary Department, "Aldo Moro" University of Bari, 70121 Bari, Italy; francesco.inchingolo@uniba.it
4. Fondazione IRCCS Cà Granda, Ospedale Maggiore Policlinico, 20100 Milan, Italy
* Correspondence: marco.farronato@unimi.it; Tel.: +39-024693807

Abstract: The use of a new fluorescent composite can reduce some of the problems related to procedures of de-bonding orthodontic bracket (enamel damage, dentine lesions, and composite residuals). The aim of the presented study was to compare the effect of fluorescent and conventional non-fluorescent composite on dental surface and composite remnants by in vitro de-bonding tests. De-bonding of florescent composite (DFC) and the de-bonding of standard composite (DSC) were performed by operators on an in vitro sample of 48 teeth under UV light (360–370 nm min 20 mW/cm^2). Modified ARI (Adhesive Remnant Index), scored under $5.0 \times /235$ magnification, was used for evaluation of dental surface after the procedure, and the duration required for de-bonding was measured. Significant differences in ARI between the two groups were observed (Pearson two-tailed $p = 0.006$ 1.4 ± 0.1 95% C.I.), and the average duration of de-bonding was 38 s (DFC) and 77 s (DSC) per tooth, respectively (Mann–Whitney test $p = 0.015$; 57.7 ± 19.9 95% C.I.). The use of fluorescent composite could significantly improve the quality of de-bonding by reducing the quantity of composite residuals and visible enamel damage, while reducing time needed for successful procedure performance.

Keywords: composite; fluorescence; de-bonding; residuals; enamel damage; orthodontics

1. Introduction

Composite removal is a crucial step at the end of the orthodontic treatment. This procedure is fundamental to restore the functional and macroscopic aesthetic appearance; if not performed correctly, it may leads to iatrogenic damages of healthy teeth and to negative clinical outcomes such as dental sensitivity, unaesthetic enamel damage, dentine lesions, and the presence of composite residuals [1–3].

Operators lacking experience are more likely to be facing the mentioned negative outcomes related to the adhesive and composite clean-up. Additionally, altered or abnormal dental anatomy can increase the difficulty of adhesive residual removal during the clean-up. Thus, it is extremely important to remove the adhesive without modifying the enamel surface with the aim to restore the original tooth appearance.

Several conventional methods are described in the literature to remove the adhesives and to polish the enamel [4]. The standard method of composite residual removal is the use of appropriate bur along with polishing discs and polishing paste. Ultrasonic devices and air-abrasion with aluminum oxide or other particles are an alternative. In addition, small loads of low-level laser irradiation applied during the bracket removal can eliminate most of the composite residuals on the enamel surface. However, in most cases, adhesive residuals are present on the enamel surface even after cleaning and polishing with rotary instruments [5].

A simplified de-bonding technique using a novel fluorescent composite and UV lamp was proposed. The method may significantly decrease the presence of the composite residuals, along with the risks related to the standard practice. BrackFix® composite (Voco GmbH, Cuxhaven, Germany) has fluorescent properties due to fluorescent dye mixed with the composite base. This characteristic allows the compound materials used to react under UV light and to become easily detectable. The aim of the study was to evaluate the efficacy of a novel type and simplified de-bonding procedure of fluorescent adhesive composite for orthodontic brackets and to critically analyze its advantages in comparison to the standard composite during the procedures of composite clean-up. We hypothesized that this new product could reduce the operator-depending factor and, therefore, can increase de-bonding safety and quality.

2. Materials and Methods

A study protocol was designed in accordance with CRIS (Checklist for Reporting In-vitro Studies) Guidelines [6]. The protocol described the procedures of the study, including the background, rationale, personnel, and institutions involved; data gathering; data management; specimen storage; materials and equipment; addressing potential bias; and defining the research and its aims.

Storage and utilization of used materials were in accordance with recommendations provided by the manufacturers. The study has been approved by the Ethics Committee of the University of Milan, Italy (protocol n. 314), and written consent for the use of extracted teeth was obtained from each patient.

De-bonding of BrackFix® (Voco GmbH, Cuxhaven, Germany) composite under UV light was compared to the conventional de-bonding method in a blind randomized in vitro test (Figures 1–3). Procedures were performed by postgraduate doctors with similar experience of de-bonding and by experienced operators. To investigate the efficacy of the novel composite, the dental surface after the de-bonding was evaluated by a single experienced operator.

Figure 1. Bracket and composite observed under UV light (360–370 nm 20 mW/cm^2).

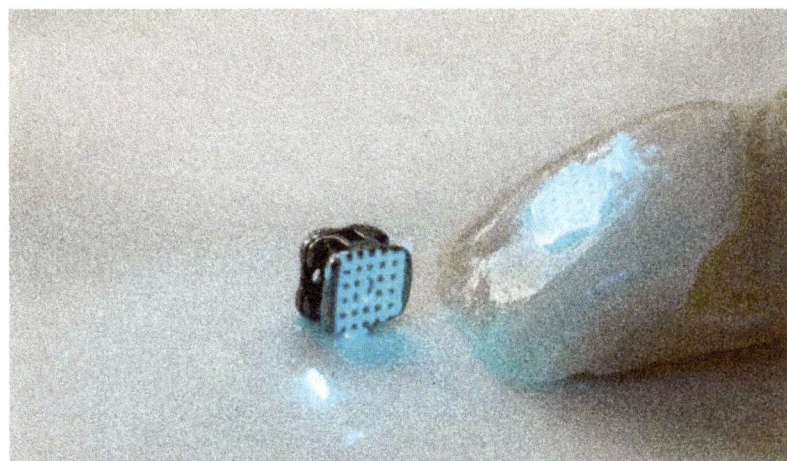

Figure 2. Bracket removal under UV light 360–370 nm 20 mW/cm^2.

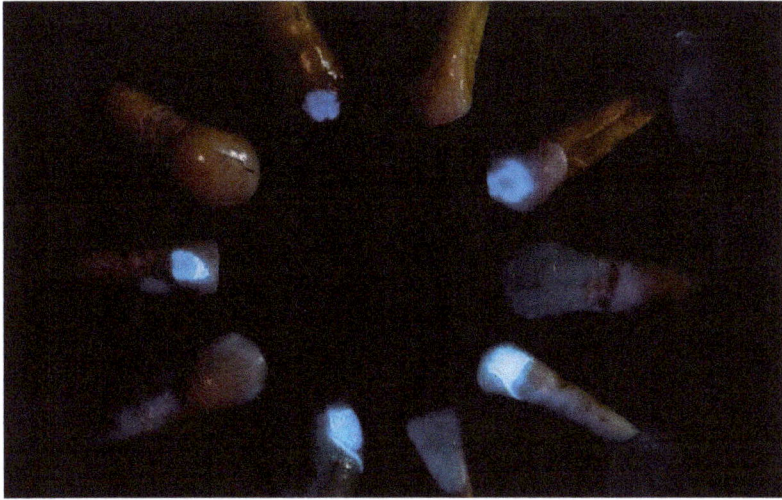

Figure 3. Visibility of Composite in two study groups under UV light (360–370 nm 20 mW/cm^2).

Operators involved in the study were recruited from the same postgraduate class, from the University of Milan, Italy, with no vision problems. The operators were randomly chosen to perform two types of de-bonding on two different extracted human teeth, the tests were also performed with experienced operators from the same institution. Each of them executed both the new de-bonding procedure of fluorescent composite (DFC) and "standard" de-bonding of non-fluorescent composite (DSC) in randomized, blinded order.

The sample consisted of 48 human teeth, extracted for various reasons. Inclusion criteria were as follows: good preservation state, integrity, absence of caries, no prior exposure to chemical agents, absence of extraction force generated cracks, and low levels or absence of demineralization. Teeth with minor cracks and small spots of demineralization were included as they are useful for the operator to evaluate enamel integrity in the process of adhesive clean-up. Such cases can be randomly found in patients undergoing or finishing orthodontic therapy. Exclusion criteria included: major cracks, lesions or dental restorations, anatomical abnormalities, or extraction signs on the crown. The sample of 48 human teeth included all teeth types in equal proportions—10 incisors, 10 canines, 14 premolars, and 14 molars. During all procedures, teeth were stored in isotonic solution at 4 °C with the solution being changed daily for a maximum of 5 days. All the teeth were selected and the inclusion/exclusion criteria were evaluated by an experienced operator prior to the study.

The teeth were etched with 37% phosphoric acid gel (Vococid, Voco GmbH, Cuxhaven, Germany) for 30 s, rinsed with water, and air-dried as recommended by the manufacturer. Stainless-steel brackets (Leone S.p.A, Sesto FiorentinoItaly) were applied to the teeth by a single operator according to manufacturer instructions. Composites (fluorescent and standard) were applied in similar quantities and cured with a light-curing unit with a brightness of at least 1000 mW/cm^3 for 20 s. The novel Composite BrackFix® (Voco GmbH, Cuxhaven, Germany) was used for the DFC group. BrackFix® primer (Voco GmbH, Cuxhaven, Germany) was applied before application of the composite BrackFix®. Fluorescent dye added to the composite base of BrackFix® allows it to be detectable and seen under the UV light (Figures 1–3). The control group (DSC) was bonded under similar conditions using a non-fluorescent composite Transbond XT (3M, Saint Paul, MN, USA).

Teeth were numbered and classified, and 24 teeth pairs were randomly assigned. Each Operator was given one teeth pair embedded in an acrylic resin block consisting of one tooth from the DSC and one from the DFC group, de-bonding instruments, and instructions to remove brackets and composite using orthodontic de-bonding pliers under assistance (aspiration of the residuals and holding of the UV lamp). The scopes of the research were blinded so the operators performed the de-bonding without knowing the effects of the UV lamp used on the composite of both DFC and DSC. The use of UV light to evidence the presence of composite remnants, even without fluorescent particles, has previously been evidenced as a positive outcome factor in past research [7–11]; therefore, blinding was necessary to avoid bias. The UV lamp used in the study had the following characteristics: 360–370 nm min 20 mW/cm^2 (which is harmless for biological tissues but requires eyes protection). It was held a maximum of 50 cm from the tooth in order not to dissipate the light and not to be in contrast with the environmental light to decrease potential risk of bias of light change due to different times of the day and weather conditions. Operators wore protective eyeglasses to avoid damage related to the use of UV light.

The simplified de-bonding procedure was performed and composite was removed with the aid of a 12-flute tungsten carbide bur under UV lamp. The procedure was performed under the same conditions for both teeth from the two sample groups. The duration of the removal was measured for a subgroup of 20 teeth with similar anatomic structures (canines and incisors) right after the removal of the orthodontic bracket at the start of the removal with burs performed by similarly experienced operators. The duration of the procedure was measured only for a subgroup (n = 20) of frontal teeth with similar anatomy (10 incisors and 10 canines) to decrease the risk of bias related to the anatomical variance (Figure 4).

- Grade 0: visible composite residuals OR significant damage to the enamel surface visible without 5× magnification from any view OR any anatomical change to the tooth;
- Grade 1: minor enamel scratching or damage not exposing the dentine, which was partially visible without 5× magnification from some views or/and composite residuals visible using 5× magnification only;
- Grade 2: absence of scratches or presence of minor scratches in the enamel surface, visible only with the use of 5× magnification.

All the collected data were analyzed using statistical software (SPSS 20, IBM) by calculation of descriptive statistics and Pearson Two-Tailed test, and Mann-Whitney U tests (independent samples) for small sample sizes were used for group comparison of ARI and duration of procedure; p-value < 0.05 was considered statistically significant (Figure 5).

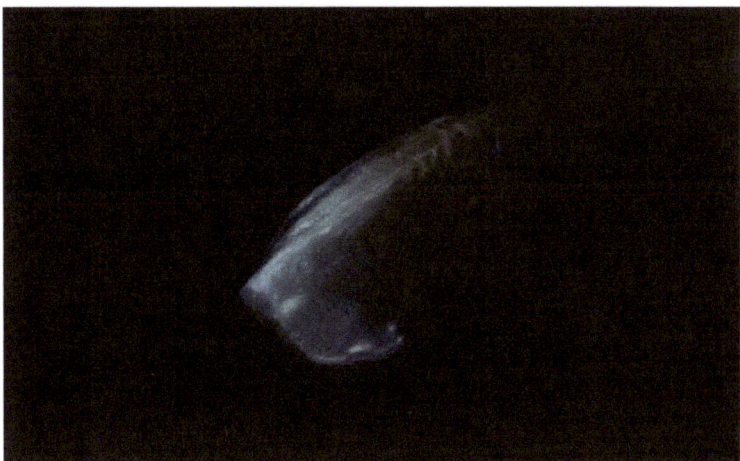

Figure 4. After de-bonding tooth surface. After the de-bonding, all the teeth were grouped, and de-bonding was evaluated by a blinded single operator. Each tooth was classified using a modified ARI (Adhesive Remnant Index) scale from 0 to 2 with the use of 5.0×/235 telescopic head-worn magnifier as follows.

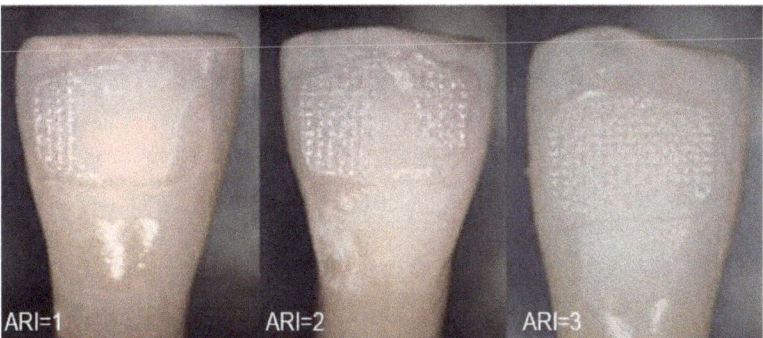

Figure 5. Illustration of Adhesive Remnant Index (ARI): ARI 0, no adhesive on the tooth; ARI 1, less than 1/2 adhesive on the tooth; ARI 2, more than 1/2 of the adhesive on the tooth; ARI 3, all of the adhesive on the tooth.

3. Results

All the operators performing de-bonding procedures with fluorescent composite found the use of this novel composite easier and therefore faster in comparison to the conventional composite used in the DSC group. The mean duration of composite removal in the DFC group (visible under UV light) was 38 s, and for the DSC group (conventional composite) it was 77 s (Table 1). The differences in the duration was significant (Mann–Whitney test $p = 0.015$ 57.7 ± 19.9 95% C.I.) under the study conditions.

Table 1. Duration of de-bonding among similarly experienced operators and similar anatomy dental elements.

	DFC	DSC
Operator #1	40 s	234 s
Operator #2	60 s	87 s
Operator #3	36 s	54 s
Operator #4	23 s	56 s
Operator #5	17 s	31 s
Operator #6	37 s	67 s
Operator #7	40 s	80 s
Operator #8	53 s	27 s
Operator #9	37 s	69 s
Operator #10	41 s	66 s
SD	12.4	58.3
mean	38 s	77 s
maximum	60 s	234 s
minimum	17 s	27 s
Mann–Whitney	$p = 0.015$	
95% C.I.	19.9	

Significant differences were also observed in the ARI evaluation ($p = 0.006$, Pearson Two-Tailed 1.4 ± 0.1 95% C.I.). In the DSC group, 16.7% (4 from 24) of teeth were assessed as Grade 0; 50% (12 from 24) as Grade 1; and 33.3% (8 from 24) as Grade 2. In the DFC group, no tooth was evaluated as Grade 0; 33.3% (8 from 24) were evaluated as Grade 1; and 66.6% (16 from 24) as Grade 2 (Table 2).

Table 2. Modified ARI evaluation.

Operator	A.R.I Grade DFC	A.R.I Grade DSC	Grades Description
Operator #1	2	1	0 grade: visible composite remnants OR significant damage to the enamel surface visible without loupes 5× from any projection of the observer OR any anatomical change to the tooth.
Operator #2	1	1	1 grade: minor enamel scratching or damage with no exposition of the dentine partially visible without loupes 5× from a limited number of visible projections of the observer or/and composite remnants visible with loupes 5× only.
Operator #3	2	1	2 grade: absence or presence of minor scratches to the enamel surface visible only with the use of head-worn loupe 5×.
Operator #4	2	0	
Operator #5	2	0	
Operator #6	2	1	
Operator #7	2	2	
Operator #8	2	2	
Operator #9	1	2	
Operator #10	2	1	

Table 2. Cont.

Operator	A.R.I Grade		Grades Description
	DFC	DSC	
Operator #11	2	2	
Operator #12	1	1	
Operator #13	1	1	
Operator #14	2	2	
Operator #15	1	1	
Operator #16	2	0	
Operator #17	2	2	
Operator #18	1	1	
Operator #19	1	1	
Operator #20	1	0	
experienced op	2	1	
experienced op	2	1	
experienced op	2	2	
experienced op	2	2	
st. dev.	0.48	0.70	
average	1.67	1.17	
MAX	2	2	
MIN	1	0	
Pearson	$p = 0.006$		
95% C.I.	0.182997		

4. Discussion

As recently described in the literature, the operator's experience during the de-bonding procedure affects the quality of the results [1–3,5,7–10]. The design of the proposed study also involved inexperienced operators. Each of the postgraduate doctors was instructed in a pre-operative session by experienced operators. This study design was chosen to minimize bias related to high experience of the operators, and also to permit repetitiveness of the test under the same conditions (by having the same experience levels) and compared to experienced professionaly.

Likewise, all procedures were done under the same lighting conditions due to the fact that changing weather and changing lighting can highly affect and compromise the reproducibility of the work. In fact, no direct sunlight was affecting the study, and the UV light was held at a minimum distance of 50 cm in both groups. This allowed the composite to have the same optical reaction during all de-bonding procedures. UV light was used under the same conditions during the DSC procedure to discard UV advantages not related to the fluorescent characteristics of the novel fluorescent composite, as described by Ribeiro et al. [11].

Montasser et al. demonstrated that ARI grades are significantly different when testing is carried out with the naked eye and 10–20× magnification; but they are similar when using 10× magnification and naked-eye evaluation [12]. The evaluation was carried out using grade scale 0 to 2 of the modified ARI. Originally, 4 grades of ARI were described by Årtun et al., or alternatively modified 5 grades by Bishara et al. [13,14]. In our study, the ARI grades were modified specifically for the purpose of macroscopic evaluationTherefore, the use of magnifying glasses can be fundamental in the phase of bracket placement and cleaning of excess composite during bonding. However, the use of Adhesive Remnant

Index remains a controversial topic [1]. Other authors evaluated the assessment of the confidence of ARI score with other methods such as photography, use of the naked eye, and 20× magnifications, resulting in no significant differences [15–23].

The simplified grades of ARI provided the teeth evaluation with a simplified procedure and less risk of bias [8,12–14].

Recently, new de-bonding techniques were developed, or existing methods were improved, for example, Taha et al. proposed the use of a novel bioactive glass via air abrasion [22,24,25].

Currently, no technique has proven to be capable of complete and efficient removal of residual adhesives without inducing even a minor amount of enamel damage [5].

The new methodology using UV light and UV florescent composite might improve the safety and decrease the iatrogenic damage of the enamel and dentine during the clean-up processes after de-bonding in the future. It might result in an improvement in the health for all patients undergoing orthodontic treatment due to the decrease of macroscopic composite residuals, which could decrease plaque retention, even though it is not a resolutive procedure. The restoration of patient's pre-treatment dental health is a priority to every orthodontic procedure, and more efforts should be made to help the clinician as well as to develop effective protocols. We can also speculate that recent advancements and popularity in clear aligners could benefit from the same technology during attachment removals [26]. The duration of the procedure is also important during this kind of procedure. The new methodology seems to highly decrease the time required to effectively remove the composite, probably because the composite remnant's magnitude and position can be recognized easily and faster due to their strong fluorescent proprieties and bright color. The main limitation of the study is that the results produced should be tested on a larger sample, and would be even better if carried out in vivo. Further in vivo studies with professionals are needed to determine if this new method requires less operating time.

Due to the nature of the study, polishing and clean-up procedures were excluded as, rarely, they can produce harm to enamel tissue; therefore, they were considered out of the scope of the research. It should, however, be considered that the ARI can be affected by this last phase.

5. Conclusions

This study suggests that the aid of UV lamps and the use of fluorescent composite might decrease macroscopic composite residuals and visible scratches after de-bonding procedures performed by postgraduate doctors. The de-bonding procedure is faster under the study circumstances. Further in vivo and larger sample studies are needed.

Author Contributions: Conceptualization, M.F. and F.I.; methodology, D.F.; software, L.G.; validation, V.L.; formal analysis, F.I.; investigation, L.G.; resources, C.M.; data curation, M.F. and D.F.; writing—original draft preparation, V.L. and C.M.; supervision, V.L.; project administration, M.F.; funding acquisition, D.F. All authors have read and agreed to the published version of the manuscript.

Funding: This research received no external funding.

Institutional Review Board Statement: The study was conducted according to the guidelines of the Declaration of Helsinki and approved by the Institutional Review Board (or Ethics Committee) of University of Milan, Italy. Protocol number 314.

Informed Consent Statement: Informed consent was obtained from all subjects involved in the study.

Data Availability Statement: Supplementary data will be made available by the official institution (www.unimi.it) (accessed on 10 May 2021).

Acknowledgments: The study was carried out without any commitment or financial support from the manufacturing company Voco GmbH, Cuxhaven, Germany. The University of Milan requested samples without any personal or institutional interest or expenses. The company kindly provided the material without having any prior information about the prepared study: Composite: BrackFix

(Voco GmbH, Cuxhaven, Germany); UV lamp 360–370 nm 20 mW/cm^2; Etching: Vococid (Voco GmbH, Cuxhaven, Germany); Primer: Brackfix primer (Voco GmbH, Cuxhaven, Germany).

Conflicts of Interest: The authors declare no conflict of interest.

References

1. Mohebi, S.; Shafiee, H.-A.; Ameli, N. Evaluation of enamel surface roughness after orthodontic bracket debonding with atomic force microscopy. *Am. J. Orthod. Dentofac. Orthop.* **2017**, *151*, 521–527. [CrossRef]
2. Bollen, C.M.; Lambrechts, P.; Quirynen, M. Comparison of surface roughness of oral hard materials to the threshold surface roughness for bacterial plaque retention: A review of the literature. *Dent. Mater.* **1997**, *13*, 258–269. [CrossRef]
3. Goel, A.; Singh, A.; Gupta, T.; Gambhir, R.S. Evaluation of surface roughness of enamel after various bonding and clean-up procedures on enamel bonded with three different bonding agents: An in-vitro study. *J. Clin. Exp. Dent.* **2017**, *9*, e608–e616. [CrossRef] [PubMed]
4. Attin, R.; Stawarczyk, B.; Kecik, D.; Knosel, M.; Wiechmann, D.; Attin, T. Shear bond strength of brackets to demineralize enamel after different pretreatment methods. *Angle Orthod.* **2012**, *82*, 56–61. [CrossRef] [PubMed]
5. Janiszewska-Olszowska, J.; Szatkiewicz, T.; Tomkowski, R.; Tandecka, K.; Grocholewicz, K. Effect of orthodontic debonding and adhesive removal on the enamel–current knowledge and future perspectives—A systematic review. *Med. Sci. Monit. Basic Res.* **2014**, *20*, 1991–2001.
6. Krithikadatta, J.; Gopikrishna, V.; Datta, M. CRIS Guidelines (Checklist for Reporting In-vitro Studies): A concept note on the need for standardized guidelines for improving quality and transparency in reporting in-vitro studies in experimental dental research. *J. Conserv. Dent.* **2014**, *17*, 301–304. [CrossRef] [PubMed]
7. Fan, X.-C.; Chen, L.; Huang, X.-F. Effects of various debonding and adhesive clearance methods on enamel surface: An in vitro study. *BMC Oral Health* **2017**, *17*, 58. [CrossRef] [PubMed]
8. Kim, S.-S.; Park, W.-K.; Son, W.-S.; Ahn, H.-S.; Ro, J.-H.; Kim, Y.-D. Enamel surface evaluation after removal of orthodontic composite remnants by intraoral sandblasting: A 3-dimensional surface profilometry study. *Am. J. Orthod. Dentofac. Orthop.* **2007**, *132*, 71–76. [CrossRef] [PubMed]
9. Maspero, C.; Giannini, L.; Galbiati, G.; Nolet, F.; Esposito, L.; Farronato, G. Titanium orthodontic appliances for allergic patients. *Minerva Stomatol.* **2014**, *63*, 403–410.
10. Dubey, C.; Prakash, A.; Sharma, A.; Jain, U. Enigma of Debonding. *Orthod. J. Nepal* **2016**, *5*, 37–41. [CrossRef]
11. Ribeiro, A.A.; Almeida, L.F.; Martins, L.P.; Martins, R.P. Assessing adhesive remnant removal and enamel damage with ultraviolet light: An in-vitro study. *Am. J. Orthod. Dentofac. Orthop.* **2017**, *151*, 292–296. [CrossRef]
12. Montasser, M.A.; Drummond, J.L. Reliability of the adhesive remnant index score system with different magnifications. *Angle Orthod.* **2009**, *79*, 773–776. [CrossRef] [PubMed]
13. Årtun, J.; Bergland, S. Clinical trials with crystal growth conditioning as an alternative to acid-etch enamel pretreatment. *Am. J. Orthod. Dentofac. Orthop.* **1984**, *85*, 333–340. [CrossRef]
14. Bishara, S.E.; Trulove, T.S. Comparisons of different debonding techniques for ceramic brackets: An in vitro study. *Am. J. Orthod. Dentofac. Orthop.* **1990**, *98*, 145–153. [CrossRef]
15. Oz, A.A.; Yazicioglu, S.; Arici, N.; Akdeniz, B.S.; Murat, N.; Arıcı, S. Assessment of the Confidence of the Adhesive Remnant Index Score with Different Methods. *Turk. J. Orthod.* **2014**, *26*, 149–153. [CrossRef]
16. Cehreli, S.B.; Polat-Ozsoy, O.; Sar, C.; Cubukcu, H.E. A comparative study of qualitative and quantitative methods for the assessment of adhesive remnant after bracket debonding. *Eur. J. Orthod.* **2011**, *34*, 188–192. [CrossRef] [PubMed]
17. Arima, S.; Namura, Y.; Tamura, T.; Shimizu, N. Easy Debonding of Ceramic Brackets Bonded with a Light-Cured Orthodontic Adhesive Containing Microcapsules with a CO_2 Laser. *Photomed. Laser Surg.* **2018**, *36*, 162–168. [CrossRef]
18. Dumbryte, I.; Linkeviciene, L.; Linkevicius, T.; Malinauskas, M. Does orthodontic debonding lead to tooth sensitivity? Comparison of teeth with and without visible enamel microcracks. *Am. J. Orthod. Dentofac. Orthop.* **2017**, *151*, 284–291. [CrossRef] [PubMed]
19. D'Apuzzo, F.; Perillo, L.; Delfino, I.; Portaccio, M. Monitoring early phases of orthodontic treatment by means of Raman spectroscopies. *J. Biomed. Opt.* **2017**, *22*, 1–10. [CrossRef] [PubMed]
20. Grassia, V.; Gentile, E.; Di Stasio, D.; Jamilian, A.; Matarese, G.; D'Apuzzo, F.; Lucchese, A. In vivo confocal microscopy analysis of enamel defects after orthodontic treatment: A preliminary study. *Ultrastruct. Pathol.* **2016**, *40*, 317–323. [CrossRef]
21. Farronato, G.; Giannini, L.; Galbiati, G.; Cannalire, P.; Martinelli, G.; Tubertini, I.; Maspero, C. Oral tissues and orthodontic treatment: Common side effects. *Minerva Stomatol.* **2013**, *62*, 431–446. [PubMed]
22. Taha, A.; Hill, R.G.; Fleming, P.S.; Patel, M.P. Development of a novel bioactive glass for air-abrasion to selectively remove orthodontic adhesives. *Clin. Oral Investig.* **2017**, *22*, 1839–1849. [CrossRef] [PubMed]
23. Farronato, M.; Maspero, C.; Lanteri, V.; Fama, A.; Ferrati, F.; Pettenuzzo, A.; Farronato, D. Current state of the art in the use of augmented reality in dentistry: A systematic review of the literature. *BMC Oral Health* **2019**, *19*, 1–15. [CrossRef]
24. Ferreira, J.T.L.; Borsatto, M.C.; Saraiva, M.C.P.; Matsumoto, M.A.N.; Torres, C.P.; Romano, F.L. Evaluation of Enamel Roughness in Vitro After Orthodontic Bracket Debonding Using Different Methods of Residual Adhesive Removal. *Turk. J. Orthod.* **2020**, *33*, 43–51. [CrossRef]

25. Pinho, M.; Manso, M.C.; Almeida, R.F.; Martin, C.; Carvalho, O.; Henriques, B.; Silva, F.; Ferreira, A.P.; Souza, J.C.M. Bond Strength of Metallic or Ceramic Orthodontic Brackets to Enamel, Acrylic, or Porcelain Surfaces. *Materials* **2020**, *13*, 5197. [CrossRef]
26. Tartaglia, G.; Mapelli, A.; Maspero, C.; Santaniello, T.; Serafin, M.; Farronato, M.; Caprioglio, A. Direct 3D Printing of Clear Orthodontic Aligners: Current State and Future Possibilities. *Materials* **2021**, *14*, 1799. [CrossRef] [PubMed]

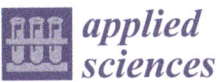

Article

Retrospective Analysis on Inferior Third Molar Position by Means of Orthopantomography or CBCT: Periapical Band-Like Radiolucent Sign

Young-Sam Kim [1], Young-Min Park [1], Saverio Cosola [2], Abanob Riad [3,*], Enrica Giammarinaro [2], Ugo Covani [2,4] and Simone Marconcini [2]

1. Gangam Dental Office, Seoul 06614, Korea; doctorkimys@gmail.com (Y.-S.K.); min1810@hotmail.com (Y.-M.P.)
2. Department of Stomatology, Tuscan Stomatologic Institute, Foundation for Dental Clinic, Research and Continuing Education, 55042 Forte dei Marmi, Italy; s.cosola@hotmail.it (S.C.); e.giammarinaro@gmail.com (E.G.); covani@covani.it (U.C.); simosurg@gmail.com (S.M.)
3. Department of Public Health, Faculty of Medicine, Masaryk University, Kamenice 5, 625 00 Brno, Czech Republic
4. Oral Surgery and Implantology, Unicamillus International Medical University, 00131 Rome, Italy
* Correspondence: abanoub.riad@med.muni.cz

Abstract: Background: Orthopantomography (OPG) is usually used as a primary diagnostic radiological exam in the planning of third molar surgery because it is deeply available in dental clinics and has lower radiation doses compared to Cone-beam computed tomography (CBCT). The OPG provides a bi-dimensional image, but several radiological signs have been proposed to study the position of the lower third molar and to predict surgical risks. Methods: Patients were divided into two groups, the OPG with a radiolucent area (D-group) and the OPG without any sign (C-group) in correspondence of inferior wisdom tooth roots. Results: The mean distance between the inferior third molar root and the lingual cortical mandibular bone was -1.09 ± 1.5 mm. The nearness of the root that is less than 1 mm was more frequent in the D-group (84.85%) compared to the C-group (14.58%) with statistical significance (Odd ratio: 32.8) using the Chi-square test. Conclusions: When the root of the impacted inferior third molar is impacted into the lingual cortical plate, a periapical band-like radiolucent sign may appear in the OPG image. It could be useful for the prediction of root position and surgical risks.

Keywords: radiolucent sign; OPG; CBCT; third molar; oral surgery; periapical sign

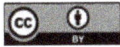

1. Introduction

Do dental clinicians need to extract all third molars? On May 2000 in the UK, National Institute for Health and Care Excellence (NICE) published the guidelines about the extraction of third molars. The NICE guidelines recommended that third molar extraction should be limited to teeth with pathologies such as caries lesion, peri-apical lesions, recurrent pericoronitis, lesion to the second molar, cyst/neoplastic lesions, etc. [1].

Still, in the last decades, the frequency of third molar extraction by oral surgeons and general dentists has been increasing [2]. Some cohort studies reported that between 30% and 60% of people who have retained their asymptomatic, unerupted wisdom teeth will need of at least one extraction in the next future (4–12 years after their first evaluation). In fact, third molars tend to change position towards the coronal and mesial direction, resulting in the damage of second molars or becoming partially erupted, thus meaning at a higher risk of caries or pericoronitis [3].

It is believed that the presence of the third molar is a phenomenon of human vestigiality so that the prevalence is very high and various according to population and familiarity [4].

In Sweden, 72% of the young population aged between 20 to 30 years has, at least, one impacted lower third molar and, in the UK, it is estimated that every year, 4 people out of 1000 will need a third molar extraction [5].

A retrospective cohort study of De Bryyn L et al. (2020) including 1682 patients reported that the common reasons to avoid third molars extraction are: right eruption with function in occlusion (31.9%), patient preference (31.5%), and absence of symptom in patients >30 years old (17.5%) [6]. Compromised health status and advanced age were often included in the decision regarding whether to retain the third molars or not. One-third of the referred patients had reasons to retain one or more third molars. These findings might facilitate the future development of a consensus statement.

Prevalent literature indicates that wisdom teeth surgery is often performed by general dentists, however, the cost-benefit relationship and the complication rate should be carefully considered before initiating any treatment plan [2].

A retrospective study of Sarica and co-workers (2019) suggested that impacted teeth with no pathologies could be left in site monitoring the evolution. In those cases, Orthopantomography (OPG) is very useful to monitor the evolution of impacted third molar but cone-beam computed tomography (CBCT) is needed to predict the surgical risk [7].

It is well reported that Orthopantomography (OPG) is routinely used as a primary diagnostic exam in third molar surgery, and it is useful in the initial decision-making process [1,8]. Typical radiological signs of high risk of inferior alveolar nerve (IAN) damage are the darkening of the roots; a deflected root; narrowing of the root; diversion or loop of the inferior alveolar canal [9].

Despite this knowledge, some studies reported that there is an incidence of 17% of transitory nerve damage in patients who presented these signs in OPG plus 2% of permanent nerve damage [10].

The present retrospective study was performed to assess whether specific OPG findings could predict the risk level of a third molar extraction and, therefore, the putative need for further patients X-ray exposure to CBCT to have a better understanding of the anatomy.

The aim was to evaluate the pre-operative position of wisdom teeth as seen on OPGs and to compare this position with the one found on CBCT. The null hypothesis was that the radiolucent area at the apical portion of third molar roots as observed on OPG-(Y-sign)-does not match with the impaction of the root into the lingual cortical bone on the CBCT of the same patient.

2. Materials and Methods

2.1. Study Design

This is a monocentric retrospective comparative study approved by the Gangnam Academy of Wisdom tooth Extraction (GAWE), Seoul, South Korea.

Patients, admitted to "Gangam Dental Office" (Seoul, South Korea) to remove an inferior third molar between January 2015 and December 2019, were retrospectively enrolled for the present study.

The subjects were searched on the database of the dental clinic using the following inclusion criteria:

- Patients who received both an OPG and CBCT before inferior third molar extraction following the guidelines: CBCT was performed after OPG because the inferior alveolar canal appeared near (or superimposed) to the root with high pre- or post-surgical risk [1];
- Patients who received the inferior third molar surgery by the director of the clinic (Kim YS.);
- Consecutive patients aged between 25 to 35 years old (this range because people with more than 40 years could have other pathologies or compliances and because the complete root development in the third molars may occur up to 24 years but with individual variation according to the studies) [11].

Evaluating the moment of the surgery, the search was pursued according to the following exclusion criteria:

- subject with severe systemic or genetic disease affecting the bone metabolism;
- subject in radiotherapy or chemotherapy or bisphosphonates;
- subject with not completely formed root of the third;
- subject with a fracture of mandibula.

2.2. Collection of Data

OPG and CBCT were performed by a CBCT machine (Vatech, South Korea).

Images of fundamental structures of CBCT in axial, panorex, and cross-sections planes and 3D were captured and reformatted in JPG-image. These screenshots were saved in the same chart of OPG for each patient with anamnestic data. The measurement of the minimum distance between the root and the lingual cortical bone of the mandibula was performed with the same program used to read the CBCT, a computer-assisted stereological analysis system (Vatech, South Korea) [12].

The chosen landmark in the lingual cortical bone was the most buccal one: if the roots overcame the buccal surface of the lingual cortical bone, the assigned value was negative because the surgery became riskier; on the contrary, if the root was inside of the trabecular bone, the value assigned was positive as represented in Figure 1 and the surgery could have less risk of complications such as fracture of cortical bone or roots. [12,13].

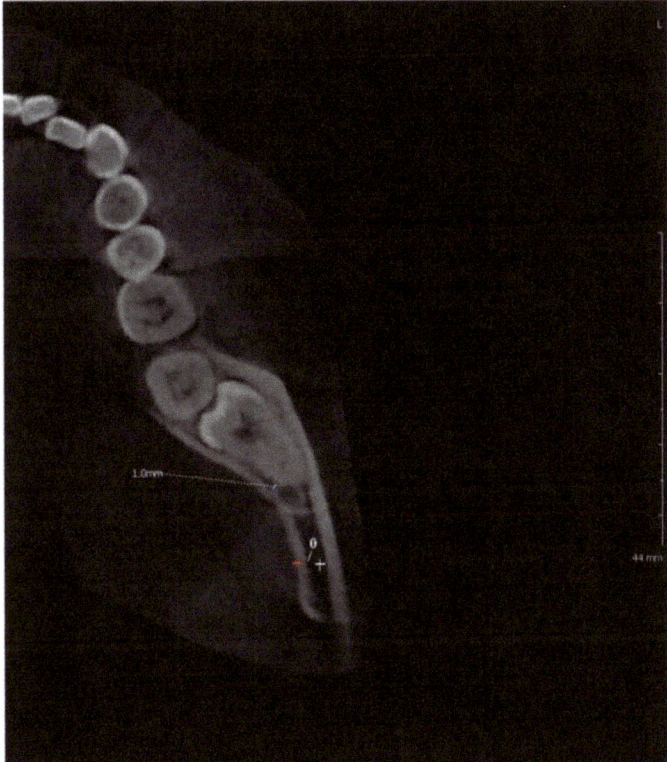

Figure 1. The distance is directly proportional to the root position. If the root is distant from the lingual cortical bone the measurement is considered positive when the root is in contact with the cortical lingual bone the distance is 0 and into the lingual cortical bone, the distance is negative. As reported in the figure the landmark for zero value is the buccal portion of the lingual cortical bone. The distance in the trabecular bone is positive (white) and the distance into the cortical bone is negative (red). The distance for this third molar is 1 mm (green).

The screenshot of this minimum distance was saved for each patient in CBCT.

Anamnestic data consisted of the following information: age, gender, smoking habits, a reason to require the extraction.

All wisdom teeth extractions were performed using the ESSE (Easy Simple Safe Efficient) surgical technique [2,13].

2.3. Modern Radiological Material for Clinicians

Modern technology such as digital OPG and CBCT in the dental field offers to clinicians several tools for diagnosis and research. The OPG and CBCT used in the present study followed the principle of justification and optimization. CBCT had a low-dose protocol with large FOV, but normal resolution and normal quality images (80 kVp, 5 mA). The acquisition time used to be 15 s corresponding to the effective dose of 35 µSv [14].

The effective dose indicates the evaluation risk of the patients, meaning the unit of energy absorbed by the unit of mass (J/Kg) [8].

PaX-i3D Smart is an advanced digital dental diagnostic software that incorporates Panoramic, Cephalometric, and CBCT imaging capabilities into a single system of Vatech, (Hwaseong-si, Korea) used in the present study.

2.4. Groups of Patients

The entire cohort of patients was divided into 2 main groups according to a first OPG examination of the inferior teeth needed for extraction.

- Dark-group (D-group): The pre-operative OPG of patients who had a dark area at the apical portion of the root/roots of the inferior third molar;
- Control-group (C-group): The pre-operative OPG of patients who did not present a radiolucent area at the apical portion of the root/roots of the inferior third molar.

2.5. Statistical Analysis

The data were evaluated using Statistical Package for the Social Sciences SPSS®® 26 (Java, May 2019, USA). Descriptive statistic was used to describe the population frequency, mean and standard deviation (SD).

D-group and C-group were compared using CBCT to check if the apical portion of the inferior third molar was distant from the lingual cortical bone of the mandibula. These two groups were compared using Student's t-test at a 0.05 significance level.

On evaluating the distance between the nearest portion of the root/roots and the buccal portion of the lingual cortical bone, the authors used a cut-off point of -1 mm. If the root is completely in the cortical bone the distance will be ≤ -1 mm and the third molar is classified as "impacted" or if the distance is > -1 mm the tooth is "non-impacted". This cut-off point of -1 mm was established for clinical reasons because, if the root is impacted completely in the lingual cortical bone (less than -1 mm), the surgery could be more difficult and the surgical risks such as fracture may be more frequent [15]. The comparisons between groups were performed using Chi-square for these parameters.

In the D-group a stratification of patients was performed according to a differential diagnosis observing the OPG and CBCT and 2 subgroups were created:

2.6. Pathological Signs

- No-group: No sign of pathologies that could explain the radiolucent area in the apical portion of the root of the inferior wisdom tooth;
- Yes-group: Some signs of pathologies that could explain the radiolucent area in the apical portion of the root of the inferior wisdom tooth, such as caries and cystitis.

The Chi-squared test was used to assess differences and correlation between variables at a 0.05 significance level.

In the D-group a stratification of patients was performed according to a differential diagnosis observing the OPG and CBCT in the second subgroup to distinguish the exact cause of the radiolucent area around the root:

3. Results

Two hundred and forty-nine patients met the inclusion criteria of this study; however, twenty-one patients were excluded after reviewing clinical and radiographic records due to. Demographic data of two hundred and twenty-eight are reported in Table 1. The mean age of patients was 30.47 ± 0.5 (30–31, n = 228) years old with 120 (52.6%) male and 108 (49,4%) female patients. While 100 (43.86%) of the extracted molars were from the right side, 128 (56.14%) were from the left side with similar distribution between groups. According to the OPG, 132 (57.89%) patients had a radiolucent area at the apical portion of the third molar in need for extraction (D-group), while 96 (42.11%) patients did not present any relevant sign (C-group). In the entire cohort, the mean distance between the nearest portion of the root/roots to the buccal portion of the lingual cortical bone was −1.09 ± 1.5 mm. While 126 (55.26%) patients had impacted third molars with at least-1 mm of root in the lingual cortical plate, 102 (44.74%) had non-impacted third molars. The impaction of the root of 1 mm resulted more frequently with statistical significance (Odd ratio: 32.8) using Chi-square in the D-group (84.85%) compared to C-group (14.58%) as showed in Figure 2. Stratification of patients was performed according to a differential diagnosis observing both OPG and comparing the presence of the "Periapical Band-Like Radiolucent Sign" in the CBCT too:

- True sign (Y-sign): the pre-operative OPG shows a band-like radiolucent sign corresponding to the apical portion of the root of the inferior third molar with no sign of other reason that could explain this. On CBCT image lingual impaction of the root is observed.
- False sign (F-sign): OPG image shows a band-like radiolucent area corresponding to the apical portion of the root of the inferior third molar and determining causes of the radiolucent area visible on OPG and CBCT such as Juxta-Apical Radio-Translucency, peri-apical lesion, immature apex, impaction of the inferior alveolar nerve into the lingual plate, apex impaction into the buccal plate.

Table 1. demographic and clinical characteristics of D-group vs. C-group patients. N = number, SD = standard deviation, Sig = statistical significance using Chi-square and One-way ANOVA. *= p value with significance level.

	C-Group (N = 96)	D-Group (N = 132)	Total (N = 228)	Sig.
Age (mean ± SD)	30.53 ± 0.5	30.43 ± 0.5	30.47 ± 0.5	0.14
Gender (Female/Male)	52/44	56/76	108/120	0.47
Side (Left/Right)	47/39	81/61	128/100	0.17
Impaction <−1 mm (Yes/Tot.)	14/96 14.58%	112/132 84.85%	126/208 60.58%	<0.001 *
Radiolucency due to a pathology/non-pathology	/	11/121		
Juxta-apical Radiolucency (JAR)	/	4/132		
Inferior Alveolar Nerve (IAN) impaction	/	10/132		

The most frequent reasons for extraction were pericoronitis with or without resorption on the adjacent lower second molar (75%), caries of the wisdom tooth (13.6%), and caries of the lower second molar (9.2%).

As reported in Table 2, the mean distance between the root and cortical bone was not significantly different between male and female patients, left side and right side of mandibula. One-way ANOVA test revealed that there was a highly significant difference in mean distance between D-group (−1.89 ± 1.26 mm) and C-group (0 ± 1.6 mm) with $p < 0.001$. Analyzing CBCT, within D-group, the dark area was related to pathology in 11 cases (subgroup Yes-pathology), no sign of pathology in 121 cases (subgroup No-pathology). Four cases within No-pathology were false Y-sign because they had juxta-apical radiolucency (JAR) and in ten CBCT an Inferior Alveolar Nerve (IAN) impaction was observed.

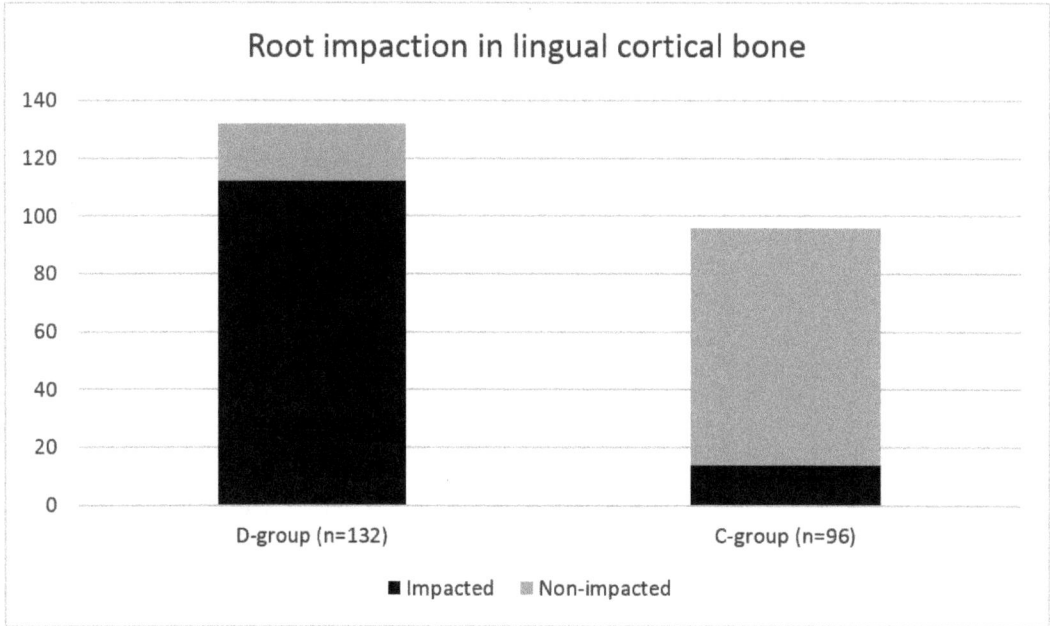

Figure 2. A graphic representation of the distribution of patients with impaction of the root in the lingual cortical bone of at least 1 mm (in black) in D-group (84.85%, 112/132) and C-group (14.58%, 14/96).

Table 2. Mean distance across the study groups. SD = standard deviation, Sig = statistical significance using One-way ANOVA and T-test. *= p value with significance level.

	Mean Distance (Mean ± SD) in Millimeter		Sig.
Total Group (n = 228)	−1.09 ± 1.5 mm		
Group	C-group (0 ± 1.6) (n = 96)	D-group (−1.89 ± 1.26) (n = 132)	<0.001 *
Pathological Sign in D-group	Yes (−0.22 ± 1.54 mm) (n = 11)	No (−2.04 ± 1.12) (n = 121)	<0.001 *
Juxta-apical Radiolucency (JAR)		(0.77 ± 0.84 mm) (n = 4)	Not detectable
Inferior Alveolar Nerve (IAN) impaction		(0.81 ± 0.44 mm) (n = 10)	Not detectable

Within D-group (n = 132), the difference between patients without pathological signs (n = 121, −2.04 ± 1.12 mm) and patients with pathological signs (n = 11, −0.22 ± 1.54 mm) was statistically significant p< 0.001 in term of mean distance. In D-group, the impaction of the root of 1 mm resulted more frequently in the No-Pathology group (110/121; 90.91%) compared to the Yes-Pathology group (2/11; 18.18%) with no statistical significance using Chi-square because of the short sample of patients with pathology in D-group.

Similarly, there was an important difference between False Y-sign due to IAN-impaction (n = 10, 0.81 ± 0.44 mm) or to JAR (n = 4, 0.77 ± 0.84 mm) compared to D-group, but it was not possible to statistically compare these subgroups due to the short samples. Within the D-group, 112 (84.84%) patients had true Y-sign, corresponding to the same value of tooth impacted in the lingual plate (2 patients belong to subgroup Yes-pathology group).

4. Discussion

If the OPG is interpreted correctly, numerous signs may help clinicians to predict the wisdom tooth position decreasing the risk of injury to the IAN. Sometimes, the signs are confirmed by CBCT and the risk of complications during or after surgery is too high so that a coronectomy technique is recommended [16,17].

Complications after third molar extractions are reported to be more frequent than complications for other teeth extractions, particularly for wound infection and loss of sensibility [18].

A correct pre-surgical planning and a proper knowledge of the teeth's' position and its contact with other anatomic structures could prevent these complications reducing the incidence, particularly of nerve damage, for these reasons CBCT may help surgeons because it is a [19,20].

When the third molar root is impacted into the cortical portion of the lingual side of the inferior jaw, the incidence of complications may increase such as the lingual nerve could be damaged, the portion of the root impacted in the bone could fracture and/or even the lingual cortical bone may fracture [21]. According to the results of the present study, the root is more frequently positioned near the lingual portion of the bone or in direct contact with it when the OPG shows a band like radiolucent area corresponding to the apical portion of the inferior third molar root with an odds ratio of 32.8 (Figure 3) confuting the null hypothesis proposed. The distance between these two structures in the control group is in line with other studies [12,22,23].

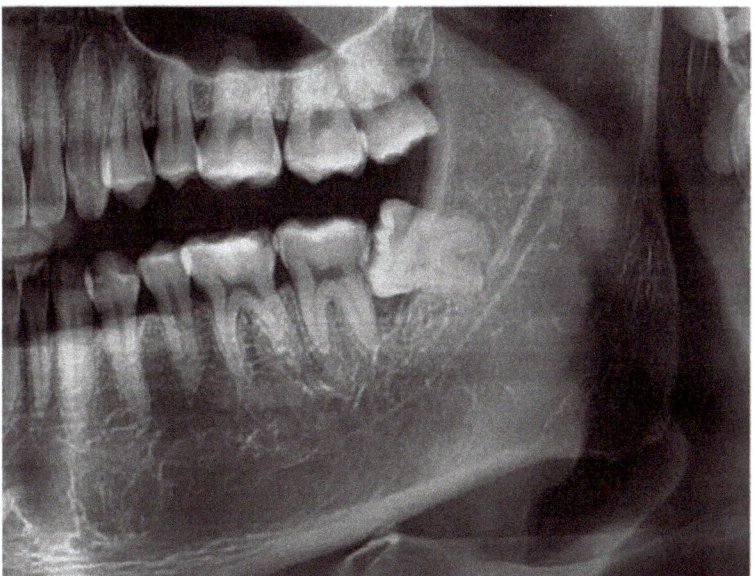

Figure 3. Patient 1801222 with a Y-sign corresponding to wisdom tooth 3.8 in the OPG.

Still, a radiolucent area does not always correspond to the proximity between root and cortical lingual bone. For these reasons, CBCT may be useful to verify the anatomic position of the third molar (Figure 4). The stratification of patients in the D-group (with a dark sign in OPG) was performed using CBCT to make a differential diagnosis and help clinicians to have as much information as possible OPG classifying subjects with no sign of pathologies that could explain the radiolucent area in the apical portion of the root of the inferior wisdom tooth, and subjects with possible pathologies.

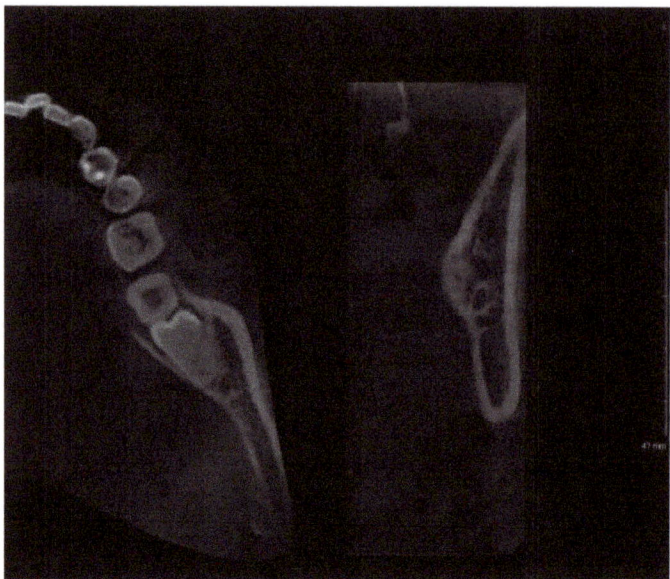

Figure 4. Patient 1801222, the CBCT confirms the nearness of the root of the wisdom tooth with the lingual cortical plate with an impaction of −1 mm. Axial plan on the left and cross-section plan on the right.

This radiolucency in "Y-sign" occurs because if the third molar root is positioned in proximity with the cortical bone, in fact, we could name this sign as "Periapical Band-Like Radiolucent Sign" possible due to its periodontal ligament impacts the lingual plate and the bone in that slight area resorbs. When this is visible in OPG, the probability to have a closeness between root and lingual cortical bone is extremely high.

After the stratification of the D-group according to the presence of Pathology (Yes) or not (No), the results significantly showed that, in 90.91% of suspected dark areas, third molar roots are close to the lingual cortical bone if there are no other pathologies. When the periapical band-like radiolucent sign is identified in OPG, there are useful clinical implications, instead, a dark area in OPG usually can also represent a pathology of the tooth or surrounding tissue.

There are other OPG signs reported in the literature strongly associated with nerve damages and surgical risks such as JAR; Peri-apical lesion; Immature apex; Inferior Alveolar Nerve (IAN) impaction into the lingual plate; apex impaction into the buccal plate [24]. This last case is reported to be very similar in OPG because it interests the buccal cortical bone, but it was not evidenced in CBCT in the present study in 228 patients, so that may be extremely rare. In some cases, the pathology is evident, and the differential diagnosis of Y-sign must be done with JAR translucency and IAN impaction.

JAR is a radiolucent area positioned laterally to the root or the apex of inferior third molars [25]. This radiological aspect of bone has been reported to be related to a variation of trabecular bone, or an ectasia of periodontal ligament and its relations with surrounding structures using CBCT.

Clinical studies showed a significant relationship between the JAR and the mandibular canal, but it is most commonly detected superiorly to the mandibular canal (59% of cases). It is reported to be mostly mesial to the tooth (43%) and above the third molars (55%), extremely rare lingual to the tooth (3%), and at the disto-angular third molar (3%) ($p = 0.005$) [26].

In these last cases, it could be misunderstood with "Y-sign" which is mostly an apical radiolucency and without pathologies. The presence of pathology is one other important variable in the differential diagnosis because this sign could be misinterpreted as a periapical lesion. Some authors reported the diagnostic accuracy of OPG and CBCT for the detection of apical periodontal lesions, even though clinical confirmation is always needed [27].

Of 249 OPG meeting the inclusion criteria of this study, twenty-one were excluded due to radiological artifacts and exclusion criteria, this aspect could be one limitation of the present analysis that makes this retrospective study less exploitable in daily practice.

One other limitation of the present study could be that the cut-off points of −1 mm were a merely clinical decision because less impaction is not a surgical risk, and it could be no appreciable in OPG. Future studies could change the results of Y-sign if the definition of impaction is different. Moreover, in the D-group the stratification Yes (pathology) and No (no pathologies) showed that in some cases also pathological teeth could be strictly near to the lingual plate and have the "Y-sign" too and it may be difficult to highlight the sign. The dark sign seems to be strongly associated with the root impaction on the lingual cortical bone, but the absence of any dark sign could bring to a false negative because in 14.58% of C-group cases there was a nearness between these two structures.

The present study highlighted the importance of evaluating all radiological signs in OPG, a tool particularly useful for making diagnoses and reducing the use of CBCT and, in line with previous studies when there are these radiolucent signs of uncertain causes (JAR, or this sign proposed), a CBCT is the only instrumental examination for dental surgeons to analyze wisdom tooth position OPG [28,29].

In some countries, it could be a medical-legal issue to not require the CBCT in case of doubts before third molars extraction, especially if complications occur. In other countries, the CBCT is not mandatory for dental implant placement in mandible or wisdom tooth extraction [30].

Nevertheless, for general dentists, the CBCT may be still more difficult to be read than the OPG, CBCT has a higher radiation dose, it is more expensive, and not all dental clinics are equipped to offer this service. Each time a patient receives has a radiological exam carried out, millions of photons transit through the body and may bring a series of reactions that in some cases can be very dangerous. Before performing any OPG/CBCT, the relationship between risk to the patients and potential benefit must be taken into account. These findings may be useful for new guidelines to reduce CBCT prescription in inferior third molar surgery planning considering the previously mentioned principles of justification and optimization, respectively.

5. Conclusions

A new periapical band-like radiolucent sign in OPG seems to be associated with the proximity of the mandibular third molar root to the lingual cortical bone. This sign could help clinicians in the decision-making process to prescribe or not a CBCT exam to predict the real position of wisdom teeth in space and anatomic rapport. Other prospective clinical studies with larger examples are needed to confute this finding.

Author Contributions: Conceptualization, S.C. and Y.-S.K.; methodology, S.C. and Y.-M.P.; software, Y.-M.P. and Y.-S.K.; validation, S.M. and U.C.; formal analysis, A.R. and Y.-M.P.; investigation, Y.-S.K. and Y.-M.P.; Surgery Y.-S.K.; resources, A.R. and Y.-S.K.; data curation, Y.-M.P. and A.R.; writing—original draft preparation, S.C. and Y.-M.P.; writing—review and editing, S.C. and E.G.; visualization, E.G. and S.M.; supervision, U.C.; project administration, S.M.; funding acquisition, Y.-S.K. All authors have read and agreed to the published version of the manuscript.

Funding: This research was supported by Tuscan Stomatologic Institute and Young Sam Kim. The work of A.R. was supported by Masaryk University grants: MUNI/IGA/1543/2020 and MUNI/A/1608/2020.

Institutional Review Board Statement: The study was conducted according to the guidelines of the Declaration of Helsinki. This is a monocentric retrospective comparative study approved by the Gangnam Academy of Wisdom tooth Extraction (GAWE).

Informed Consent Statement: Written informed consent was obtained from all subjects involved in the study to analyze retrospectively the radiographs. Written informed consent has been obtained from the patient(s) to publish this paper.

Data Availability Statement: Restrictions apply to the availability of these data. Data was obtained from [third party] and are available [from the authors / at URL] with the permission of [third party].

Acknowledgments: The authors would like to acknowledge "Istituto Stomatologico Toscano" and its director Ugo Covani, who allowed this study, setting this international team and the Young Sam Kim to have this large number of cases of wisdom teeth.

Conflicts of Interest: The authors declare no conflict of interest.

Abbreviations

CBCT	Cone-Beam Computed Tomography
ESSE	Easy Simple Safe Efficient
GAWE	Gangnam Academy of Wisdom tooth Extraction
IAN	Inferior Alveolar Nerve
JAR	Juxta-Apical Radiolucency
MR	Magnetic resonance
NICE	National Institute for Health and Care Excellence
OAC	Oroantral Communication
OPG	Orthopantomography
OR	Odds Ratio
SD	Standard Deviation
Y-sign	Periapical band-like radiolucent sign introduced by Young Sam Kim

References

1. Barraclough, J.; Power, A.; Pattni, A. Treatment planning for mandibular third molars. *Dent. Updat.* **2017**, *44*, 221–228. [CrossRef] [PubMed]
2. Kim, Y.S. *Extraction of Third Molars: Easy Simple Safe Efficient Minimally Invasive & Atraumatic*; Koonja Publishing Inc.: Seoul, Korea, 2018.
3. Dodson, T.B.; Susarla, S.M. Impacted wisdom teeth. *BMJ Clin. Evid.* **2014**, *2014*, 1302. [PubMed]
4. Rozkovcová, E.; Marková, M.; Dolejší, J. Studies on agenesis of third molars amongst populations of different origin. *Sb. Lek.* **1999**, *100*, 71–84.
5. Worrall, S.; Riden, K.; Haskell, R.; Corrigan, A. UK National Third Molar project: The initial report. *Br. J. Oral Maxillofac. Surg.* **1998**, *36*, 14–18. [CrossRef]
6. De Bruyn, L.; Vranckx, M.; Jacobs, R.; Politis, C. A retrospective cohort study on reasons to retain third molars. *Int. J. Oral Maxillofac. Surg.* **2020**, *49*, 816–821. [CrossRef]
7. Derindağ, G.; Sarica, I.; Kurtuldu, E.; Naralan, M.E.; Caglayan, F. A retrospective study: Do all impacted teeth cause pathology? *Niger. J. Clin. Pr.* **2019**, *22*, 527–533. [CrossRef] [PubMed]
8. Di Dino, B. *Atlas of Cone Beam: Volumetric 3d Images: Safety in Implantology and General Dentistry*; BDD: Monsumano Terme–Pistoia, Italy, 2011; pp. 1–275.
9. Rood, J.; Shehab, B.N. The radiological prediction of inferior alveolar nerve injury during third molar surgery. *Br. J. Oral Maxillofac. Surg.* **1990**, *28*, 20–25. [CrossRef]
10. Renton, T.; Hankins, M.; Sproate, C.; McGurk, M. A randomised controlled clinical trial to compare the incidence of injury to the inferior alveolar nerve as a result of coronectomy and removal of mandibular third molars. *Br. J. Oral Maxillofac. Surg.* **2005**, *43*, 7–12. [CrossRef] [PubMed]
11. Jung, Y.-H.; Cho, B.-H. Radiographic evaluation of third molar development in 6- to 24-year-olds. *Imaging Sci. Dent.* **2014**, *44*, 185–191. [CrossRef] [PubMed]
12. Vidya, K.C.; Mallik, A.; Waran, A.; Rout, S.K. Measurement of lingual cortical plate thickness and lingual position of lower third molar roots using cone beam computed tomography. *J. Int. Soc. Prev. Community Dent.* **2017**, *7*, S8–S12. [CrossRef]
13. Steed, M.B. The indications for third-molar extractions. *J. Am. Dent. Assoc.* **2014**, *145*, 570–573. [CrossRef] [PubMed]
14. Feragalli, B.; Rampado, O.; Abate, C.; Festa, F.; Stromei, F.; Caputi, S.; Guglielmi, G.; Macrì, M. Cone beam computed tomography for dental and maxillofacial imaging: Technique improvement and low-dose protocols. *La Radiol. medica* **2017**, *122*, 581–588. [CrossRef] [PubMed]
15. Stacchi, C.; Daugela, P.; Berton, F.; Lombardi, T.; Andriulionis, T.; Perinetti, G.; Di Lenarda, R.; Juodžbalys, G. A classification for assessing surgical difficulty in the extraction of mandibular impacted third molars: Description and clinical validation. *Quintessence Int.* **2018**, *49*, 745–753. [PubMed]

16. Cosola, S.; Kim, Y.; Park, Y.; Giammarinaro, E.; Covani, U. Coronectomy of Mandibular Third Molar: Four Years of Follow-Up of 130 Cases. *Med.* **2020**, *56*, 654. [CrossRef]
17. Cervera-Espert, J.; Pérez-Martínez, S.; Cervera-Ballester, J.; Peñarrocha-Oltra, D.; Peñarrocha-Diago, M. Coronectomy of impacted mandibular third molars: A meta-analysis and systematic review of the literature. *Med. Oral Patol. Oral Cir. Bucal* **2016**, *21*, e505–e513. [CrossRef]
18. Miclotte, I.; Agbaje, J.; Spaey, Y.; Legrand, P.; Politis, C. Incidence and treatment of complications in patients who had third molars or other teeth extracted. *Br. J. Oral Maxillofac. Surg.* **2018**, *56*, 388–393. [CrossRef]
19. Harada, N.; Vasudeva, S.; Joshi, R.; Seki, K.; Araki, K.; Matsuda, Y.; Okano, T. Correlation between panoramic radiographic signs and high-risk anatomical factors for impacted mandibular third molars. *Oral Surg.* **2013**, *6*, 129–136. [CrossRef]
20. Glera-Suárez, P.; Soto, D.; Peñarrocha-Oltra, D.; Peñarrocha-Diago, M. Patient morbidity after impacted third molar extraction with different flap designs. A systematic review and meta-analysis. *Medicina Oral Patología Oral y Cirugia Bucal* **2020**, *25*, e233–e239. [CrossRef]
21. Aydın, Z.U.; Bulut, D.G. Relationship between the anatomic structures and mandibular posterior teeth for endodontic surgery in a Turkish population: A cone-beam computed tomographic analysis. *Clin. Oral Investig.* **2019**, *23*, 3637–3644. [CrossRef] [PubMed]
22. Kim, S.-Y.; Yang, S.-E. Cone-Beam Computed Tomography Study of Incidence of Distolingual Root and Distance from Distolingual Canal to Buccal Cortical Bone of Mandibular First Molars in a Korean Population. *J. Endod.* **2012**, *38*, 301–304. [CrossRef] [PubMed]
23. Zhang, X.; Xu, N.; Wang, H.; Yu, Q. A Cone-beam Computed Tomographic Study of Apical Surgery–related Morphological Characteristics of the Distolingual Root in 3-rooted Mandibular First Molars in a Chinese Population. *J. Endod.* **2017**, *43*, 2020–2024. [CrossRef] [PubMed]
24. Nascimento, E.H.L.; Oenning, A.C.C.; Nadaes, M.R.; Ambrosano, G.M.B.; Haiter-Neto, F.; Freitas, D.Q. Juxta-apical radiolucency: Relation to the mandibular canal and cortical plates based on cone beam CT imaging. *Oral Surgery, Oral Med. Oral Pathol. Oral Radiol.* **2017**, *123*, 401–407. [CrossRef] [PubMed]
25. Nascimento, E.H.L.; Oenning, A.C.C.; Nadaes, M.R.; Ambrosano, G.M.B.; Haiter-Neto, F.; Freitas, D.Q. Juxta-Apical Radiolucency: Prevalence, Characterization, and Association With the Third Molar Status. *J. Oral Maxillofac. Surg.* **2018**, *76*, 716–724. [CrossRef] [PubMed]
26. Yalcin, E.; Artas, A. Juxta-apical radiolucency and relations with surrounding structures on cone-beam computed tomography. *Br. J. Oral Maxillofac. Surg.* **2020**, *58*, 309–313. [CrossRef] [PubMed]
27. Nardi, C.; Calistri, L.; Pradella, S.; Desideri, I.; Lorini, C.; Colagrande, S. Accuracy of Orthopantomography for Apical Periodontitis without Endodontic Treatment. *J. Endod.* **2017**, *43*, 1640–1646. [CrossRef] [PubMed]
28. Nardi, C.; Talamonti, C.; Pallotta, S.; Saletti, P.; Calistri, L.; Cordopatri, C.; Colagrande, S. Head and neck effective dose and quantitative assessment of image quality: A study to compare cone beam CT and multislice spiral CT. *Dentomaxillofacial Radiol.* **2017**, *46*, 20170030. [CrossRef] [PubMed]
29. Nascimento, E.H.L.; Oenning, A.C.C.; Freire, B.B.; Gaêta-Araujo, H.; Haiter-Neto, F.; Freitas, D.Q. Comparison of panoramic radiography and cone beam CT in the assessment of juxta-apical radiolucency. *Dentomaxillofacial Radiol.* **2018**, *47*, 20170198. [CrossRef] [PubMed]
30. Luangchana, P.; Pornprasertsuk-Damrongsri, S.; Kiattavorncharoen, S.; Jirajariyavej, B. Accuracy of linear measurements using cone beam computed tomography and panoramic radiography in dental implant treatment planning. *Int. J. Oral Maxillofac. Implant.* **2015**, *30*, 1287–1294. [CrossRef] [PubMed]

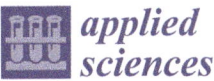 **applied sciences** MDPI

Article

Healing Capacity of Bone Surrounding Biofilm-Infected and Non-Infected Gutta-Percha: A Study of Rat Calvaria

Daniel Moreinos [1,2,†], Ronald Wigler [3,†], Yuval Geffen [4], Sharon Akrish [5] and Shaul Lin [1,2,6,*]

1. Endodontics and Dental Trauma Department, School of Graduate Dentistry, Rambam Health Care Campus, P.O. Box 9602, Haifa 3109601, Israel; d_moreinos@rambam.health.gov.il
2. Ruth and Bruce Rappaport Faculty of Medicine, Israel Institute of Technology—Technion, Haifa 3525433, Israel
3. Department of Endodontology, The Goldschleger School of Dental Medicine, Tel Aviv University, Tel Aviv 6100000, Israel; dr.wigler@gmail.com
4. Department of Pathology, Rambam Health Care Campus, Haifa 3500000, Israel; y_geffen@rambam.health.gov.il
5. Clinical Microbiology Laboratory, Rambam Health Care Campus, Haifa 3500000, Israel; s_akrish@rambam.health.gov.il
6. The Israeli National Center for Trauma and Emergency Medicine Research Gertner Institute, Tel Hashomer 5262000, Israel
* Correspondence: sh_lin@rambam.health.gov.il; Tel.: +972-4-8370752
† Equal contribution.

Featured Application: It has been suggested that some root canal treatments fail because of non-microbial factors, including extruded root canal filling materials, which may cause a reaction to a foreign body. This study shows that overextension of sealing material, without other clinical or roentgen signs or symptoms, should not be considered an indication for endodontic surgery.

Abstract: This paper aims to evaluate the healing capacity of bony lesions around biofilm-infected and non-infected gutta-percha (GP) points. Bony defects were created in the calvaria of 28 Wistar rats. The rats were divided into three groups: Group 1—Implantation of infected GP particles in the bony defect; Group 2—Positive control implantation of non-infected GP particles in the bony defect; and Group 3—Negative control, in which no GP particles were implanted. The biofilm consisted of three strains of bacteria: Enterococcus faecalis, Streptococcus sanguis, and Porphyromonas gingivalis. The animals were sacrificed 60 days postoperation, and histological assessments were performed. In Group 1, the biofilm-infected group, we observed a mild foreign body reaction with a few inflammatory cells adjacent to the capsule and a newly woven bone matrix surrounded by osteoblasts and mature bone. In Group 2, the non-infected GP particles group, minimal inflammatory cell reactions were observed in the adjacent tissue, and a newly woven bone matrix was surrounded by osteoblasts. This study shows that bone healing is possible around both sterile and infected GP points. This contradicts the claim that some root canal treatments fail because of non-microbial factors, including extruded root canal filling materials, which may cause foreign body reactions. The healing observed suggests that overextension should not be considered an indication for endodontic surgery.

Keywords: biofilm; bone healing capacity; infected gutta-percha; rat calvarium

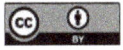

1. Introduction

Gutta-percha (GP) is the most popular root canal filling material [1]. The widely held view that GP has low toxicity and is therefore well tolerated by human tissues is inconsistent with the observations of outcome studies in which extruded GP is associated with the delayed healing of apical tissues [2–6]. According to Ng et al. (2008), the presence of the apical extent of root filling is a significant prognostic factor of endodontic treatment success [2].

There is consensus that microorganisms, mainly bacteria, cause primary apical periodontitis, but the reasons for persistent apical periodontitis lesions are debatable [7,8]. Secondary factors, such as foreign material in the periapical area of a tooth with apical periodontitis, may contribute to additional irritation and/or inflammatory reactions [8]. Nair (2008) claimed that extruded root canal filling might cause a foreign body reaction [9], but Haapasalo et al. (2008) suggested that a primary role for such factors, without the continued presence of bacteria, is lacking [8].

It has been suggested that this adverse effect (i.e., the foreign body reaction) could be a result of over-instrumentation and the subsequent transportation of contaminated debris periapically [10–12]. Siqueira (2001) stated that failure associated with overfilled teeth is usually caused by a concomitant intraradicular and/or extraradicular infection [10]. Over-instrumentation usually precedes overfilling and induces the displacement of infected debris into apical tissues in teeth with infected necrotic pulps [10–13].

The prevention of contamination becomes a problem when GP cones are used since this material does not readily lend itself to sterilization by moist or dry heat [14]. A one-minute immersion in 5.25% sodium hypochlorite may be used in clinical practice to sterilize GP cones and avoid this possible source of exogenous contamination [15]. Bacteria adherent to GP and growing as a biofilm may play a role in the delayed healing of apical tissues, but few studies have examined the biofilm potential on GP points as a cause for persistent apical periodontitis after endodontic treatment [16,17].

This study aimed to examine the healing capacity of bony lesions around biofilm-infected and non-infected GP points in a rat calvaria model. Our main hypothesis was that biofilm and GP would induce bone destruction, whereas bone defects alone would not.

2. Materials and Methods

2.1. Biofilm Culture on GP

GP points 40/0.04 (VDW GmbH, Munich, Germany) were sterilized with plasma gas (low-temperature hydrogen peroxide gas plasma, Kingsport, TN, USA) and divided into two groups:

Sterile GP points—The GP points were cut into 1 × 1 mm GP particles using a sterile scalpel (no. 11) and an endodontic ruler under 2.5× magnification (Orascoptic Inc., Madison, WI, USA).

Infected GP points—The formation of biofilm on GP points was carried out according to Takemura et al. (2004). Three strains of bacteria, i.e., *Enterococcus faecalis* (E.F.) ATCC 29212, *Streptococcus sanguis* (S.S.) ATCC 10556, and *Porphyromonas gingivalis* (P.G.) ATCC 33277, were cultured in equal amounts on GP points. The infected GP points were suspended in a growth medium containing varying percentages of human serum [14]. Each bacterial strain was harvested during the stationary phase, and 100 µL of each bacterial suspension was inoculated into 900 µL of cell culture medium, 900 µL of human serum (Biological Industries, Israel), or 900 µL of cell culture medium supplemented with 5% or 50% (vol/vol) human serum. Formalin fixation was performed at the end of the incubation process (Tissue-Tek ® O.C.T. ™ Compound, Sakura, The Netherlands). The GP points were sliced at 20–40 µm (Leica CM1900 Cryostat, Germany). Several segments were stained according to the Strathmann et al. (2002) protocol [15]. Briefly, extracellular polymeric substances (EPS) were stained red with concanavalin. A conjugate to tetramethyl rhodamine isothiocyanate (TRITC) was used as a marker for biofilm, and DNA-binding stain SYTO 9 (green color) was used to visualize live bacterial cells. Slices were observed under a laser scanning confocal microscope (Carl Zeiss CLSM (LSM 510 META) with an Apo 60 × 1.40 objective) to confirm the generated biofilm. Then, 3D depth images of the biofilm generated over the GP were taken (Figure 1).

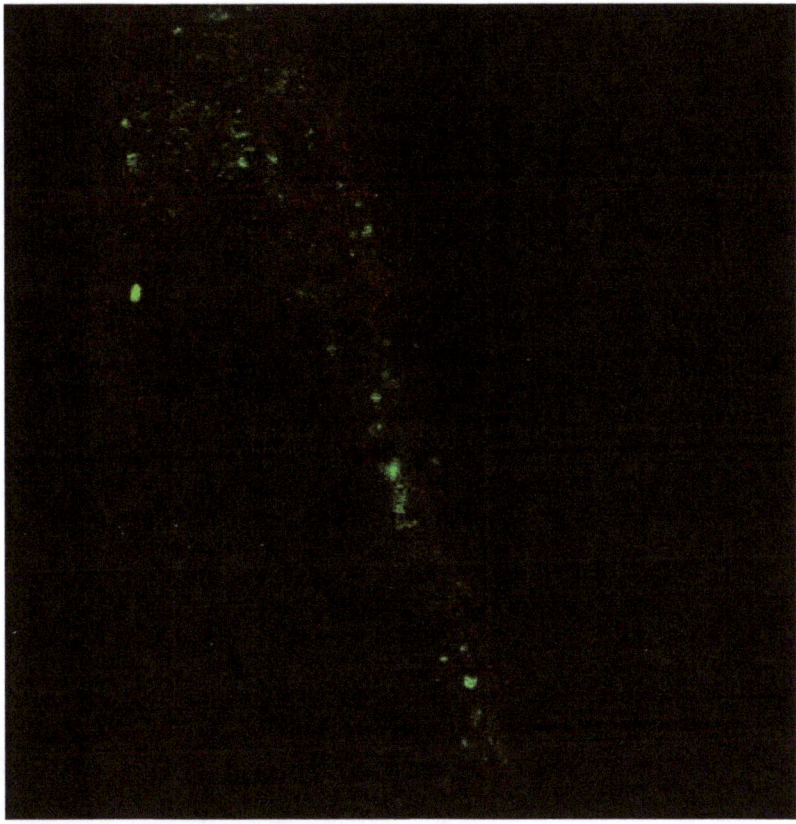

Figure 1. Confocal laser scanning microscopy image of bacteria and biofilm generated over a gutta-percha segment.

Non-infected and infected GP were incubated in primary fixative containing 2.5% GA and 2% PFA in 0.1 M sodium cacodylate buffer at pH 7.4 for 1 h at RT. Following washes in 0.1 M cacodylate buffer, the samples underwent a second fixation in 1% OsO4 for 20 min. The specimens were then dehydrated through a graded ethanol series, and the critical points were dried and coated with 10 nm chromium. A Zeiss ULTRA plus field emission scanning electron microscope was used to observe the samples (Figure 2A,B).

After slicing the infected GP points, several segments were transferred into 2 mL sterile tubes. The vials were then shaken on a Retsch MM401 bead mill for 2.5 min at 30 Hz. Aliquots of the bead-milled suspensions were collected and then inoculated into blood culture bottles. Additional aliquots were spread on blood agar plates and PolyViteX chocolate agar plates, both of which were incubated for 5 days at 37 °C in 5% CO_2 and at 37 °C in an anaerobic atmosphere. Isolated bacteria were identified according to standard laboratory procedures. In all cases, viable E.F., S.S., and P.G. isolates were recovered from the infected GP points. The remaining GP points were cut using the same technique as the sterile GP points.

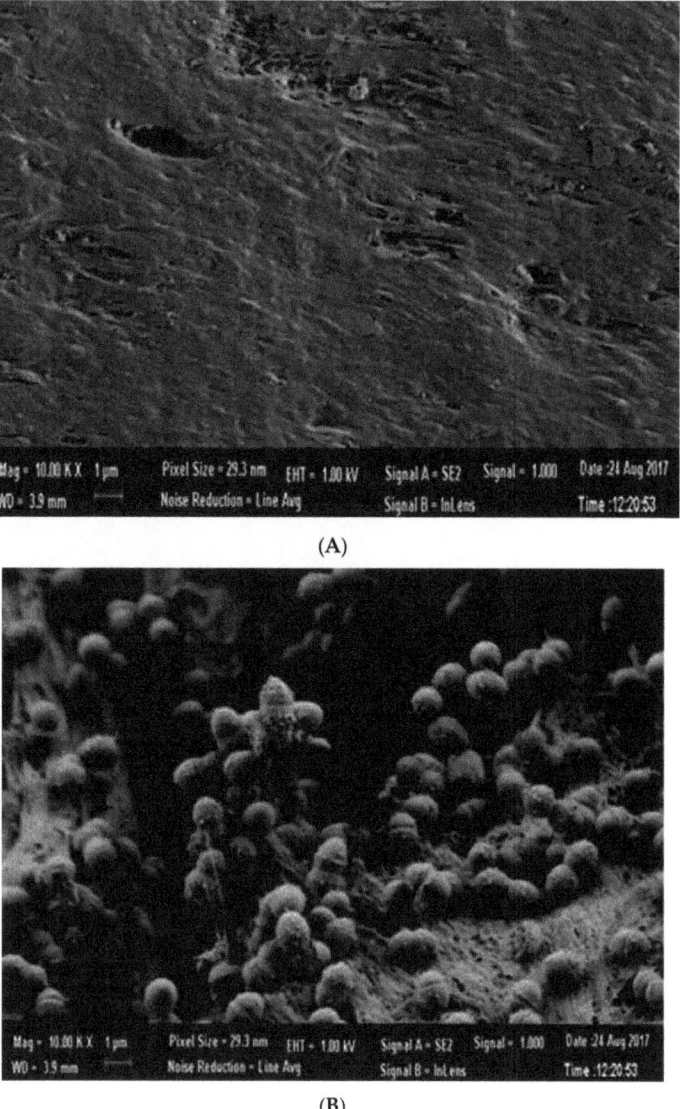

Figure 2. (**A**) Scanning electron microscope image of biofilm on infected GP. (**B**) Scanning electron microscope image of sterilized GP.

2.2. Animals and Surgery

The study consisted of 28 female, 8-month-old Wistar rats that were maintained in a room with a 12 h light/dark cycle. The animals had free access to tap water and standard laboratory food. The Animal Research Council approved this research (il-071-06-2009).

The rats were divided into 3 groups:

Group 1 (n = 12): Implantation of infected GP particles in the bony defects;

Group 2 (n = 12): Positive control group implantation of non-infected GP particles in the bony defects;

Group 3 (n = 4): Negative control group, in which no GP particles were implanted in the bony defects.

The animals were weighed and anesthetized with an intramuscular injection of ketamine chlorhydrate (90 mg/kg) and xylazine (2%** 10 mg/kg body weight), and then their heads were shaved.

A modification of Turnbull and Freeman's (1974) original surgical approach was used [18]. A U-shaped incision was made in the scalp between the eyebrows that caudally connected two sagittal incisions extending posteriorly over the parietal bone to enable the elevation of a full-thickness flap and expose the soft tissues covering the calvarium. The fascia overlying the bone was dissected to expose the periosteum (Figure 3). A high-speed, water-cooled, diamond wheel-shaped bur was used under 2.5× magnification (Orascoptic, Middleton, WI, USA) to create a bony defect measuring 3 mm in diameter and 1 mm in depth while avoiding damage to the dura mater or puncturing the sagittal sinus.

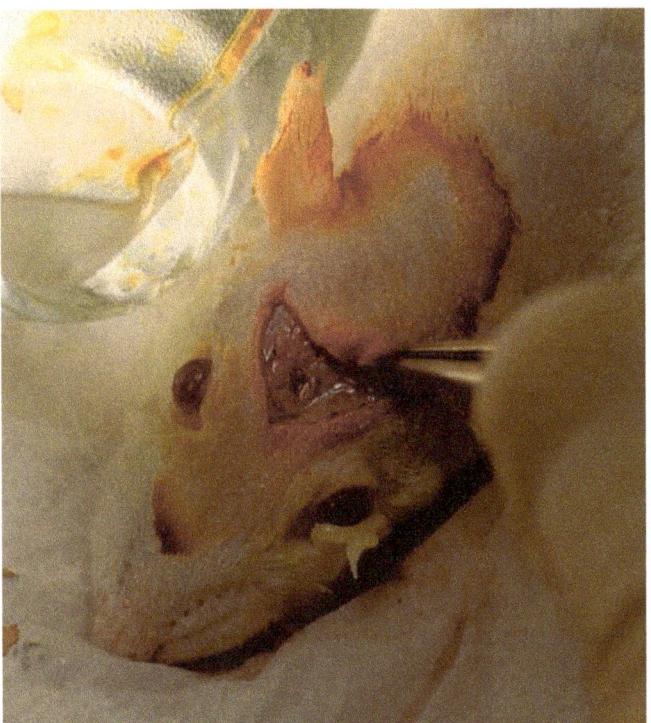

Figure 3. Intra-operative view of the rat caldarium operation.

Resorbable collagen membranes (4BONE Resorbable Collagen Membrane, MIS Implants Technologies Ltd., Bar Lev Industrial Park, Israel) were cut into 28 membrane discs (4 mm in diameter) and used to cover each bony defect.

The flaps were repositioned and sutured using 3–0 vicryl absorbable sterile surgical suture (Ethicon, Inc., Somerville, NJ, USA).

The animals were sacrificed at 60 days postoperation, then the calvariae were resected, fixed in 10% neutral buffered formalin, washed, dehydrated in ethanol and xylene, embedded in paraffin, and cut into transverse 5 mm sections. Sections were stained with hematoxylin and eosin (H&E) for examination under light microscopy.

The histological appearance was assessed regarding the degree and type of inflammation and the thickness of the connective tissue capsule surrounding GP particles.

The level of inflammation was classified as none/mild or moderate/severe, with the former describing an absence of inflammation or scattered inflammatory cells surrounding the particles. An intense concentration of inflammatory cells indicated a moderate/severe reaction to the GP particles. The inflammation types were defined as acute or chronic. Acute inflammation represented a predominance of polymorphonuclear leukocytes with few chronic inflammatory cells (e.g., macrophages, lymphocytes, or plasma cells), and chronic inflammation consisted of a predominance of chronic inflammatory cells with few polymorphonuclear neutrophils.

3. Results

3.1. Control (n = 4)

No remnants of the resorbable collagen membranes were found at the surgical site at 60 days. Fibrous connective tissue containing fibroblasts and blood vessels, a few inflammatory cells, and a newly woven bone matrix surrounded by osteoblasts were noted.

3.2. Non-Infected GP Points (n = 12)

No remnants of the resorbable collagen membranes were found at the surgical site at 60 days. The GP particles were surrounded by a fine thin fibrous capsule, fibroblasts, and a few chronic inflammatory cells. In adjacent tissues, minimal inflammatory cell reactions were observed. In some specimens, a newly woven bone matrix surrounded by osteoblasts was noted, similar to findings in the control group (Figure 4).

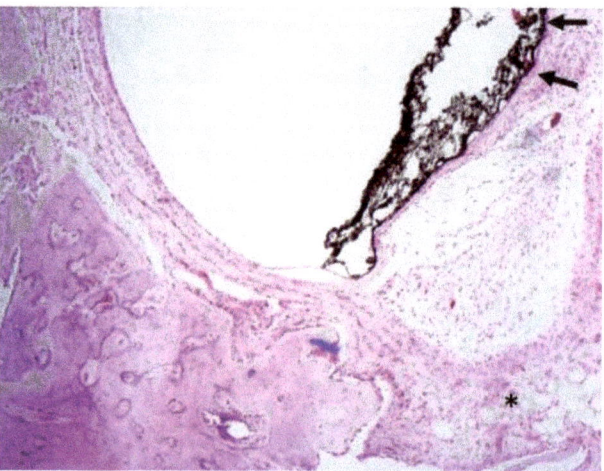

Figure 4. Histologic micrograph showing foreign material surrounded by a thin fibrous connective tissue capsule (arrows) and mild chronic inflammatory cell infiltrate composed primarily of lymphocytes (asterisk).

A newly woven bone matrix surrounded by active osteoblasts was also noted. H&E: hematoxylin & eosin stain, ×100.

3.3. Infected GP Points (n = 12)

No remnants of the resorbable collagen membranes were found at the surgical site at 60 days. Two rats in Group 1 were excluded from the experiment. Adjacent to the capsule, a mild foreign body reaction with a few inflammatory cells was noted. In some specimens, a newly woven bone matrix surrounded by osteoblasts and mature bone was observed at 60 days (n = 10) (Figures 5 and 6).

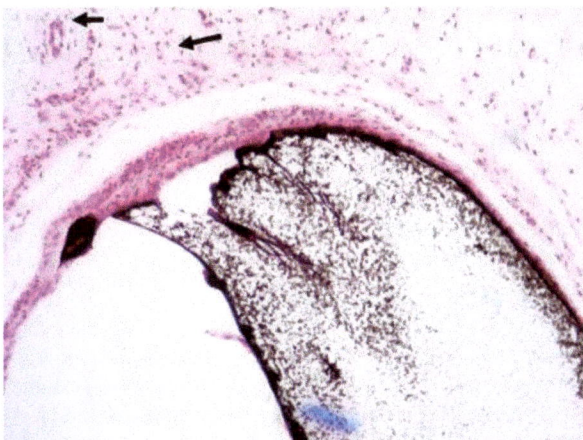

Figure 5. Histologic micrograph of foreign material surrounded by a thin fibrous connective tissue capsule. The matrix contained mild inflammatory cell infiltrate composed primarily of lymphocytes and few scattered small blood vessels (arrows). H&E: hematoxylin & eosin stain, ×200.

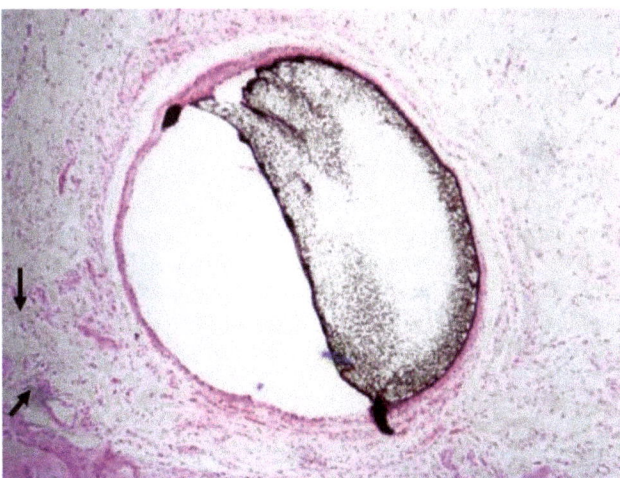

Figure 6. Magnified view showing mild inflammatory cell infiltrate composed primarily of lymphocytes and few scattered small blood vessels (arrows). H&E: hematoxylin & eosin stain, ×200.

4. Discussion

Previous studies have shown that foreign bodies, such as GP (infected and noninfected), prevent wound healing and bone formation [19]. The aim of this pilot study was to test the hypothesis that biofilm and GP would induce bone destruction, whereas bone defects alone would not, using a rat calvarium model known in periodontology for its ability to show bone formation [20,21]. To the best of our knowledge, this is the first study testing this hypothesis using the methodology described above.

Root canal treatment aims to eliminate infection from the root canal and prevent reinfection by filling the root [22]. Despite the highest standards of care, some cases still result in failure due to persistent or secondary intraradicular infection or extraradicular infection [10]. It has been claimed that failures in other cases are due to non-microbial factors, such as extruded root canal filling materials; this may cause a foreign body reaction [10,23].

Contrary to our hypotheses, GP, per se, did not cause bone destruction at the calvaria, and surprisingly, biofilm-infected GP also did not cause bone destruction. Likewise, a mild inflammatory reaction was observed in the adjacent tissue in the non-infected group, and a newly woven bone matrix surrounded by osteoblasts was noted in some specimens. In the infected group, a mild foreign body reaction with a few inflammatory cells was observed adjacent to the capsule. A newly woven bone matrix surrounded by osteoblasts and mature bone was detected at 60 days.

GP points consist of approximately 65% zinc oxide, 20% GP, 10% radiopacifiers, and 5% plasticizers [24]. Wolfson and Seltzer (1975) studied the reaction of rat connective tissue to some formulations of GP in common use for up to 64 days and noticed that most of the specimens initially showed an acute response, followed by fibrous tissue encapsulation [25].

Sjogren et al. (1995) claimed that the size of the GP particles determines how the tissues react to the material [26]. These investigators studied the tissue reaction to various GP sizes subcutaneously implanted in guinea pigs and found that large particles (1–2 mm in size) were well encapsulated while the surrounding tissue was free of inflammation [26]. However, fine particles (50–100 µm in size) evoked an intense, localized tissue response characterized by the presence of macrophages and multinucleated giant cells [25]. Nair (2008) claimed that GP particles in apical tissue might gradually fragment into fine particles that induce a foreign body reaction [8]. In this research, we used a rat calvarium model, which is known in periodontology for its ability to evaluate bone formation [20,21]. The aim was to assess the ability of a foreign body, such as GP (infected and non-infected), in preventing wound healing and bone formation. GP, per se, did not cause bone destruction at the calvaria, but more surprisingly, infected GP with biofilm was also incapable of causing bone destruction. It seems this biofilm alone could not cause bone destruction unless there is a connection between the infected root and the periapical lesion. "It is possible that other types of bacteria are capable of causing such isolated infection; the independent extraradicular infection probably does not occur often and is usually associated with apical actinomycosis" [27]. Further research is warranted regarding GP fragmentation into fine particles in apical tissues and the response of apical tissues to fine particles.

The connection, or lack thereof, between the presence of GP particles in apical tissues and biofilm accumulation on GP points has not been sufficiently studied. Outcome studies showing associations between extruded GP and delayed apical tissue healing do not refer to this issue [2–6]. However, some studies state that over-instrumentation and apical transportation of contaminated debris might cause this adverse effect [2,10–12]. This might also be the result of an unusual root apex form or apical zipping that might leave residual bacteria around the apex.

The most common cause of failure is persistent intraradicular infection. Therefore, retreating failed teeth prior to surgery is recommended to exclude this possibility [10]. Retreatment of a failed root canal treatment requires the complete removal of the root canal filling. Poorly condensed GP fillings can be easily removed, but GP fragments may remain in the periapical tissue during attempts to remove overextended fillings [28]. Our findings suggest that healing was noticed in the non-infected and infected groups, even when GP particles remained in the apical tissue. Therefore, clinicians should not initiate surgical procedures as long as the tooth is functional, with no radiographic evidence of enlargement of apical rarefication. Note that the biofilm in this study was formed by two strains of Gram-positive facultative anaerobic bacteria (E.F. and S.S.) and one Gram-negative anaerobic bacterium (P.G.) that were capable of colonizing and forming extracellular matrices on GP. To the best of our knowledge, this is the first study on the biofilm-forming ability of these species on GP points. E.F. is the most frequently isolated strain from root-filled teeth with apical periodontitis [29]. Few species can overcome host defense mechanisms, flourish in the inflamed periapical tissues, and establish an extraradicular infection. Actinomyces and

Propionibacterium propionicum participate in extraradicular infections that cause apical actinomycosis, which can be successfully treated only by periapical surgery [30–32].

Earlier studies suggested that some root canal treatments fail because of non-microbial factors, such as extruded root canal filling materials, which may cause foreign body reactions. In this study, healing was noticed in both the non-infected and infected groups, suggesting that overextension should not be considered an indication for endodontic surgery.

5. Conclusions

Our results contradict the hypothesis of this study. We have shown, contrary to common knowledge, that gutta-percha (both infected and non-infected) does not obstruct the healing of bony defects. Further study is needed to better understand the effect of different concentrations and strains of bacteria on intrabony wound healing.

Author Contributions: Conceptualization, S.L.; methodology, S.L.; investigation, Y.G., S.A., R.W. and S.L.; writing—original draft preparation, D.M., S.L. and R.W.; writing—review and editing, D.M. and S.L. All authors have read and agreed to the published version of the manuscript.

Funding: This study was funded in part by MIS Company Implants Technologies Ltd., (Bar Lev Industrial Park, Israel).

Institutional Review Board Statement: The Animal Research Council approved this research (il-071-06-2009).

Informed Consent Statement: Not applicable.

Data Availability Statement: Not applicable.

Acknowledgments: The authors would like to thank MIS Company Implants Technologies Ltd., (Bar Lev Industrial Park, Israel) for funding and supporting scientific research in Israel.

Conflicts of Interest: The authors declare that there were no conflicts of interest in this research.

References

1. Johnson, W.; Kulild, J. *Obturation of the Cleaned and Shaped Root Canal System*; Elsevier: St. Louis, MO, USA, 2011; pp. 349–388.
2. Ng, Y.L.; Mann, V.; Gulabivala, K. Outcome of secondary root canal treatment: A systematic review of the literature. *Int. Endod. J.* **2008**, *41*, 1026–1046. [CrossRef]
3. Fristad, I.; Molven, O.; Halse, A. Nonsurgically retreated root filled teeth—Radiographic findings after 20–27 years. *Int. Endod. J.* **2004**, *37*, 12–18. [CrossRef] [PubMed]
4. Bergenholtz, G.; Lekholm, U.; Milthon, R.; Engstrom, B. Influence of apical overinstrumentation and overfilling on re-treated root canals. *J. Endod.* **1979**, *5*, 310–314. [CrossRef]
5. Bergenholtz, G.; Lekholm, U.; Milthon, R.; Heden, G.; Odesjö, B.; Engström, B. Retreatment of endodontic fillings. *Scand. J. Dent. Res.* **1979**, *87*, 217–224. [CrossRef] [PubMed]
6. Van Nieuwenhuysen, J.P.; Aouar, M.; D'Hoore, W. Retreatment or radiographic monitoring in endodontics. *Int. Endod. J.* **1994**, *27*, 75–81. [CrossRef]
7. Nair, P.N. On the causes of persistent apical periodontitis: A review. *Int. Endod. J.* **2006**, *39*, 249–281. [CrossRef]
8. Haapasalo, M.; Shen, Y.A.; Ricucci, D. Reasons for persistent and emerging post-treatment endodontic disease: Reasons for persistent and emerging post-treatment endodontic disease. *Endod. Top.* **2008**, *18*, 31–50. [CrossRef]
9. Ingle, J.I.; Bakland, L.K.; Baumgartner, J.C. *Ingle's Endodontics 6*; BC Decker: Raleigh, NC, USA, 2008.
10. Siqueira, J.F., Jr. Aetiology of root canal treatment failure: Why well-treated teeth can fail. *Int. Endod. J.* **2001**, *34*, 1–10. [CrossRef]
11. Friedman, S. Prognosis of initial endodontic therapy. *Endod. Top.* **2002**, *2*, 59–88. [CrossRef]
12. Farzaneh, M.; Abitbol, S.; Lawrence, H.P.; Friedman, S. Treatment outcome in endodontics-the Toronto Study. Phase II: Initial treatment. *J. Endod.* **2004**, *30*, 302–309. [CrossRef]
13. Yusuf, H. The significance of the presence of foreign material periapically as a cause of failure of root treatment. *Oral Surg. Oral Med. Oral Pathol.* **1982**, *54*, 566–574. [CrossRef]
14. Senia, E.S.; Marraro, R.V.; Mitchell, J.L.; Lewis, A.G.; Thomas, L. Rapid sterilization of gutta-percha cones with 5.25% sodium hypochlorite. *J. Endod.* **1975**, *1*, 136–140. [CrossRef]
15. Takemura, N.; Noiri, Y.; Ehara, A.; Kawahara, T.; Noguchi, N.; Ebisu, S. Single species biofilm-forming ability of root canal isolates on gutta-percha points. *Eur. J. Oral Sci.* **2004**, *112*, 523–529. [CrossRef] [PubMed]
16. Strathmann, M.; Wingender, J.; Flemming, H.C. Application of fluorescently labelled lectins for the visualization and biochemical characterization of polysaccharides in biofilms of Pseudomonas aeruginosa. *J. Microbiol. Methods* **2002**, *50*, 237–248. [CrossRef]

17. George, S.; Basrani, B.; Kishen, A. Possibilities of gutta-percha-centered infection in endodontically treated teeth: An in vitro study. *J. Endod.* **2010**, *36*, 1241–1244. [CrossRef]
18. Turnbull, R.S.; Freeman, E. Use of wounds in the parietal bone of the rat for evaluating bone marrow for grafting into periodontal defects. *J. Periodontal. Res.* **1974**, *9*, 39–43. [CrossRef]
19. Ramachandran Nair, P.N. Light and electron microscopic studies of root canal flora and periapical lesions. *J. Endod.* **1987**, *13*, 29–39. [CrossRef]
20. Moses, O.; Vitrial, D.; Aboodi, G.; Sculean, A.; Tal, H.; Kozlovsky, A.; Artzi, Z.; Weinreb, M.; Nemcovsky, C.E. Biodegradation of three different collagen membranes in the rat calvarium: A comparative study. *J. Periodontol.* **2008**, *79*, 905–911. [CrossRef]
21. Kozlovsky, A.; Aboodi, G.; Moses, O.; Tal, H.; Artzi, Z.; Weinreb, M.; Nemcovsky, C.E. Bio-degradation of a resorbable collagen membrane (Bio-Gide) applied in a double-layer technique in rats. *Clin. Oral Implant. Res.* **2009**, *20*, 1116–1123. [CrossRef]
22. Peters, O.A.; Peters, C.I. Chapter 9—Cleaning and Shaping of the Root Canal System. In *Cohen's Pathways of the Pulp*, 10th ed.; Hargreaves, K.M., Cohen, S., Eds.; Mosby: St. Louis, Mo, USA, 2011; pp. 283–348.
23. Nair, P.N.; Sjögren, U.; Krey, G.; Sundqvist, G. Therapy-resistant foreign body giant cell granuloma at the periapex of a root-filled human tooth. *J. Endod.* **1990**, *16*, 589–595. [CrossRef]
24. Friedman, C.E.; Sandrik, J.L.; Heuer, M.A.; Rapp, G.W. Composition and physical properties of gutta-percha endodontic filling materials. *J. Endod.* **1977**, *3*, 304–308. [CrossRef]
25. Wolfson, E.M.; Seltzer, S. Reaction of rat connective tissue to some gutta-percha formulations. *J Endod.* **1975**, *1*, 395–402. [CrossRef]
26. Sjögren, U.; Sundqvist, G.; Nair, P.N. Tissue reaction to gutta-percha particles of various sizes when implanted subcutaneously in guinea pigs. *Eur. J. Oral Sci.* **1995**, *103*, 313–321. [CrossRef]
27. Lin, L.M.; Huang, G.T.J. Chapter 14—Pathobiology of the Periapex. In *Cohen's Pathways of the Pulp*, 10th ed.; Hargreaves, K.M., Cohen, S., Eds.; Mosby: St. Louis, Mo, USA, 2011; pp. 529–558.
28. Metzger, Z.; Ben-Amar, A. Removal of overextended gutta-percha root canal fillings in endodontic failure cases. *J. Endod.* **1995**, *21*, 287–288. [CrossRef]
29. Molander, A.; Reit, C.; Dahlén, G.; Kvist, T. Microbiological status of root-filled teeth with apical periodontitis. *Int. Endod. J.* **1998**, *31*, 1–7. [CrossRef] [PubMed]
30. Happonen, R.P. Periapical actinomycosis: A follow-up study of 16 surgically treated cases. *Endod. Dent. Traumatol.* **1986**, *2*, 205209. [CrossRef] [PubMed]
31. Siquera, J.F., Jr. Periapical Actinomycosis and infection with Propionibacterium Propionicum. *Endod. Top.* **2003**, *6*, 78–95. [CrossRef]
32. Lin, S.; Sela, G.; Sprecher, H. Periopathogenic bacteria in persistent periapical lesions: An in vivo prospective study. *J. Periodontol.* **2007**, *78*, 905–908. [CrossRef]

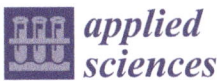

Article

Radiation-Induced Stable Radicals in Calcium Phosphates: Results of Multifrequency EPR, EDNMR, ESEEM, and ENDOR Studies

Fadis F. Murzakhanov [1,*], Peter O. Grishin [2], Margarita A. Goldberg [3], Boris V. Yavkin [1], Georgy V. Mamin [1], Sergei B. Orlinskii [1], Alexander Yu. Fedotov [3], Natalia V. Petrakova [3], Andris Antuzevics [4], Marat R. Gafurov [1] and Vladimir S. Komlev [3]

[1] Institute of Physics, Kazan Federal University, 18 Kremlevskaya Str., 420008 Kazan, Russia; boris.yavkin@gmail.com (B.V.Y.); George.Mamin@kpfu.ru (G.V.M.); orlinskii@list.ru (S.B.O.); marat.gafurov@kpfu.ru (M.R.G.)
[2] Dentistry Faculty, Kazan State Medical University, 49 Butlerova Str., 420000 Kazan, Russia; phlus8@mail.ru
[3] A.A. Baikov Institute of Metallurgy and Materials Science, Russian Academy of Sciences, 49 Leninsky pr., 119334 Moscow, Russia; margo.goldberg@yandex.ru (M.A.G.); antishurik@mail.ru (A.Y.F.); petrakova.nv@mail.ru (N.V.P.); komlev@mail.ru (V.S.K.)
[4] Institute of Solid State Physics, University of Latvia, Kengaraga str. 8, 1000 Riga, Latvia; andris.antuzevics@cfi.lu.lv
* Correspondence: murzakhanov.fadis@gmail.com; Tel.: +7-9270395512

Abstract: This article presents the results of a study of radiation-induced defects in various synthetic calcium phosphate (CP) powder materials (hydroxyapatite—HA and octacalcium phosphate—OCP) by electron paramagnetic resonance (EPR) spectroscopy at the X, Q, and W-bands (9, 34, 95 GHz for the microwave frequencies, respectively). Currently, CP materials are widely used in orthopedics and dentistry owing to their high biocompatibility and physico-chemical similarity with human hard tissue. It is shown that in addition to the classical EPR techniques, other experimental approaches such as ELDOR-detected NMR (EDNMR), electron spin echo envelope modulation (ESEEM), and electron-nuclear double resonance (ENDOR) can be used to analyze the electron–nuclear interactions of CP powders. We demonstrated that the value and angular dependence of the quadrupole interaction for ^{14}N nuclei of a nitrate radical can be determined by the EDNMR method at room temperature. The ESEEM technique has allowed for a rapid analysis of the nuclear environment and estimation of the structural positions of radiation-induced centers in various crystal matrices. ENDOR spectra can provide information about the distribution of the nitrate radicals in the OCP structure.

Keywords: calcium phosphate; radiation-induced center; hyperfine interaction; EDNMR; ESEEM; ENDOR

Citation: Murzakhanov, F.F.; Grishin, P.O.; Goldberg, M.A.; Yavkin, B.V.; Mamin, G.V.; Orlinskii, S.B.; Fedotov, A.Y.; Petrakova, N.V.; Antuzevics, A.; Gafurov, M.R.; et al. Radiation-Induced Stable Radicals in Calcium Phosphates: Results of Multifrequency EPR, EDNMR, ESEEM, and ENDOR Studies. *Appl. Sci.* **2021**, *11*, 7727. https://doi.org/10.3390/app11167727

Academic Editor: Vittorio Checchi

Received: 10 July 2021
Accepted: 20 August 2021
Published: 22 August 2021

Publisher's Note: MDPI stays neutral with regard to jurisdictional claims in published maps and institutional affiliations.

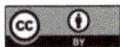

Copyright: © 2021 by the authors. Licensee MDPI, Basel, Switzerland. This article is an open access article distributed under the terms and conditions of the Creative Commons Attribution (CC BY) license (https://creativecommons.org/licenses/by/4.0/).

1. Introduction

Nowadays, bone diseases, which are mainly caused by infections, defects, tumors, and injuries, are among the most common pathologies in clinical practices. It is certain that these defects require an appropriate bone treatment, without which irreversible consequences up to invalidity can occur. One of the most difficult but effective methods of treatment is surgery, with the subsequent replacement of the damaged area. One of the main aspects of bone treatment is the type and quality of materials used as a base for implants, which will determine the future successful healing of patients. Therefore, the creation and investigation of novel synthesized materials is gaining increasing interest in physics, biology, chemistry, and medicine [1–4].

Currently, there are a number of suitable materials for bone substitution such as inert metals (titanium- and tantalum-based alloys), polymers (polycaprolactone, cellulose, collagen), and ceramics (bioglass, gypsum, calcium carbonate) [2,5,6]. However, it is considered that calcium phosphate (CP)-based compounds are the most favorable choice for the reliable restoration of human hard-tissue defects due to their chemical stability and compositional similarities to the inorganic, mineral phase of the bone. At the same time, processes of biomineralization have attracted scientific and technological attention for a long time in view of creating personalized, non-toxic materials for bone and dental tissue engineering [7–9], myocardial tissue regeneration [10], bioimaging and drug delivery [11,12], tumor hypothermal treatment [13], tracking of the course of pathological calcification [14], etc. Several inorganic phases are involved in biomineralization, generally presented as non-stoichiometric carbonate-substituted calcium phosphates, among which the following are of the most importance: hydroxyapatite (HA, chemical formula $Ca_{10}(PO_4)_6(OH)_2$), tricalcium phosphate (TCP, chemical formula Ca_3PO_4), dicalcium phosphate dihydrate (DCPD, $CaHPO_4 \times 2H_2O$, brushite), and octacalcium phosphate (OCP, $Ca_8H_2(PO_4)_6 \times 5H_2O$).

At present, CP-based materials are commonly used in medicine and dentistry since they have shown excellent biocompatibility, osteoconductivity, and suitable mechanical properties. All of these CP materials provide the conditions for inducing osteoblast differentiation and improving the viability and proliferation of the bone cells [15,16]. Such suitable properties have contributed to the use of these materials in a wide range of other biological applications, e.g., drug and gene delivery, as a filler for biocomposites, transfection processes, as fluorescing probes and biomarkers in nanomedical applications [17,18].

At the same time, there are a lot of emerging applications in addition to the biomedical ones. For example, OCP has demonstrated a good capacity for the defluorization of water [19], which has previously been demonstrated for HA [20]. HA has also been applied as a catalyst and catalyst support [21]. HA and cation-doped HA in the form of nanoparticles were used for the environmentally friendly oxidative desulfurization of oil [22] and light gas oil [23]. Likewise, HA was presented as an efficient and reusable catalyst for the epoxidation of olefins and α, β-unsaturated ketones using hydrogen peroxide under relatively mild conditions [24]. Recently, the nitrate doping of CP nanoparticles was proposed for potential use as (P,N) nanofertilizers in agricultural applications [25], and EPR was recognized as one of the fastest methods of evaluating the presence and amount of nitrates. It is also known that HA is applied as an adsorbent for water purification [26], including the removal of nitrate due to its adsorption onto CP surfaces [27].

An extremely deep understanding of the physical, chemical, or biological processes that occur in crystal structures is required to develop or promote any field of materials science. This is especially important for new or poorly studied materials that have recently been obtained with a new chemical composition. However, it often happens that for a certain type of material, one distinct method is not sufficient to get the whole set of structural information. For disordered materials such as CPs, all available experimental tools are required to determine the more interesting features of doped materials. The magnetic resonance approach is a suitable experimental means that significantly complements and expands the knowledge of doped materials. Magnetic resonance-based methods can provide an insight into interatomic interactions, define their origin/mechanisms, and study the local environment of impurity centers, which cannot be directly analyzed by other techniques.

Calcium phosphate materials have been thoroughly studied by various experimental techniques. Most of the published CP-related articles can be categorized into studies of the morphology of nanoparticles, the structure of the crystal lattice, and the biological properties of the synthesized materials [1,2]. To solve problems with the structural analysis of CP powders, combinational approaches are utilized by applying Fourier transform infrared spectroscopy, scanning electron microscopy, X-ray diffraction, differential thermal and thermogravimetric analysis, Raman spectroscopy, as well as in vivo/in vitro analysis for the study of biological properties [28]. The abovementioned methods allow for the determination of the size and shape of nanoparticles, the presence of different functional groups, and additional crystalline phases as well as the lattice structure, depending on the type/concentration of impurity ions [3,5]. However, questions concerning the magnetic behavior/origin of defects and their electron–nuclear interactions with the local ionic environment remain unexplored, requiring additional experimental methods.

One of the analytical, non-destructive tools for the investigation of CPs of both biogenic and synthetic origins is electron paramagnetic resonance (EPR) [29–43]. The increased sensitivity, spectral and temporal resolution, along with the improved stability of modern commercial EPR spectrometers has opened new possibilities in the study of CPs during the last decade, taking a step towards in situ EPR imaging (EPRI) [44]. Pure, non-substituted CPs are EPR-silent. Consequently, conventional EPR can be used for the purity check of CP materials, for example, the presence of metal impurities [31]. A standard way of studying EPR-silent CPs is through the creation of certain types of defects with ionizing radiation such as X-, β-, γ-rays or ultraviolet light, and the investigation of their spectroscopic properties. Several radiation-induced paramagnetic species (anion radicals) located at hydroxyl or phosphate sites have been identified in synthetic HA, depending mainly on the nature of the biogenic materials and synthesis route/treatment of the artificial compounds as well as on the radiation conditions [45–49]. Among them, oxygen radicals O^-, trapped atomic hydrogen centers, holes trapped on OH^- and PO_4^{2-}, carbonate radicals CO_2^-, CO_3^-, CO_3^{3-}, and color centers have been observed. In burnt bones, coal-type C-radicals have been identified [41,50]. Besides material characterization, the spectroscopic and relaxation parameters of the observed paramagnetic centers can be used to track the radiation dose in HA-containing dental enamel [41], to follow the processes of calcification [29] and the doping/co-doping of synthetic materials with various ions [35,38]. The effect of diverse amino acids on the local microstructure of calcium-deficient hydroxyapatite was also tracked/confirmed by EPR spectroscopy [51].

As mentioned above, the EPR method is a well-established approach for the study of disordered materials such as CPs. However, we should accept the fact that this method has several limitations (low spectral resolution and technical restrictions) that do not allow us to resolve weak hyperfine interactions. The main problems arise from line broadening and signal overlapping. Therefore, important information about the local nuclear environment remains unexplored. More complicated approaches in hardware and better physical understanding have led to the advancement of magnetic resonance techniques. However, methods based on double resonance techniques for the study of disordered materials are still not used as widely as would be expected. In this article, we will demonstrate that there are a number of interesting techniques, which are targeted to the study of weak hyperfine splittings, allowing us to study local atomic (nuclear) surroundings. Such methods as electron spin echo envelope modulation (ESEEM), electron nuclear double resonance (ENDOR), and electron–electron double resonance (ELDOR) detected NMR (EDNMR) provide information that is related to the NMR spectroscopy approach and obviously cannot be obtained by conventional EPR. The corresponding experimental data (Larmor frequencies of nuclei, the values of hyperfine and quadrupole interactions with angular-selected measurements) significantly complement and deepen the existing understanding of the structural behavior of CP materials.

The diverse field of pulse EPR spectroscopy allows us to obtain a complete set of spectroscopic and dynamic parameters for the radiation-induced centers in calcium phosphate materials. The parameters of the spin Hamiltonian (anisotropic g-factor, hyperfine A and quadrupole P interaction matrices) reflect the local symmetry of the defect position. The extent of anisotropy and principal values of the tensors depend on the electron density, the distribution of nearby ions, and the local gradients of electric fields. Additional quantum chemical methods can be employed to calculate the listed energy characteristics, which are determined by the structural features of defects as well as the localization of impurity ions in the vicinity. Thus, a comparative analysis of experimental data from pulse EPR spectroscopy with further theoretical calculations is crucial for a more complete understanding of the structural features of the crystal lattice of calcium phosphate materials. The explicit identification of certain paramagnetic centers is important for biphasic materials (HA + TCP), which are now generating great interest in dentistry [52]. For the successful characterization of biphasic compounds, a comprehensive understanding of structural nuances in single-phase materials is required.

The experimentally obtained data in this article (anisotropic g-factors, hyperfine A and quadrupole P interaction values) for different impurity centers can be used as a reference point for further theoretical calculations based on quantum chemistry (e.g., the density functional theory—DFT approach), which would allow for the acquisition of additional structural information about the features of the doped crystal lattice.

2. Materials and Methods

2.1. Sample Synthesis

HA powders were synthesized by precipitation from aqueous solutions according to the reaction (Equation (1)), using reactants of analytical grade (Labtech, Russia) and deionized water:

$$10Ca(NO_3)_2 + 6(NH_4)_2HPO_4 + 8NH_4OH \rightarrow Ca_{10}(PO_4)_6(OH)_2 + 20NH_4NO_3 + 6H_2O \quad (1)$$

The ammonium phosphate solution was added dropwise into a calcium nitrate solution during the stirring. The pH of the reaction mixture was maintained at a value of 11.0–12.0 by adding aqueous ammonia. After the synthesis, the mixture was ripened for 21 days for the crystallization of the precipitate [53].

The powder of OCP was synthesized by hydrolysis of the initial DCPD powder in a buffer solution. A total of 10 g of DCPD powder was immersed in 1000 mL of 1.5 M sodium acetate aqueous solution, with a pH value of 8.8 ± 0.2. The powder was kept in the solution for 24 h, with a constant stirring rate at 35 °C, and then thoroughly washed in distilled water and dried overnight at 37 °C.

The jawbone material of a Vietnamese mini-pig (a mineral phase that consists mainly of hydroxyapatite) was extracted by removing an implant with small bone fragments of peri-implant tissues. The corresponding preparation of the jawbone sample for EPR measurements was carried out by separating it from the implant and sawing it into blocks. All requirements and relevant ethical standards for interventionary studies involving animals were rigorously followed according to the Local Ethics Committee of the Federal State Budgetary Educational Institution "Kazan State Medical University" of the Ministry of Health of the Russian Federation.

The studied samples were in dry powder form, which facilitated sample preparation before experiments. Standard quartz flasks were used for all types of EPR spectroscopy measurements at different frequency ranges. Since the Bruker Elexsys spectrometers use a resonator system (the dimensions of which are proportional to the microwave length), the sizes of the flasks (cylindrical sample holders) for each range were different: 7 mm, 3 mm, and 0.6 mm for the X, Q, and W-bands, respectively. The volume/mass of each sample corresponded to a fully filled resonator, ensuring a fill factor of K = 1. A quantitative assessment of the radiation-induced center concentration was not carried out; therefore, the specific mass of the samples was not relevant. For X-ray and γ irradiation, the powder samples were packaged in plastic containers and plastic bags, and irradiated in air at room temperature.

2.2. Experimental Setup

Conventional (continuous wave—CW) and pulsed EPR measurements were performed, exploiting the abilities of Bruker Elexsys 580/680 spectrometer in X- (ν_{MW} = 9–10 GHz), Q- (ν_{MW} = 33–34 GHz), and W-band (ν_{MW} = 94–95 GHz) ranges. At CW mode, experimental parameters (amplitude modulation, power of mw-source, and integration times) were chosen to avoid any distortion and saturation of absorption signals. Electron spin echo (ESE)-detected EPR spectra were recorded using a standard Hahn echo sequence with π = 32 ns and τ = 300 ns for the X-band, and π = 64 ns and τ = 240 ns for the W-band, unless otherwise specified in the text. Relaxation time measurements were taken using a 2-pulse

Hahn echo sequence and an inversion-recovery 3-pulse sequence for the spin–spin T_2 and spin–lattice T_1 relaxation times, respectively.

Electron Spin Echo Envelope Modulation (ESEEM) was implemented using a well-known two-pulse Hahn sequence: $\pi/2 - \tau - \pi$, where the length of π was 32 ns, and τ was equal to 200 ns. In this method, the integral intensity of the electron spin echo (ESE) was recorded, depending on the time interval τ between two pulses at a fixed magnetic field. This parameter was increased to the required value (before the loss of information on nuclear modulations). To increase the sensitivity and spectroscopic resolution, the smallest possible step, t = 4 ns, was chosen and the ESE was integrated only at its peak with an integration time of t = 4 ns. Further spectral analysis of obtained results involved a Fourier transform using the program OriginPro.

Electron nuclear double resonance (ENDOR) experiments were conducted using special (for nuclei and electron) cavities and a scheme of simultaneous electron-nuclear excitations called the Mims pulse sequence: $\pi/2 - \tau - \pi/2 - T - \pi/2$, with an additional radiofrequency (RF) π-pulse inserted between the second and third microwave $\pi/2$ pulses, where the length of $\pi/2$ was 64 ns, τ = 250 ns, T = 20 µs, and for the RF pulse, π = 18 µs. Since the Larmor frequency of the nuclei is less than for an electron by about 2000 times, and is consequently in the radio frequency range, an additional RF-source with a wide frequency range (1–200 MHz) was used to stimulate the NMR transitions. To increase the spectroscopic resolution and separate close nuclear frequencies or overlapping splitting from each other in the RF-scale, experiments were performed in the high-field part of the spectrometer (W-band, ν_{MW} = 94 GHz). Due to method requirements for T_1 time measurements, the experiments were performed at a low temperature, T = 50 K.

The ELDOR-detected NMR (EDNMR) method for the electron-nuclear study is based on the electron–electron double resonance (ELDOR) approach. The additional ELDOR module E580-400U, and a dielectric ring resonator ER 4118X-MD5, were used to investigate double electron–electron transitions. In this case, the initial (main) source of microwave radiation acts as the observation frequency (ν_{mw1} or ν_{obs}) at a fixed value (ν_{MW} = 9.59 GHz). At the same time, module E580-400U is necessary for generating and varying the second independent microwave frequency (ν_{mw2} or ν_{pump}) in the range from 9.3 to 10 GHz. Owing to its adjustable Q-factor, the ER 4118X-MD5 resonator allows for the optimization of the bandwidth of resonant frequencies in accordance with the specific requirements of the experiment. The duration of the selective pulse t_{sel} was chosen to be 6 µs, which corresponds to the excitation band in the EPR spectrum, with ΔB = 7.2 µT and the length of the detection pulse equal to 300 ns (ΔB = 144 µT). All of these tuning parameters allow for the recording of the spectra at a high resolution.

To create stable paramagnetic centers in the nominal pure material, X-ray irradiation of the synthesized powders was provided by a URS-55 source (U = 55 kV, I = 16 mA, W anticathode) at room temperature for 30 min, with the estimated dose of 10 kGy.

γ-ray irradiation was performed on a cyclic electron accelerator for 15 and 90 min (with the estimated doses of 4 and 25 kGy, respectively) at room temperature. Irradiation was carried out on a cyclic electron accelerator "Microtron-cT". The irradiation parameters were as follows: the electron energy was 21 MeV, the electron beam current was up to 5 µA, the pulse repetition rate was 200 Hz, the pulse duration was 3 µs, the gamma–quantum flux was 5×10^{13} s^{-1} cm^{-2}. The duration of sample irradiation was 15 and 90 min at an electron beam current of 4 µA, with the estimated absorbed doses of about 4 and 25 kGy, respectively. The details of irradiation are provided in our paper [54].

3. Results and Discussion

3.1. EPR Spectroscopy

There are no paramagnetic centers in nominally pure samples (HA and OCP); therefore, no EPR signals in CP materials can be observed. An X-ray or γ-irradiation procedure performed on the samples leads to the formation of radiation centers that can be successfully detected by EPR (Figure 1). As we can see, the acquired EPR spectra from the irradiated samples have quite a strong anisotropy, with a characteristic splitting into hyperfine structures. Powder spectra of the radiation-induced centers (nitrate radicals) in CPs are very often described by a Spin-Hamiltonian of axial symmetry:

$$H = g_{||}\beta B_z S_z + g_\perp \beta (B_x S_x + B_y S_y) + A_{||} S_z I_z + A_\perp (S_x I_x + S_y I_y) \quad (2)$$

where $g_{||}$ and $g_\perp$ are the main components of the g tensor, $A_{||}$ and $A_\perp$ are the main components of the hyperfine tensor, B_i, S_i, and I_i are the projections of the external magnetic field strength, electronic ($S = 1/2$), and nuclear ($I = 1$) spins, respectively, onto the $i = \{x, y, z\}$ coordinate axis, and β is the Bohr magneton.

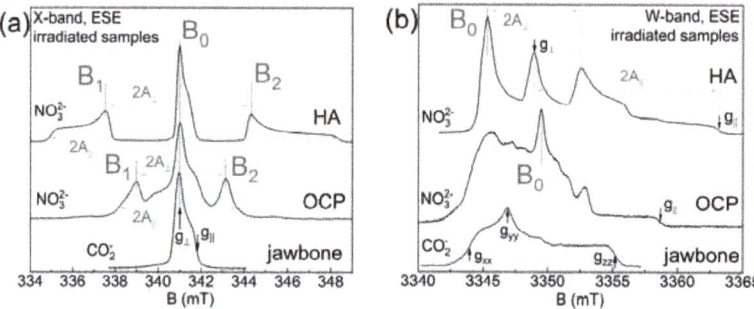

Figure 1. EPR spectra of the irradiated samples in pulse mode for the (**a**) X-band and (**b**) W-band frequency ranges at T = 297 K.

The Spin-Hamiltonian parameters for the same center may differ significantly, depending on the type of sample. The spectra of the CP samples synthesized from the nitrogen-containing reagents (see Equation (1)) can be described with the parameters that are shown in Table 1.

Table 1. The Spin-Hamiltonian parameters of the X-ray irradiated samples.

	g_{xx}	g_{yy}	g_{zz}	$A_\perp$ (mT)	$A_{||}$ (mT)
jawbone	2.0026 (2)	2.0008 (2)	1.996 (1)	-	-
HA	2.006 (1)	2.006 (1)	2.002 (1)	3.37 (5)	6.65 (4)
OCP	2.0014 (3)	2.0014 (3)	2.0035 (5)	2.08 (5)	2.50 (5)

The shape of the EPR line and the splitting values for HA and OCP are very different. This may be due to the different atomic environments, the degree of distortion of the crystal lattice, or the level of delocalization of the paramagnetic center [55]. Differences in the parameters of the Spin-Hamiltonian should be useful for further analysis of crystal structures of samples doped with various cations.

It should be noted that the EPR spectra of CP samples differ in the degree of anisotropy in the experiment on the high-frequency part of the spectrometer (Figure 1b). Experimental measurements in two or more different frequency ranges allow for a description of the obtained results more accurately, i.e., unequivocally identify the paramagnetic centers and determine the parameters of the main interactions. The W-band EPR spectrum of OCP is more difficult to interpret, despite the fact that the values of the hyperfine interaction ($A_{||}$ or $A_\perp$) are the smallest for the calcium phosphates group. It was concluded that in the irradiated HA samples, EPR is mainly due to the stable NO_3^{2-} ions, preferably substituting one distinct PO_4^{3-} position in the HA structure (substitution of the B-type), while there are several non-equivalent positions for the nitrate radical in the OCP structure. In our paper [55], we found that the distribution of $A_\perp$ for TCP is larger than that of the HA. We suggested that it could be due to the three different positions for PO$_4$ group substitution in the TCP structure, as well as due to the various mechanisms for charge compensation.

Since hydroxyapatite is an inorganic mineral component of bone tissue, we studied the biogenic material after X-ray irradiation. As an example, the jawbone of a Vietnamese mini-pig was chosen for the EPR study. This sample, like synthetic hydroxyapatite, does not contain its own paramagnetic centers. However, after X-ray exposure, radiation-induced centers are formed. The EPR spectra of samples in two frequency ranges are shown in Figure 1. The signal is attributed to the stable carbonate radical, which is identified by the degree of rhombic anisotropy (shape of line) and the values of the g-factor (see Table 1). As we can see, all three values of the g-factor can be accurately determined due to the high spectroscopic resolution (at W-band), while for the X-band, it is possible to distinguish only perpendicular ($g_{xx} = g_{yy} = g_\perp$) and parallel orientations ($g_{zz} = g_{||}$). At the same time, there is no evidence of a nitrate radical. Figure 1 clearly shows that the presence of free radicals in the irradiated sample depends on the type of biomaterial under study.

Relaxation characteristics were also investigated for the CP samples. The obtained data are shown in Table 2. As we can see, the relaxation times T_1 (spin–lattice or longitudinal relaxation) and T_2 (spin–spin or transverse relaxation) differ depending on the type of CP material. This difference may indicate that the radiation-induced centers occupy various positions in the crystal lattices of HA, OCP, and biogenic compounds (jawbone of a Vietnamese mini-pig). Because of the difference in spin–spin relaxation times, we can conclude that there is an unequal distribution of free radicals for various CP materials. Therefore, a full set of spectroscopic values and dynamic characteristics of radiation-induced centers will allow us to unambiguously determine the nature of EPR signals in poorly studied CP materials (amorphous, biphasic, and doped materials).

Table 2. Relaxation characteristics of radiation-induced paramagnetic centers in different matrices at room temperature T = 297 K, in the X-band frequency range ν_{MW} = 9.6 GHz. Values for CP materials were measured at B$_0$ (see Figure 1a).

Type of Material	Spin–Lattice Relaxation T_1 (µs)	Spin–Spin Relaxation T_2 (µs)
HA	28.5(5)	3.0(1)
OCP	60.7(8)	0.68(5)
jawbone of a mini-pig	17.7(2)	1.31(8)

Samples irradiated by X-ray and γ-radiation were additionally explored in the Q-band microwave range. Experimental results are presented only in continuous wave mode at room temperature. Figure 2 shows the difference in the EPR spectra between the types of irradiation for the same type of material. The nature of the paramagnetic centers can be dependent on the type of radiation exposure. The influence of the type of radiation (and other radiation characteristics) on the EPR spectrum was extensively discussed in the literature [56,57]. However, for the OCP sample, the difference in the EPR spectra according to the type of irradiation is not observed. It may serve as additional proof to the conclusion made in ref. [54] that, in contrast to HA, the radiation-induced radicals in OCP are stabilized not in the apatite, but in the hydrated layers of OCP.

The results obtained in the Q-band frequency range provide additional information about the spectroscopic values of the spin system. But as we can see in the case of irradiated calcium phosphates, not all available frequency ranges are suitable for the analysis of powdered materials. The anisotropy of the g-factor for nitrate radicals in high magnetic fields is comparable to or even greater than the hyperfine interaction splitting, while at the X-band, the converse can be observed. Therefore, measurements of the nitrogen radical in an intermediate frequency range lead to the formation of a complex EPR spectrum that is difficult to interpret. Nevertheless, in other cases, a comparison of the EPR spectra makes it possible to clearly determine the origin of the radiation-induced paramagnetic centers and calculate the parameters of the Spin-Hamiltonian.

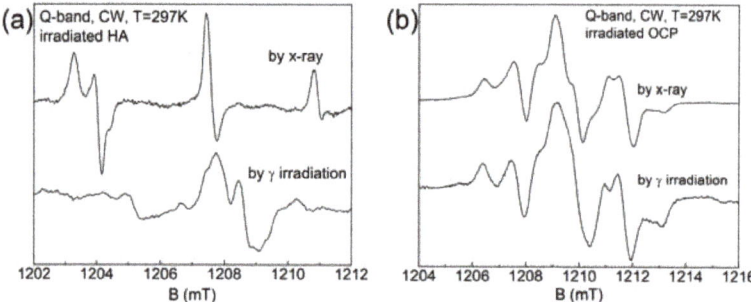

Figure 2. EPR spectra of the nitrate radical in (**a**) HA and (**b**) OCP in the Q-band frequency range at room temperature.

3.2. EDNMR Spectroscopy Analysis

The significant anisotropy of g- and A-tensors and a relatively long transverse relaxation time ($T_2 = 3$ μs) of the NO_3^{2-} radical (see Figure 1a) allows us to carry out angular-selected EDNMR measurements at room temperature in the X-band frequency range.

Signals corresponding to the Larmor frequencies of ^{31}P (± 6 MHz) and ^{1}H (± 14.8 MHz) nuclei are shown on the overview spectra at $B_0 \approx 0.34$ T (Figure 3). These signals are expected because hydrogen and phosphorus ions are structural elements of the HA and indicate that the studied nitrogen radical is located in the HA crystal lattice. The lack of additional structures (or splitting) for these nuclei indicates an insufficient spectral resolution of the EDNMR method (at least at room temperature in the X-band). The most interesting signals are those observed at $\nu = \pm 47.5$ and ± 95 MHz. Given the theoretical calculations [58,59] for various electron–electron transitions as well as the known values of hyperfine structure A from EPR measurements (Figure 1a), it follows that these transitions are caused by the anisotropic hyperfine interaction from nitrogen nuclei. Due to the fact that the value of A exceeds the Larmor frequency of ^{14}N nuclei (I = 1, $\nu_{Larmor} = 1.04$ MHz for $B_0 \approx 0.34$ T), this leads to the localization of the EDNMR signal in the range of the half (for single-quantum transitions with $\Delta M_I = \pm 1$) and whole (for double-quantum transitions with $\Delta M_I = \pm 2$) values of A.

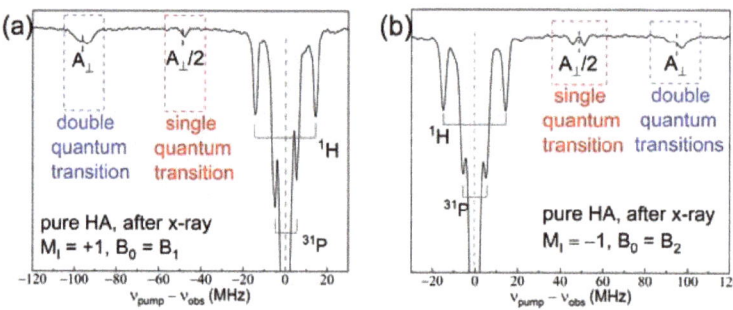

Figure 3. Total EDNMR spectra of HA according to the quantum number M_I: (**a**) $M_I = +1$ at $B_0 = B_1$, (**b**) $M_I = -1$ at $B_0 = B_2$ (see Figure 1a).

A more detailed analysis of the spectrum at $\Delta \nu > 0$ ($M_I = -1$) shows an additional splitting for the single-quantum transition exactly localized at the value $A_\perp/2$ (Figure 4). Using the expression for single-quantum transitions [58]:

$$\Delta = 2\nu_{Larmor} \pm 3P \quad (3)$$

where Δ is the splitting value of single-quantum transitions, and a choice of the sign "±" depends on the quantum number of M_I ("+" for $M_I = -1$ and "−" for $M_I = +1$), we concluded that the observed splitting occurs due to the presence of a quadrupole interaction of the ^{14}N nuclei with a gradient of crystal field. Assuming that the tensors A and P are collinear, the value (and sign) of the quadrupole splitting can be calculated quite easily. Thus, we could establish that the value of quadrupole splitting $P = 1.2$ MHz. Due to the fact that the P value is comparable to the Larmor frequency of ^{14}N at $B_0 = 340$ mT, splitting in the same orientation for $M_I = +1$ is not observed. Additionally, EDNMR measurements were performed for an aluminum-doped hydroxyapatite within the frequency range of the single-quantum transitions. Although the substitution degree by aluminum ions was extremely high (up to 20%), the value of quadrupole splitting was not changed. This means that the local environment of the nitrogen radical, i.e., the electric (crystal) field gradient, does not change significantly. Consequently, aluminum-doped hydroxyapatite up to 20% retains its initial space group.

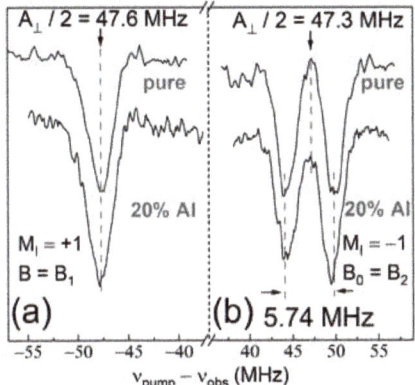

Figure 4. EDNMR spectra for the single quantum transition according to the quantum number M_I: (a) $M_I = +1$ at $B_0 = B_1$, (b) $M_I = -1$ at $B_0 = B_2$ (see Figure 1a).

One of the proofs that the splitting of the line for the single-quantum transition is actually caused by a quadrupole interaction is the presence of an angular dependence of the P value:

$$P(\theta) = P(3\cos^2\theta - 1) \qquad (4)$$

The anisotropic EPR spectrum of the nitrate radical (Figure 1a) and a rather narrow microwave excitation band make it possible to conduct angular selected measurements of the quadrupole splitting. Indeed, in our experiments, we can clearly observe that the value of splitting significantly depends on the B_0, confirming the aforementioned assumption (see Table 3). Therefore, the presence of the splitting in the EDNMR spectrum (by quadrupole interaction for a single quantum transition and by $2\nu_{Larmor}$ Larmor frequency of ^{14}N for a double quantum transition), as well as the localization of obtained signals near A, clearly indicate that the radiation-induced center is related to the nitrogen radical NO_3^{2-}. Furthermore, this nitrogen radical can surely be used as a spin probe.

However, it should be noted that the hyperfine A and quadrupole P tensors are not collinear (the principal/canonical axes of the tensors do not match), which are based on the simple calculation and analysis of the angular dependencies of the A and P values. Earlier, a similar mutual behavior of tensors was observed in oil samples [60]. The possibility of detecting resolved EDNMR spectra is due to the good localization of the nitrogen center (in the position of phosphate, see [37,38]), which leads to the absence of local variations of g, A, and the electric field gradient. Such measurements make it possible to establish unequivocally the presence of a nitrogen atom in the free radical. The EDNMR method easily copes with cases when A is much larger than $2\nu_{Larmor}$, which is almost impossible to achieve with other methods (ESEEM and ENDOR).

Table 3. Quantitative values of quadrupole interaction, depending on the external magnetic field values.

B_0	$\Delta = |\nu_{sq2} - \nu_{sq1}|$, (MHz)	
	$B_1 - \Delta B; \Delta\nu < 0\ (M_I = +1)$	$B_2 + \Delta B; \Delta\nu > 0\ (M_I = -1)$
$B_0 = B_{1,2}$	0	5.7
$B_0 = B_{1,2} \pm 0.25$ mT	≈0.5	4.1
$B_0 = B_{1,2} \pm 0.5$ mT	3.83	2.5
$B_0 = B_{1,2} \pm 1$ mT	5.53	0
$B_0 = B_{1,2} \pm 1.5$ mT	5.58	0

3.3. Hyperfine Interaction Spectroscopy (ESEEM and ENDOR Methods)

There are several approaches for the analysis of hyperfine interactions that cannot be registered in EPR spectra due to the small value of splitting. This section is dedicated to ESEEM (X-band) and ENDOR (X- and W-band) spectra recorded at the field positions corresponding to the maximum of echo intensity. Taking into account the wide excitation bandwidth of short microwave pulses (approx. 50 MHz) and significant spectra overlapping between signals of different paramagnetic centers, current X-band ENDOR measurements cannot be used to selectively address the paramagnetic centers. Nevertheless, important information can be gathered from the analysis.

The crystal lattice of CP samples contains ions with magnetic nuclei (^{1}H and ^{31}P both with $I = 1/2$). Therefore, if the radiation-induced center is localized near these ions, we can register the corresponding signal of the electron–nuclear interaction. In the spectrum for the X-ray irradiated HA sample (Figure 5a), only signals from phosphorus nuclei (^{31}P, $\nu_z \approx 5.9$ MHz at $B_0 = 340$ mT) are observed, although the material also contains hydrogen atoms. This result may indicate that for the HA material, the carbonate radical occupies positions near the phosphorus groups PO_4. The ESEEM spectrum of the irradiated OCP sample (Figure 5b) was registered for the nitrate radical at $B_0 = 341.8$ mT (see Figure 1a). The ESEEM spectrum contains a complete set of signals from all magnetic nuclei (^{1}H, $\nu_z \approx 14.2$ MHz), which indicates the position of the nitrate radical directly in the crystal lattice of the OCP sample. Consequently, in further investigations, the nitrate radical can be successfully used as a spin probe for analyzing the concentration dependences of samples doped with various impurity ions. However, the presence of a sufficiently intense signal from the hydrogen nuclei and the existence of the second harmonic of ^{1}H ($2\nu_z$) may indicate the localization of the nitrate radical near the hydrogen layers of OCP. The nitrogen radical in the CP structure can also provide the possibility of using the ENDOR method for a more detailed analysis of the nuclear environment. It is worth noting that due to the insufficient spectroscopic resolution of the method, we could not observe the additional splitting of the lines.

In contrast to other methods of measuring hyperfine interactions with neighboring magnetic ligands, the ENDOR method allows for the direct registration of NMR transitions, which significantly increases the spectral resolution. In the ENDOR spectrum of the irradiated OCP with fixed $B_0 = 341$ mT, signals at the Zeeman frequencies corresponding to protons ($\nu_z \approx 14.8$ MHz) and phosphorous ^{31}P ($\nu_z \approx 5.9$ MHz) nuclei are observed (Figure 6). Only one broad signal for ^{31}P is detected, which can be simulated as a convolution of Gaussian and Lorentzian lines with the line widths of 1.6 MHz and 0.4 MHz; however, in HA, a ^{31}P splitting of 0.5–1.0 MHz can be observed [35,36,58]. The absence of well-structured ENDOR and ESEEM signals from phosphorous and hydrogen nuclei may be explained by the irregularity of the incorporation of several distinct (R1-R3) defects [54] into the lattice (it is either because of preferential localization in the disordered hydrated layer or due to a large variety of incorporation sites in the apatite layer). Most probably, in line with the discussion on the EPR parameters given above, this means that the radical(s) are not located in the majority of apatite crystallites (A- or B-type substitution) but in the hydrated layers [61].

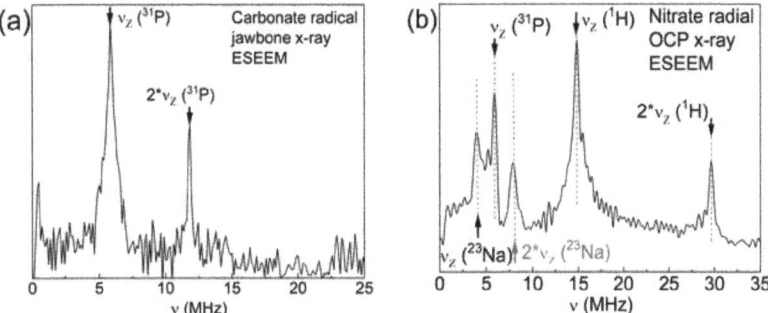

Figure 5. ESEEM spectra of irradiated jawbone containing HA (a) and OCP (b) samples registered in a perpendicular orientation (B_0) of carbonate and nitrate radicals, respectively (see Figure 1a).

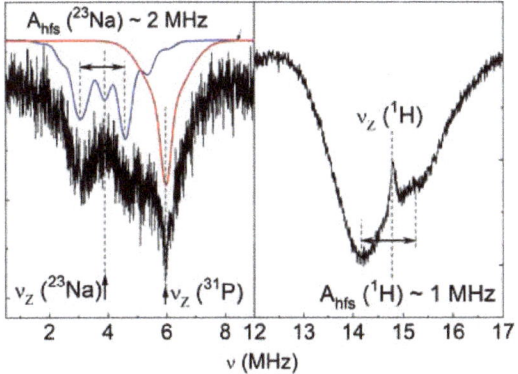

Figure 6. X-band ENDOR spectra detected at B_0 (see Figure 1a) and T = 100K of the OCP sample after X-ray irradiation.

Other features of the ESEEM and ENDOR spectra can be ascribed to the interaction with ^{23}Na nuclei ($\nu_z \approx 3.9$ MHz at $B_0 = 340$ mT, $I = 3/2$ and, therefore, quadrupolar). The presence of a signal from ^{23}Na nuclei is probably due to the incorporation of sodium into the OCP lattice during the synthesis stage. Similar results without deep analysis have been reported in some papers devoted to apatite investigations (see [61], for example). Frequently, the quadrupolar interaction makes the ^{23}Na spectra too complicated for analysis. Using the EasySpin procedure *salt* for ENDOR spectra simulations and assuming an isotropic interaction, we were able to estimate $A_{23Na} = 1.5$ MHz and $e^2Qq/h = 3.3$ MHz (Figure 6).

4. Conclusions

In this paper, we studied calcium phosphate materials using diverse magnetic resonance approaches. The powders under study were exposed to X-ray/gamma radiation to create paramagnetic centers (free radicals). The EPR method makes it possible to distinguish the types of radiation-induced paramagnetic centers in different samples through the values of the Spin-Hamiltonian parameters and dynamic (relaxation) characteristics. Methods targeted to the analysis of weak hyperfine interactions (EDNMR, ESEEM, and ENDOR) demonstrated their advantage in the characterization of synthetic calcium phosphate powder samples. The EDNMR method allows for the determination of the value of the quadrupole interaction for the nitrogen radical, which is a sensitive parameter of the local gradient of the electric (crystal) field. It is possible to identify the various nuclear environments and estimate the position of the radiation-induced centers by ESEEM spectroscopy, while ENDOR provides extensive information about local structural changes caused by the introduction of even non-paramagnetic ions.

Author Contributions: The research work was performed and completed through the contributions of all authors. S.B.O., M.R.G., and V.S.K. designed and administered the experiments. F.F.M., B.V.Y., A.A., and G.V.M. conducted all EPR, ESEEM, ENDOR, and EDNMR experiments. P.O.G., F.F.M., and M.R.G. wrote the main part of the manuscript. M.A.G., N.V.P., and A.Y.F. performed the sample synthesis and characterization. All authors analyzed and discussed the data. All authors have read and agreed to the published version of the manuscript.

Funding: Authors would like to thank the Russian Foundation for Basic Research, project no. 18-29-11086. Institute of Solid State Physics, University of Latvia as the Center of Excellence received funding from the European Union's Horizon 2020 Framework Programme H2020-WIDESPREAD-01–2016-2017- TeamingPhase2 under grant agreement No. 739508, project CAMART^2.

Informed Consent Statement: Not applicable.

Data Availability Statement: Data can be available upon request from the authors.

Conflicts of Interest: The authors declare no conflict of interest.

References

1. Habibovic, P.; Barralet, J.E. Bioinorganics and biomaterials: Bone repair. *Acta Biomater.* **2011**, *7*, 3013–3026. [CrossRef] [PubMed]
2. Habraken, W.; Habibovic, P.; Epple, M.; Bohner, M. Calcium phosphates in biomedical applications: Materials for the future? *Mater. Today* **2016**, *19*, 69–87. [CrossRef]
3. Epple, M.; Ganesan, K.; Heumann, R.; Klesing, J.; Kovtun, A.; Neumann, S.; Sokolova, V.J.J.C. Application of calcium phosphate nanoparticles in biomedicine. *J. Mater. Chem.* **2010**, *20*, 18–23. [CrossRef]
4. Insley, G.; Suzuki, O. *Octacalcium Phosphate Biomaterials: Understanding of Bioactive Properties and Application*, 1st ed.; Woodhead Publishing: Cambridge, UK, 2019.
5. Bazin, D.; Daudon, M. Physicochemistry in medicine: Some selected examples. *J. Spectr. Imaging* **2019**, *8*, a16. [CrossRef]
6. Bohner, M. Resorbable biomaterials as bone graft substitutes. *Mater. Today* **2010**, *13*, 24–30. [CrossRef]
7. Goldberg, M.A.; Smirnov, V.V.; Teterina, A.Y.; Barinov, S.M.; Komlev, V.S. Trends in development of bioresorbable calcium phosphate ceramic materials for bone tissue engineering. *Polym. Sci. Ser. D* **2018**, *11*, 419–422. [CrossRef]
8. de Groot, K. Ceramics of Calcium Phosphates: Preparation and Properties. In *Bioceramics Calcium Phosphate*, 1st ed.; CRC Press: Boca Raton, FL, USA, 2018.
9. LeGeros, R.Z. Calcium phosphate-based osteoinductive materials. *Chem. Rev.* **2008**, *108*, 4742–4753. [CrossRef]
10. Silvestri, A.; Boffito, M.; Sartori, S.; Ciardelli, G. Biomimetic materials and scaffolds for myocardial tissue regeneration. *Macromol. Biosci.* **2013**, *13*, 984–1019. [CrossRef] [PubMed]
11. Ridi, F.; Meazzini, I.; Castroflorio, B.; Bonini, M.; Berti, D.; Baglioni, P. Functional calcium phosphate composites in nanomedicine. *Adv. Colloid Interface Sci.* **2017**, *244*, 281–295. [CrossRef] [PubMed]
12. Victor, S.P.; Paul, W.; Sharma, C.P. Calcium phosphate nanoplatforms for drug delivery and theranostic applications. In *Drug Delivery Nanosystems for Biomedical Applications*, 1st ed.; Elsevier: Amsterdam, The Netherlands, 2018.
13. Haider, A.; Haider, S.; Han, S.S.; Kang, I.K. Recent advances in the synthesis, functionalization and biomedical applications of hydroxyapatite: A review. *RSC Adv.* **2017**, *7*, 7442–7458. [CrossRef]
14. Epple, M. Review of potential health risks associated with nanoscopic calcium phosphate. *Acta Biomater.* **2018**, *77*, 1–14. [CrossRef] [PubMed]
15. Lu, J.; Yu, H.; Chen, C. Biological properties of calcium phosphate biomaterials for bone repair: A review. *RSC Adv.* **2018**, *8*, 2015–2033. [CrossRef]
16. Zhou, C.; Hong, Y.; Zhang, X. Applications of nanostructured calcium phosphate in tissue engineering. *Biomater. Sci.* **2013**, *1*, 1012–1028. [CrossRef] [PubMed]
17. Šupová, M. Substituted hydroxyapatites for biomedical applications: A review. *Ceram. Int.* **2015**, *41*, 9203–9231. [CrossRef]
18. Hui, J.; Wang, X. Hydroxyapatite nanocrystals: Colloidal chemistry, assembly and their biological applications. *Inorg. Chem. Front.* **2014**, *1*, 215–225. [CrossRef]
19. Idini, A.; Frau, F.; Gutierrez, L.; Dore, E.; Nocella, G.; Ghiglieri, G. Application of octacalcium phosphate with an innovative household-scale defluoridator prototype and behavioral determinants of its adoption in rural communities of the East African Rift Valley. *Integr. Environ. Assess. Manag.* **2020**, *16*, 856–870. [CrossRef]

20. Sundaram, C.S.; Viswanathan, N.; Meenakshi, S. Defluoridation chemistry of synthetic hydroxyapatite at nano scale: Equilibrium and kinetic studies. *J. Hazard. Mater.* **2008**, *155*, 206–215. [CrossRef] [PubMed]
21. Sebti, S.; Tahir, R.; Nazih, R.; Saber, A.; Boulaajaj, S. Hydroxyapatite as a new solid support for the Knoevenagel reaction in heterogeneous media without solvent. *Appl. Catal. A* **2002**, *228*, 155–159. [CrossRef]
22. Saha, B.; Yadav, S.K.; Sengupta, S. Synthesis of nano-Hap prepared through green route and its application in oxidative desulfurisation. *Fuel* **2018**, *222*, 743–752. [CrossRef]
23. Riad, M.; Mikhail, S. Oxidative desulfurization of light gas oil using zinc catalysts prepared via different techniques. *Catal. Sci. Technol.* **2012**, *2*, 1437–1446. [CrossRef]
24. Pillai, U.R.; Sahle-Demessie, E. Epoxidation of olefins and α, β-unsaturated ketones over sonochemically prepared hydroxyapatites using hydrogen peroxide. *Appl. Catal. A* **2004**, *261*, 69–76. [CrossRef]
25. Carmona, F.J.; Dal Sasso, G.; Bertolotti, F.; Ramírez-Rodríguez, G.B.; Delgado-López, J.M.; Pedersen, J.S.; Masciocchi, N.; Guagliardi, A. The role of nanoparticle structure and morphology in the dissolution kinetics and nutrient release of nitrate-doped calcium phosphate nanofertilizers. *Sci. Rep.* **2020**, *10*, 12396. [CrossRef]
26. Wijesinghe, W.P.S.L.; Mantilaka, M.M.M.G.P.G.; Peiris, T.N.; Rajapakse, R.M.G.; Wijayantha, K.U.; Pitawala, H.M.T.G.A.; Premachandra, T.N.; Herath, H.M.T.U.; Rajapakse, R.P.V.J. Preparation and characterization of mesoporous hydroxyapatite with non-cytotoxicity and heavy metal adsorption capacity. *New J. Chem.* **2018**, *42*, 10271–10278. [CrossRef]
27. Islam, M.; Mishra, P.C.; Patel, R. Physicochemical characterization of hydroxyapatite and its application towards removal of nitrate from water. *J. Environ. Manag.* **2010**, *91*, 1883–1891. [CrossRef]
28. Raza, M.; Zahid, S.; Asif, A. Analytical tools for substituted hydroxyapatite. In *Handbook of Ionic Substituted Hydroxyapatites*; Elsevier: Amsterdam, The Netherlands, 2020; pp. 21–51.
29. Abdul'Yanov, V.A.; Galiullina, L.; Galyavich, A.; Izotov, V.G.; Mamin, G.; Orlinskii, S.; Rodionov, A.A.; Salakhov, M.K.; Silkin, N.I.; Sitdikova, L.M.; et al. Stationary and high-frequency pulsed electron paramagnetic resonance of a calcified atherosclerotic plaque. *JETP Lett.* **2008**, *88*, 69–73. [CrossRef]
30. Gafurov, M.; Chelyshev, Y.; Ignatyev, I.; Zanochkin, A.; Mamin, G.; Iskhakova, K.; Kiiamov, A.; Murzakhanov, F.; Orlinskii, S. Connection Between the Carotid Plaque Instability and Paramagnetic Properties of the Intrinsic Mn^{2+} Ions. *BioNanoScience* **2016**, *6*, 558–560. [CrossRef]
31. Gabbasov, B.; Gafurov, M.; Starshova, A.; Shurtakova, D.; Murzakhanov, F.; Mamin, G.; Orlinskii, S. Conventional, pulsed and high-field electron paramagnetic resonance for studying metal impurities in calcium phosphates of biogenic and synthetic origins. *J. Magn. Magn. Mater.* **2019**, *470*, 109–117. [CrossRef]
32. Murzakhanov, F.; Gabbasov, B.; Iskhakova, K.; Voloshin, A.; Mamin, G.; Putlyaev, V.; Klimashina, E.; Fadeeva, I.; Fomin, A.; Barinov, S.; et al. Conventional electron paramagnetic resonance for studying synthetic calcium phosphates with metal impurities (Mn^{2+}, Cu^{2+}, Fe^{3+}). *Magn. Reson. Solids* **2017**, *19*, 17207–17210.
33. Fadeeva, I.V.; Gafurov, M.R.; Kiiaeva, I.A.; Orlinskii, S.B.; Kuznetsova, L.M.; Filippov, Y.Y.; Fomin, A.S.; Davydova, G.A.; Selezneva, I.I.; Barinov, S.M. Tricalcium phosphate ceramics doped with silver, copper, zinc, and iron (III) ions in concentrations of less than 0.5 wt.% for bone tissue regeneration. *BioNanoScience* **2017**, *7*, 434–438. [CrossRef]
34. Chelyshev, Y.; Gafurov, M.; Ignatyev, I.; Zanochkin, A.; Mamin, G.; Sorokin, B.; Sorokina, A.; Lyapkalo, N.; Gizatullina, N.; Mukhamedshina, Y.; et al. Paramagnetic Manganese in the Atherosclerotic Plaque of Carotid Arteries. *BioMed Res. Int.* **2016**, *2016*, 3706280. [CrossRef] [PubMed]
35. Goldberg, M.; Gafurov, M.; Makshakova, O.; Smirnov, V.; Komlev, V.; Barinov, S.; Kudryavtsev, E.; Sergeeva, N.; Achmedova, S.; Mamin, G.; et al. Influence of Al on the structure and in vitro behavior of hydroxyapatite nanopowders. *J. Phys. Chem. B* **2019**, *123*, 9143–9154. [CrossRef] [PubMed]
36. Gafurov, M.; Biktagirov, T.; Mamin, G.; Orlinskii, S. A DFT, X-and W-band EPR and ENDOR study of nitrogen-centered species in (nano) hydroxyapatite. *Appl. Magn. Reson.* **2014**, *45*, 1189–1203. [CrossRef]
37. Gafurov, M.; Biktagirov, T.; Yavkin, B.; Mamin, G.; Filippov, Y.; Klimashina, E.; Putlayev, V.; Orlinskii, S. Nitrogen-containing species in the structure of the synthesized nano-hydroxyapatite. *JETP Lett.* **2014**, *99*, 196–203. [CrossRef]
38. Biktagirov, T.; Gafurov, M.; Mamin, G.; Klimashina, E.; Putlayev, V.; Orlinskii, S. Combination of EPR measurements and DFT calculations to study nitrate impurities in the carbonated nanohydroxyapatite. *J. Phys. Chem. B* **2014**, *118*, 1519–1526. [CrossRef]
39. Yavkin, B.V.; Mamin, G.V.; Orlinskii, S.B.; Gafurov, M.R.; Salakhov, M.K.; Biktagirov, T.B.; Klimashina, E.S.; Putlayev, V.I.; Tretyakov, Y.D.; Silkin, N.I. Pb^{3+} radiation defects in $Ca_9Pb(PO_4)_6(OH)_2$ hydroxyapatite nanoparticles studied by high-field (W-band) EPR and ENDOR. *Phys. Chem. Chem. Phys.* **2012**, *14*, 2246–2249. [CrossRef]
40. Vorona, I.P.; Nosenko, V.V.; Baran, N.P.; Ishchenko, S.S.; Lemishko, S.V.; Zatovsky, I.V.; Strutynska, N.Y. EPR study of radiation-induced defects in carbonate-containing hydroxyapatite annealed at high temperature. *Radiat. Meas.* **2016**, *87*, 49–55. [CrossRef]
41. Fattibene, P.; Callens, F. EPR dosimetry with tooth enamel: A review. *Appl. Radiat. Isot.* **2010**, *68*, 2033–2116. [CrossRef] [PubMed]
42. Goldberg, M.A.; Akopyan, A.V.; Gafurov, M.R.; Makshakova, O.N.; Donskaya, N.O.; Fomin, A.S.; Polikarpova, P.P.; Anisimov, A.V.; Murzakhanov, F.F.; Leonov, A.V.; et al. Iron-Doped Mesoporous Powders of Hydroxyapatite as Molybdenum-Impregnated Catalysts for Deep Oxidative Desulfurization of Model Fuel: Synthesis and Experimental and Theoretical Studies. *J. Phys. Chem. C* **2021**, *125*, 11604–11619. [CrossRef]

43. Goldberg, M.A.; Gafurov, M.R.; Murzakhanov, F.F.; Fomin, A.S.; Antonova, O.S.; Khairutdinova, D.R.; Pyataev, A.V.; Makshakova, O.N.; Konovalov, A.A.; Leonov, A.V.; et al. Mesoporous Iron(III)-Doped Hydroxyapatite Nanopowders Obtained via Iron Oxalate. *Nanomaterials* **2021**, *11*, 811. [CrossRef] [PubMed]
44. Gustafsson, H.; Hallbeck, M.; Lindgren, M.; Kolbun, N.; Jonson, M.; Engström, M.; de Muinck, E.; Zachrisson, H. Visualization of oxidative stress in ex vivo biopsies using electron paramagnetic resonance imaging. *Magn. Reson. Med.* **2015**, *73*, 1682–1691. [CrossRef] [PubMed]
45. Gilinskaya, L.G. Organic radicals in natural apatites according to EPR data: Potential genetic and paleoclimatic indicators. *J. Struct. Chem.* **2010**, *51*, 471–481. [CrossRef]
46. Fisher, B.V.; Morgan, R.E.; Phillips, G.O.; Wardale, H.W. Radiation damage in calcium phosphates and collagen: An interpretation of ESR spectra. *Radiat. Res.* **1971**, *46*, 229–235. [CrossRef]
47. Cevc, P.; Schara, M.; Ravnik, Č. Electron paramagnetic resonance study of irradiated tooth enamel. In *Radiation Research*; Radiation Research Society: Lawrence, UK, 1972; Volume 51, pp. 581–589. [CrossRef]
48. Vanhaelewyn, G.C.A.M.; Sadlo, J.; Matthys, P.F.A.E.; Callens, F.J. Comparative X-and Q-band EPR study of radiation-induced radicals in tooth enamel. *Radiat. Res.* **2002**, *158*, 615–625. [CrossRef]
49. Vanhaelewyn, G.C.A.M.; Morent, R.A.; Callens, F.J.; Matthys, P.F.A.E. X-and Q-band electron paramagnetic resonance of CO_2^- in hydroxyapatite single crystals. *Radiat. Res.* **2000**, *154*, 467–472. [CrossRef]
50. Wencka, M.; Hoffmann, S.K.; Hercman, H. EPR dating of hydroxyapatite from fossil bones. Transient Effects after gamma and UV irradiation. *Acta Phys. Pol. A* **2005**, *108*, 331. [CrossRef]
51. Erceg, I.; Maltar-Strmečki, N.; Jurašin, D.D.; Strasser, V.; Ćurlin, M.; Lyons, D.M.; Radatović, B.; Mlinarić, N.M.; Kralj, D.; Sikirić, M.D. Comparison of the Effect of the Amino Acids on Spontaneous Formation and Transformation of Calcium Phosphates. *Crystals* **2021**, *11*, 792. [CrossRef]
52. Ebrahimi, M.; Botelho, M.; Lu, W.; Monmaturapoj, N. Synthesis and characterization of biomimetic bioceramic nanoparticles with optimized physicochemical properties for bone tissue engineering. *J. Biomed. Mater. Res. Part A* **2019**, *107*, 1654–1666. [CrossRef]
53. Gol'dberg, M.A.; Smirnov, V.V.; Ievlev, V.M.; Barinov, S.M.; Kutsev, S.V.; Shibaeva, T.V.; Shvorneva, L.I. Influence of ripening time on the properties of hydroxyapatite-calcium carbonate powders. *Inorg. Mater.* **2012**, *48*, 181–186. [CrossRef]
54. Shurtakova, D.V.; Yavkin, B.V.; Mamin, G.V.; Orlinskii, S.B.; Sirotinkin, V.P.; Fedotov, A.Y.; Shinkarev, A.; Antuzevics, A.; Smirnov, I.V.; Tovtin, V.I.; et al. X-Ray Diffraction and Multifrequency EPR Study of Radiation-Induced Room Temperature Stable Radicals in Octacalcium Phosphate. *Radiat. Res.* **2021**, *195*, 200–210. [CrossRef]
55. Shurtakova, D.; Yavkin, B.; Gafurov, M.; Mamin, G.; Orlinskii, S.; Kuznetsova, L.; Bakhteev, S.; Ignatyev, I.; Smirnov, I.; Fedotov, A.; et al. Study of radiation-induced stable radicals in synthetic octacalcium phosphate by pulsed EPR. *Magn. Reson. Solids* **2019**, *21*, 19105. [CrossRef]
56. Baran, N.P.; Vorona, I.P.; Ishchenko, S.S.; Nosenko, V.V.; Zatovskii, I.V.; Gorodilova, N.A.; Povarchuk, V.Y. NO_3^{2-} and CO_2^- centers in synthetic hydroxyapatite: Features of the formation under γ-and UV-irradiations. *Phys. Solid State* **2011**, *53*, 1891–1894. [CrossRef]
57. Nosenko, V.V.; Vorona, I.P.; Ishchenko, S.S.; Baran, N.P.; Zatovsky, I.V.; Gorodilova, N.A.; Povarchuk, V.Y. Effect of pre-annealing on NO_3^{2-} centers in synthetic hydroxyapatite. *Radiat. Meas.* **2012**, *47*, 970–973. [CrossRef]
58. Goldfarb, D. ELDOR-Detected NMR. *eMagRes* **2007**, *6*, 101–114. [CrossRef]
59. Wili, N.; Richert, S.; Limburg, B.; Clarke, S.J.; Anderson, H.L.; Timmel, C.R.; Jeschke, G. ELDOR-detected NMR beyond hyperfine couplings: A case study with Cu (ii)-porphyrin dimers. *Phys. Chem. Chem. Phys.* **2019**, *21*, 11676–11688. [CrossRef] [PubMed]
60. Gracheva, I.N.; Gafurov, M.R.; Mamin, G.V.; Biktagirov, T.B.; Rodionov, A.A.; Galukhin, A.V.; Orlinskii, S.B. ENDOR study of nitrogen hyperfine and quadrupole tensors in vanadyl porphyrins of heavy crude oil. *Magn. Reson. Solids* **2016**, *18*, 16102.
61. Moens, P.D.W.; Callens, F.J.; Boesman, E.R.; Verbeeck, R.M.H. ^1H and ^{31}P ENDOR of the isotropic CO_2^- signal at g = 2.0007 in the EPR spectra of precipitated carbonated apatites. *Appl. Magn. Reson.* **1995**, *9*, 103–113. [CrossRef]

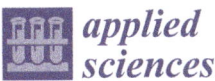

Article

Observational Study Regarding Two Bonding Systems and the Challenges of Their Use in Orthodontics: An In Vitro Evaluation

Sorana Maria Bucur [1], Anamaria Bud [2], Adrian Gligor [3,*], Alexandru Vlasa [2,*], Dorin Ioan Cocoș [1] and Eugen Silviu Bud [2]

[1] Faculty of Medicine, Dimitrie Cantemir University of Târgu Mureș, 3-5 Bodoni Sandor Str., 540545 Târgu-Mureș, Romania; bucursoranamaria@gmail.com (S.M.B.); cdorin1123@gmail.com (D.I.C.)
[2] Faculty of Dental Medicine, George Emil Palade University of Medicine, Pharmacy, Science and Technology of Târgu Mureș, 38 Gheorghe Marinescu Str., 540139 Târgu Mureș, Romania; anamaria.bud@umfst.ro (A.B.); Eugen.bud@umfst.ro (E.S.B.)
[3] Faculty of Engineering and Information Technology, George Emil Palade University of Medicine, Pharmacy, Science and Technology of Târgu Mureș, 38 Gheorghe Marinescu Str., 540139 Târgu Mureș, Romania
* Correspondence: adrian.gligor@umfst.ro (A.G.); alexandru.vlasa@umfst.ro (A.V.)

Abstract: The purpose of this in vitro study was to analyze and identify a methodology for the improvement of the shear bond strength of orthodontic brackets bonded with two orthodontic adhesive systems considered to be widely used, Transbond Plus Color Change with Transbond Plus Self-Etching Primer and Fuji Ortho LC with orthophosphoric acid under various enamel conditions: dry, moistened with water and moistened with saliva. The sample size included a group of 120 freshly extracted premolars distributed into six study groups, each one of 20 teeth. A universal testing machine was used to detach the brackets. We determined and compared the strength of the two studied adhesive systems used in different enamel surface conditions. The mean shear bond strength values in groups 1 (TPCC, TSEP, dry), 2 (TPCC, TSEP, water), 3 (TPCC, TSEP, saliva), 4 (Fuji Ortho LC, etched, dry enamel), 5 (Fuji Ortho LC, etched enamel, water) and 6 (Fuji Ortho LC, etched enamel, saliva) were 15.86, 12.31, 13.04, 15.27, 14.14 and 13.11 MPa, respectively. ANOVA test and Student's t-test showed significant differences between groups. While clinically acceptable shear bond strengths were obtained for all six studied groups, a particular outcome that to the authors' knowledge has not been documented elsewhere has been obtained: in case of water contamination, it is preferable to use Fuji Ortho LC instead of Transbond Plus.

Keywords: bond strength; brackets; dry; wet and moistened enamel; adhesion

Citation: Bucur, S.M.; Bud, A.; Gligor, A.; Vlasa, A.; Cocoș, D.I.; Bud, E.S. Observational Study Regarding Two Bonding Systems and the Challenges of Their Use in Orthodontics: An In Vitro Evaluation. Appl. Sci. 2021, 11, 7091. https://doi.org/10.3390/app11157091

Academic Editor: Vittorio Checchi

Received: 15 July 2021
Accepted: 29 July 2021
Published: 31 July 2021

Publisher's Note: MDPI stays neutral with regard to jurisdictional claims in published maps and institutional affiliations.

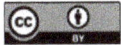

Copyright: © 2021 by the authors. Licensee MDPI, Basel, Switzerland. This article is an open access article distributed under the terms and conditions of the Creative Commons Attribution (CC BY) license (https://creativecommons.org/licenses/by/4.0/).

1. Introduction

The possibility of bonding brackets was an important step in fixed orthodontics, resulting in the shortening of working time for the orthodontist, better hygiene and fewer dental and periodontal pathological conditions after wearing the appliances, better aesthetics and the elimination of the working phase in which the interdental spaces were closed after detaching the bands [1].

The bond strength between the brackets and the tooth enamel is an extremely important issue in performing the mechanics of orthodontic treatment; the brackets' detachments cause a series of inconveniences, the reattachment being a difficult, unpleasant maneuver, besides the fact that the detachment of the brackets can cause delays of the treatment results and mechanical injuries of the neighboring soft tissues of the oral cavity [1,2].

From a chemical point of view, adhesion is the gluing of two materials that can be different by means of a chemical compound called adhesive or bonding. The difference from physical adhesion is that chemical groups which appear on both surfaces can form an intramolecular or intermolecular chemical bond. Chemical adhesion involves a chemoabsorption process in which the adhesive molecules attached by adsorption to the surface of the material can react with its active groups by forming chemical bonds [3]. In our case, the purpose of adhesion is to join the enamel surface with another substrate, represented by the materials used for bonding the brackets. The tooth enamel is the hardest tissue of the body due to its hypermineralization. Its hardness varies depending on the dental area in which the tooth is positioned; in areas with intense functional stress, it can reach 5 degrees of hardness on the Mohs scale. The tooth enamel does not retain water, being consequently easy to wash and dry [4].

Many orthodontists are accustomed to using composite resins for bonding brackets, even if those adhesive systems have high technical sensitivity because they require a completely dry surface throughout the application procedures. The number of clinical steps and the long application time require the patient's cooperation and the focus of the doctor to eliminate the possible technical errors [5].

Ekhlassi et al. [6] showed that Transbond Plus Color Change Adhesive (3M Unitek, Monrovia, CA, USA) is an improved resin that has ionized glass particles in its composition; this adhesive is described by the manufacturer as having excellent adhesion with metal and ceramic brackets. TPCC has been described as having hydrophilic properties.

Because of the chemical composition of ionized particles, Transbond Plus Color Change is an adhesive that slowly releases fluoride, which results in the reduction in enamel demineralization around the brackets' bases [7]. Its pink-colored component is activated by light-curing or by exposing it to the natural light, and during the polymerization, the initial pink color changes and turns irreversibly into a shade similar to that of the tooth enamel. The color change restores the aesthetic appearance of the bonding agent during the treatment. The initial pink color helps the doctor to remove excessive bonding material from the tooth surface before light-curing [6,8]. Excess adhesive may cause food retention, dental plaque and injuries of the superficial periodontium or the oral mucosa. Bacterial plaque with a large variety of microbial strains and food debris may produce inflammation and infection of the periodontal tissues and demineralization of the tooth enamel, especially in the cervical region of the vestibular surfaces, above the upper edge of the brackets' bases [8]. These great advantages of bonding procedures and the entire orthodontic treatment are important reasons why the use of TPCC is preferred by many orthodontists.

Self-etching primers began to be used about 20 years ago because their use was found to result in the formation of a continuum between the adhesive contained and the etched surface by simultaneous acid demineralization and penetration of the treated surface with acidic monomers. Those monomers can be then easily polymerized in situ, so the bonding technique is simplified [8]. Self-etching primers are combinations of etching acids and bonding resins that are manufactured in order to eliminate the etching step and to reduce the chairside working time and the risk of salivary contamination; using the primer reduces the adhesion process to two steps instead of three.

According to the manufacturer's (3M Unitek, Monrovia, CA, USA) datasheet, Transbond Plus Color Change adhesive when used together with Transbond Plus Self-Etching Primer (3M) provides a moisture-tolerant bonding system. Transbond Plus Self-Etching Primer (TSEP) contains methacrylate phosphoric acid esters as the main ingredients [9]. The acidic end group of the resin derivate has hydrophilic properties [10].

Contamination may occur frequently in clinical activity after application of the primer; in this case, the ability of the primer to create a chemical bond strong enough to allow the proper adhesion of the brackets is to be considered.

Another bonding material used in our study was Fuji Ortho LC, an adhesive made by GC America, Inc.; this dental material has been described by the manufacturer as a light-cured resin-reinforced glass ionomer cement. Resins have been added to ionomeric cements to improve their aesthetic and mechanical characteristics, to increase adhesion and to maintain the fluoride-releasing property [11].

Fuji Ortho LC is a viscous material that becomes hard by polymerization that occurs upon exposure to ultraviolet or natural light. In orthodontics, it has been frequently used for bonding brackets and bands.

The study described in this work aimed to evaluate the adhesion created by using two adhesive systems with a different chemical composition for bonding brackets, Transbond Plus Color Change with Transbond Plus Self-Etching Primer and pre-etched Fuji Ortho LC in three enamel conditions achievable in regular dental office activity: dry, contaminated with water and contaminated with saliva.

2. Materials and Methods

In this in vitro study, we used a total of 120 mandibular and maxillary premolars extracted for orthodontic purposes. The donor patients approved the use of their extracted teeth in the study by signing a written consent. The criteria for including teeth in the study were:

- The crown integrity, namely the absence of any structural or developmental crown defects, decays, restorations or cracks caused by the extraction procedures [12,13];
- The teeth not having undergone any chemical treatment [9].

The extracted teeth were washed in water then placed in a 0.1% thymol solution. Later, they were stored for a week in distilled water that was changed once a day. They were removed from distilled water on the day of testing and were gently cleaned with Depural Neo from Spofa Dental, a slightly abrasive fluoride-free paste that is generally used for professional teeth polishing [14].

We wanted to use only the premolar crowns for easier handling, so we separated the premolar roots and crowns at the anatomical cement–enamel junction using low-speed diamond disks and water cooling [15]. All the premolar crowns were mounted in Duracrol (a self-curing methacrylate resin produced by Spofa Dental, which now is part of Danaher Corporation, California) blocks with only their buccal surfaces exposed (Figure 1) in order to allow the brackets' bonding and testing [15]; the hard self-curing resin kept the crowns of the teeth immobile during the brackets' debonding. The cubes were prepared by putting the acrylic resin in plastic cubes previously insulated with Vaseline before starting the setting. The size of the cubes was 3.3 cm/3.3 cm/2 cm. Just before the setting, the crowns of the premolars were submerged so that only the vestibular surface remained exposed. We made sure that the vestibular surfaces were not contaminated with Duracrol [16]. For all the specimens in the study, we used Discovery brackets from DENTAURUM GmbH & Co., Ispringen, Germany.

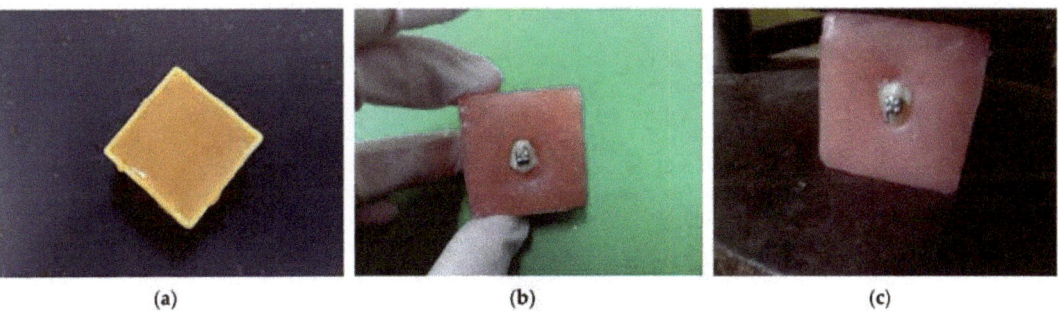

Figure 1. Sample preparation: (**a**) Duracrol cube; (**b**) before testing; and (**c**) position during the testing process.

Thus, prepared teeth were randomly divided into six groups (20 samples for each group) according to the bonding system and enamel preparation:

Group 1: Transbond Plus Color Change together with Transbond Plus Self-Etching Primer (3M). The buccal surfaces of teeth in this group were treated with Transbond Plus

Self-Etching Primer; the primer was rubbed onto the buccal surfaces for 10 s using the disposable supplied. Then, the moisture-free spray was used for 10 s in order to deliver air to the primer. We applied Transbond Plus Color Change paste to the brackets' bases which then were pressed evenly and placed on the teeth, respecting the positioning bonding rules by localizing the center of the buccal surfaces [17]. Excessive bonding material around the bracket base was then gently removed by using a sealer, and the adhesive was light-cured with a Demetron LC lamp (SDS Kerr, USA) which had a light intensity of 800 mW/cm^2. The specimens were light-cured from occlusal, gingival, mesial and distal aspects for 10 s each, for a total of 40 s [18,19].

Group 2: Transbond Plus Color Change together with Transbond Plus Self-Etching Primer (3M) moistened with distilled water. We first prepared the buccal surfaces of the teeth in this group as we did with the specimens from Group 1; the difference was that after the application of the primer and the use of the air spray, we moistened the entire buccal surfaces of the teeth in this group with water. The water was applied by using first a dental syringe and then using a microbrush. Then, we applied the bonding material Transbond Plus Color Change in the same way as we did in Group 1.

Group 3: Transbond Plus Color Change together with Transbond Plus Self-Etching Primer (3M) moistened with saliva. The working steps were the same as in Group 2, except that after applying the primer and using the air spray, a small amount of saliva was applied to the entire buccal surfaces of the group's specimens. The saliva was donated by one of the authors and applied by using a microbrush. The donor had been asked to clean their teeth well just before collecting the saliva [5].

Group 4: Fuji Ortho LC in capsules on etched and dry enamel. The specimens were first etched with 37% orthophosphoric acid for 15 s [11,16,18]. Then, the treated surfaces were rinsed thoroughly with the water spray for 15 s and air-dried with the oil-free spray for 20 s [18].

Fuji Ortho LC was applied to the bracket base. Then, the brackets were pressed evenly on the enamel surfaces, respecting the positioning bonding rules by localizing the center of the buccal surfaces [17]. In order to achieve the minimum adhesive thickness, the brackets were compressed over the tooth surface by putting a special blade in the slots. Excessive bonding material around the bracket base was then gently removed by using a common sealer. The light-curing was performed with the lamp Demetron LC. The specimens were light-cured from occlusal, gingival, mesial and distal aspects for 10 s each [18,19].

Group 5: Fuji Ortho LC in capsules on etched enamel entirely moistened with distilled water before bonding. All the stages of the teeth preparation were similar to those in Group 4. The difference was that after being treated with orthophosphoric acid, washed and dried, the buccal surfaces of the teeth were moistened by using distilled water and a microbrush.

Group 6: Fuji Ortho LC in capsules on etched enamel surfaces entirely moistened with saliva before bonding. All the stages of the teeth preparation were similar to those in Group 4. The only difference was that after being treated with orthophosphoric acid, washed and dried, the buccal surfaces of the teeth were moistened by using saliva donated by one of the authors and a microbrush in the same way as in Group 3 [5].

We used a universal testing machine (Model DDW-100, DTEC, Deity Testing Equipment Co., Ltd., Beijing, China) (Figure 2) to determine the force required to detach the brackets. For testing the bond strength, the bracket slot was positioned parallel to the horizontal plane and the surveyor blade was placed perpendicular to the bracket's base [18]. We tested the shear bond strength by applying an occlusal–cervical force to the bracket base, with a cross-head speed of 1 mm/min [5]. The force required to detach the brackets was expressed in megapascal (MPa) by using a common conversion from N/mm^2 to MPa [12], taking into account the dimension of the bracket base, i.e., 10.3 mm^2 (data obtained from the manufacturer—Dentaurum, Ispringen, Germany).

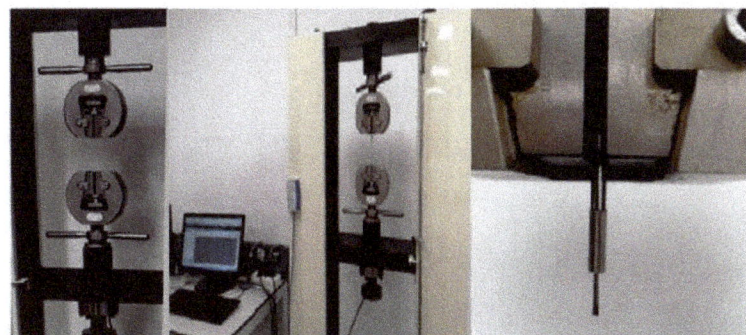

Figure 2. Device used for evaluation of the force required to detach the brackets.

Data resulting from the experimental investigation were verified to avoid outliers and considered for statistical analysis. The results are expressed as mean ± standard deviation. For testing the normality of data, we used the Kolmogorov–Smirnov test. For the parametric data, we used Student's t-test. To compare all six groups together, we used the ANOVA test. The statistically significant level was $p < 0.05$.

3. Results

The mean shear bond strength values in Groups 1–6 were 15.86, 12.31, 13.04, 15.27, 14.14 and 13.11 MPa, respectively (Table 1). The highest value of force required to remove the bracket was found when examining TPCC and TSEP in dry conditions, 15.86 MPa +/− 1.97 SD. The lowest force required to remove the brackets was found when examining TPCC and TSEP in moist conditions, 12.31 MPa +/− 2.16 SD.

Table 1. Average values of force required to remove the brackets in the study groups.

Groups	Bonding System, Enamel Conditioning	Average (MPa)	Variance
Group 1	TPCC, TSEP, dry	15.86	1.97
Group 2	TPCC, TSEP, water	12.31	2.16
Group 3	TPCC, TSEP, saliva	13.04	2.75
Group 4	Fuji Ortho LC, etched, dry	15.27	2.33
Group 5	Fuji Ortho LC, etched, water	14.14	1.54
Group 6	Fuji Ortho LC, etched, saliva	13.11	1.84

When comparing the results obtained from the study groups, significant values ($p > 0.05$) were observed (Table 2).

Table 2. Statistical comparison between studied groups.

Groups	1	2	3	4	5	6
Group 1	-	<0.0001	0.0007	0.3794	0.0093	0.0003
Group 2			0.3112	0.0003	0.0077	0.2231
Group 3				0.0058	0.112	0.9212
Group 4					0.0851	0.0036
Group 5						0.0943

When comparing the results regarding the surface of the tooth, no statistically significant differences between the study groups were recorded (Figure 3).

Significant differences in bond strength were detected between Group 1 and all the other groups ($p < 0.05$), except Group 4. Significant differences were detected between Group 4 and all the other groups ($p < 0.05$), except Groups 1 and 5. We found no significant difference between Groups 1 and 4 ($p > 0.05$) (Figure 4). Group 2 exhibited significant differences from Groups 1, 4 and 5. Group 3 exhibited significant differences from Groups 1 and 4. Significant differences were detected between Group 5 and Groups 1 and 2. Group 6 exhibited significant differences from Groups 1 and 4.

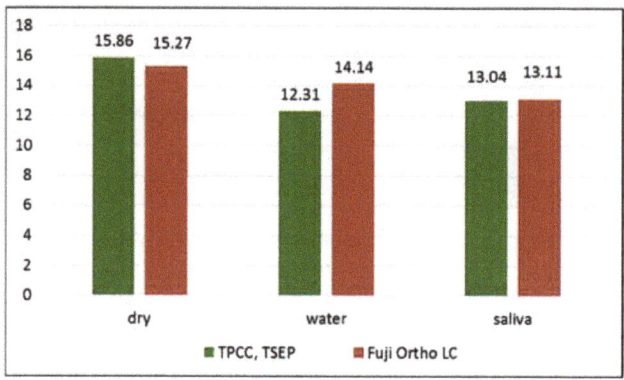

Figure 3. Comparison between the study groups regarding the surface of the tooth.

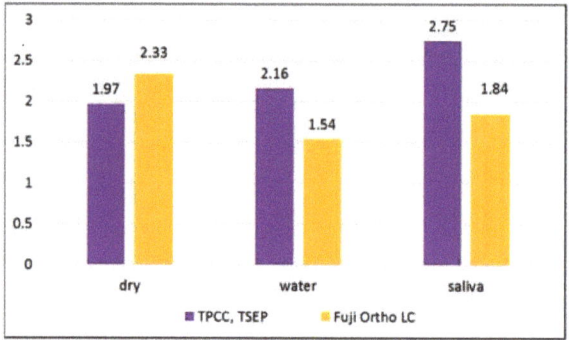

Figure 4. Comparison of the statistical variance of the averages in the study groups.

4. Discussions

We have chosen to compare these two adhesive systems because they are widely used for bonding brackets in orthodontic clinical practice [6,12,18] and it was very important to determine the difference between their bond strengths in different working conditions; still, they were uniquely studied comparatively in various enamel conditions only in this research by the time of documenting and writing of this report.

In recent decades, primers were manufactured and used for bonding resin composites to the enamel surface. Unfortunately, these coupling agents had poor hydrolytic stability, so they were chemically unstable in the oral environment where the saliva is always present and the risk of enamel contamination is high [5,12]. We wanted a good adhesion even in humid conditions, so we had to choose bonding materials with hydrophilic properties.

The studied adhesive systems in all described working conditions have demonstrated an adequate adhesion for use as bonding agents for orthodontic brackets. According to Reynolds [20], the adequate bond strength required for orthodontic needs starts from 5.9–7.8 MPa. This value of adhesion could counteract orthodontic and masticatory forces [20]. In our study, the highest bond strength was found for the group in which we used TPCC and TSEP on dry enamel, and the lowest bond strength was found for the same adhesive system on the enamel moistened with saliva. A statistically significant difference between water-moistened groups was found: Fuji Ortho LC had a higher bond strength. A very small difference without statistical significance was found between saliva-moistened groups. The ANOVA comparison of the variance of the averages demonstrated a statistically significant difference between groups ($p = 0.000002244$).

The results of our study showed that the mean bond strength of the Transbond Plus Color Change used with the primer without contamination was higher than that in the other two groups, with water and saliva contamination. Saliva contamination does not affect the strength of the bond as much as water contamination in the case of using Transbond Plus Color Change with Transbond Plus Self-Etching Primer. The reason why we chose to use the Transbond Plus Self-Etching Primer together with Transbond Plus Color Change is that it has been demonstrated that this combination with a hydrophilic resin gives a superior bond strength compared to that of the same primer used with the conventional Transbond XT, which is a hydrophobic resin, even under conditions of saliva contamination [12].

Other researchers, such as Ascensión Vicente et al. [21], found that Transbond Plus with TSEP proves better adhesion under saliva contamination than with water contamination or even without any contamination. In their study, as in ours, the contamination was performed after applying the primer, but the use of Transbond Plus instead of the Transbond Plus Color Change we used could explain the different results [21].

Mandava Prasad et al. [5] found that the groups in which they used a self-etch bonding system—TSEP—contaminated with water and saliva had significantly higher bond strength than groups bonded with a conventional bonding system in the same conditions. They found a better tolerance of TSEP in wet conditions compared to Transbond XT (3M Unitek) after acid etching in the same conditions [5].

In their in vivo study, Mariá D. Campoy et al. [22] found that saliva contamination before or after application of Transbond Plus Self-Etching primer does not significantly change the bonding strength and does not increase the risk of bond failure [22].

It has been also demonstrated by Cacciafesta et al. [23] that Transbond Plus Self-Etching Primer gives higher bonding strength values than two other primers, one conventional and one hydrophilic. It proved to be less affected by water or saliva contamination [23].

In the molecular structure of TSEP, there is a combination between a phosphoric acid and a methacrylate group. These two groups form a methacrylate phosphoric acid ester. When TSEP is applied on the hard dental structures, the phosphate group dissolves calcium and removes it. The phosphate group and calcium form a complex that is incorporated into the adhesive network during polymerization. By this mechanism, the acid etching of the enamel and the penetration of the monomer into the created microretentions are synchronized. So, the depth at which the enamel is etched coincides with the depth of penetration of the primer [5].

As a chemical composition, TSEP also has water as a solvent [9]; this could give the primer tolerance to wet conditions. TSEP's performance in such conditions could be explained by the self-etching primer's chemical composition of hydrophilic monomers.

Transbond Plus Color Change may owe its tolerance to humid conditions to the polyethylene glycol dimethacrylate (PEGDMA) and the low concentration of hydrophobic bisphenol A diglycidyl ether dimethacrylate (bis-GMA) in its composition; polyethylene glycol dimethacrylate (PEGDMA) favors the infiltration of bis-GMA adhesives into the wet enamel [9] and bonding with TSEP even in humid conditions. Saliva is an oral fluid composed of a variety of minerals and electrolytes such as calcium, sodium, magnesium, potassium, bicarbonate and phosphates. The existence of salivary ions probably multiplies the chemical bonds between TSEP and TPCC and increases the bonding strength [24].

Fuji Ortho LC can be applied on the enamel surface with or without an etching technique [18]. Because this bonding material is basically a glass ionomer luting cement with a high capacity to slowly release fluoride, it prevents the decalcification of the tooth enamel and the appearance of "white spots" after debonding brackets. Researchers have demonstrated by many studies that the use of phosphoric acid for slight demineralization of the enamel before bonding with glass ionomers improves the bond strength without affecting the mineralization of the tooth because of their ability to gradually release mineral ions [11,16].

The superior adhesion of Fuji Ortho LC in the case of acid pretreatment of the enamel with 37% phosphoric acid was even better than that created by using a self-etching adhesive system [25].

Among the groups in which we used Fuji Ortho LC, we found the highest adhesion strength when the teeth were not contaminated with anything after etching and the lowest adhesion strength when the teeth were moistened with saliva after etching. The difference was statistically significant between the dry and saliva-moistened groups and without statistical significance between the dry and water-moistened groups and water-moistened and saliva-moistened groups. In our opinion, it would be desirable to add chemical components to the composition of this material to increase its adhesion in case of salivary contamination.

Bishara et al. [26] obtained a result similar to that of our study by finding no statistically significant differences between two experimental groups of teeth, one bonded with Fuji Ortho LC with the enamel etched and moistened with water before bonding and another bonded with Fuji Ortho LC with the enamel etched and moistened with saliva before bonding [26].

Feizbakhsh et al. [18] conducted a study partially similar to ours by applying Fuji Ortho LC after etching on dry enamel, enamel moistened with distilled water and enamel moistened with saliva. They found results similar to those of our study. The bonding strength was maximum in the dry enamel group; they found a statistically significant difference between this group and the group of teeth moistened with saliva, which proved to have the lowest bonding strength value among etched groups [18]. They also found a significant difference between the group of teeth moistened with distilled water and that moistened with saliva. There was no significant difference after etching between the group of teeth moistened with water and the dry enamel group. The very similar results not as absolute values but as differences between the studied groups could be explained by the fact that these authors used acid etching and subsequent contamination with distilled water and saliva in ways similar to our research [18]. Their study demonstrated that saliva prevents micromechanical bonding between Fuji Ortho LC and tooth enamel to a great extent in the etched groups because of deposition of salivary constituents [18]; this must be the reason why we also found the lowest adhesion in the group where the contamination after etching was done with saliva.

Other studies, such as that of Cook et al. [27], demonstrated that "etching the tooth surface with phosphoric acid produced a significantly poorer bond to the enamel" [27]. Cacciafesta and Toledano have demonstrated that Fuji Ortho LC bonded without any enamel conditioning gives a significantly lower shear bond strength compared with that made by glass ionomer cement on enamel etched with 37% phosphoric acid [16,28]. Using acid etching creates a layer of porous enamel that ranges in depth from 5 to 50 µm [29], which is more suitable to achieve a stronger micromechanical adhesion by increasing the accessible areas for bonding. The acid application eliminates the organic biofilm and increases the enamel surface's free energy [30]. It is well known that the adhesion of glass ionomer cements to enamel is also one of a chemical nature [16,18].

Cacciafesta et al. [31] found that in the case of using stainless steel lingual brackets, Fuji Ortho LC had a significantly higher bond strength after application on saliva-moistened enamel, after enamel conditioning with polyacrylic acid, when compared to all other tested enamel conditions: nonetched and dry, nonetched and wet, etched with polyacrylic acid and water-moistened. The hydrophilic monomer HEMA (2-hydroxy ethyl methacrylate) which is a main component of Fuji Ortho LC, may be responsible for infiltration and hydration [18].

Many studies have been done to compare the bond strengths of glass ionomer cements and composite resins [32–34]. Reddy et al. [32] showed that the bond strength of the composite resin was better than that of glass ionomer, and the adhesion given by both bonding materials decreased after contamination with blood. Yassaei and Rix [33,34] also demonstrated that Transbond XT had a better shear bond strength than Fuji Ortho LC.

In our study, we found no significant differences between the two bonding systems on dry enamel and enamel moistened with saliva. The difference between the two bonding systems was statistically significant in their application on water-moistened enamel; Fuji Ortho LC exhibited better shear bond strength.

The laboratory conditions may greatly differ from those in vivo; the debonding forces may act in different directions. Moreover, water and saliva contamination varies in quantity and cannot be controlled as finely as in our study. It would be useful to test other parameters that reflect the adhesion of the brackets, such as the tensile bond strength [35].

5. Conclusions

Both studied bonding systems in all three different conditions yielded acceptable bond strengths in vitro. Both systems demonstrated better adhesion on dry enamel than on wet enamel moistened with distilled water or saliva. In clinical situations where there is a risk of salivary contamination, we may use both studied adhesive systems, but in the case of water contamination, it is preferable to use Fuji Ortho LC. To confirm the results of this study, we will have to test them in vivo.

Author Contributions: Conceptualization, S.M.B. and A.B.; methodology, S.M.B. and A.V.; validation, S.M.B., A.V. and E.S.B.; writing—original draft preparation, S.M.B., A.B., A.G. and D.I.C.; writing—review and editing, A.G. and A.V.; supervision, S.M.B. and E.S.B. All authors have read and agreed to the published version of the manuscript.

Funding: This research received no external funding.

Institutional Review Board Statement: The study was conducted according to the guidelines of the Declaration of Helsinki and approved by the Ethics Committee of S.C. Algocalm SRL, Târgu-Mures, Romania, protocol 898/25.01.2021.

Informed Consent Statement: Informed consent was obtained from all subjects involved in the study.

Data Availability Statement: Not applicable.

Conflicts of Interest: The authors declare no conflict of interest.

References

1. Ribeiro, G.L.U.; Jacob, H.B. Understanding the basis of space closure in Orthodontics for a more efficient orthodontic treatment. *Dent. Press J. Orthod.* **2016**, *21*, 115–125. [CrossRef] [PubMed]
2. Almosa, N.A.; Zafar, H. Incidence of orthodontic brackets detachment during orthodontic treatment: A systematic review. *Pak. J. Med Sci.* **2018**, *34*, 744–750. [CrossRef] [PubMed]
3. Von Fraunhofer, J.A. Adhesion and Cohesion. *Int. J. Dent.* **2012**, *2012*, 951324. [CrossRef]
4. Klimuszko, E.; Orywal, K.; Sierpinska, T.; Sidun, J.; Gołębiewska, M. The evaluation of zinc and copper content in tooth enamel without any pathological changes—An in vitro study. *Int. J. Nanomed.* **2018**, *13*, 1257–1264. [CrossRef] [PubMed]
5. Prasad, M.; Mohamed, S.; Nayak, K.; Shetty, S.K.; Talapaneni, A.K. Effect of moisture, saliva, and blood contamination on the shear bond strength of brackets bonded with a conventional bonding system and self-etched bonding system. *J. Nat. Sci. Biol. Med.* **2014**, *5*, 123–129. [CrossRef] [PubMed]
6. Ekhlassi, S.; English, J.D.; Ontiveros, J.C.; Powers, J.M.; Bussa, H.I.; Frey, G.N.; Colville, C.D.; Ellis, R.K. Bond strength comparison of color-change adhesives for orthodontic bonding using a self-etching primer. *Clin. Cosmet. Investig. Dent.* **2011**, *3*, 39–44. [CrossRef]
7. Eissaa, O.; El-Shourbagy, E.; Ghobashy, S. In vivo effect of a fluoride releasing adhesive on inhibition of enamel demineralization around orthodontic brackets. *Tanta Dent. J.* **2013**, *10*, 86–96. [CrossRef]
8. Maurya, R.; Tripathi, T.; Rai, P. New generation of color bonding: A comparative in vitro study. *Indian J. Dent. Res.* **2011**, *22*, 733–734. [CrossRef]
9. Goswami, A.; Mitali, B.; Roy, B. Shear bond strength comparison of moisture-insensitive primer and self-etching primer. *J. Orthod. Sci.* **2014**, *3*, 89–93. [CrossRef]
10. Liu, W.; Meng, H.; Sun, Z.; Jiang, R.; Dong, C.; Zhang, C. Phosphoric and carboxylic methacrylate esters as bonding agents in self-adhesive resin cements. *Exp. Ther. Med.* **2018**, *15*, 4531–4537. [CrossRef]
11. Jurišić, S.; Jurišić, G.; Jurić, H. Influence of Adhesives and Methods of Enamel Pretreatment on the Shear Bond Strength of Orthodontic Brackets. *Acta Stomatol. Croat.* **2015**, *49*, 269–274. [CrossRef] [PubMed]

12. Shaik, J.A.; Reddy, R.K.; Bhagyalakshmi, K.; Shah, M.J.; Madhavi, O.; Ramesh, S.V.M. In vitro evaluation of shear bond strength of orthodontic brackets bonded with different adhesives. *Contemp. Clin. Dent.* **2018**, *9*, 289–292. [CrossRef] [PubMed]
13. Sfondrini, M.F.; Fraticelli, D.; Gandini, P.; Scribante, A. Shear Bond Strength of Orthodontic Brackets and Disinclusion Buttons: Effect of Water and Saliva Contamination. *BioMed Res. Int.* **2013**, *2013*, 180137. [CrossRef]
14. Bucur, S.M.; Cocoș, D.; Saghin, A. Bond strength of three adhesive systems used for bonding orthodontic brackets. *Rom. J. Oral Rehabil.* **2020**, *12*, 162–167.
15. Shelb, E.A.; Etman, W.M.; Genaid, T.M.; Shalaby, E. Durability of bond strength of glass-ionomers to enamel. *Tanta Dent. J.* **2015**, *12*, 16–27. [CrossRef]
16. Cacciafesta, V.; Sfondrini, M.F.; Baluga, L.; Scribante, A.; Klersy, C. Use of a self-etching primer in combination with a resin-modified glass ionomer: Effect of water and saliva contamination on shear bond strength. *Am. J. Orthod. Dentofac. Orthop.* **2003**, *124*, 420–426. [CrossRef]
17. Armstrong, D.; Shen, G.; Petocz, P.; Darendeliler, M.A. A comparison of accuracy in bracket positioning between two techniques–localizing the centre of the clinical crown and measuring the distance from the incisal edge. *Eur. J. Orthod.* **2007**, *29*, 430–436. [CrossRef] [PubMed]
18. Feizbakhsh, M.; Aslani, F.; Gharizadeh, N.; Heidarizadeh, M. Comparison of bracket bond strength to etched and unetched enamel under dry and wet conditions using Fuji Ortho LC glassionomer. *J. Dent. Res. Dent. Clin. Dent. Prospect.* **2017**, *11*, 30–35. [CrossRef]
19. Naseh, R.; Afshari, M.; Shafiei, F.; Rahnamoon, N. Shear bond strength of metal brackets to ceramic surfaces using a universal bonding resin. *J. Clin. Exp. Dent.* **2018**, *10*, e739–e745. [CrossRef]
20. Reynolds, I.R. A Review of Direct Orthodontic Bonding. *Br. J. Orthod.* **1975**, *2*, 171–178. [CrossRef]
21. Vicente, A.; Mena, A.; Ortiz, A.J.; Bravo, L.A. Water and Saliva Contamination Effect on Shear Bond Strength of Brackets Bonded with a Moisture-Tolerant Light Cure System. *Angle Orthod.* **2009**, *79*, 127–132. [CrossRef]
22. Campoy, M.D.; Plasencia, E.; Vicente, A.; Bravo, L.A.; Cibrian, R. Effect of saliva contamination on bracket failure with a self-etching primer: A prospective controlled clinical trial. *Am. J. Orthod. Dentofac. Orthop.* **2010**, *137*, 679–683. [CrossRef] [PubMed]
23. Cacciafesta, V.; Sfondrini, M.F.; De Angelis, M.; Scribante, A.; Klersy, C. Effect of water and saliva contamination on shear bond strength of brackets bonded with conventional, hydrophilic, and self-etching primers. *Am. J. Orthod. Dentofac. Orthop.* **2003**, *123*, 633–640. [CrossRef]
24. Humphrey, S.P.; Williamson, R.T. A review of saliva: Normal composition, flow, and function. *J. Prosthet. Dent.* **2001**, *85*, 162–169. [CrossRef] [PubMed]
25. Pithon, M.M.; Dos Santos, R.L.; Ruellas, A.C.; Sant'Anna, E.F. One-component self-etching primer: A seventh generation of orthodontic bonding system? *Eur. J. Orthod.* **2010**, *32*, 567–570. [CrossRef]
26. Bishara, S.E.; Olsen, M.E.; Damon, P.; Jakobsen, J.R. Evaluation of a new light-cured orthodontic bonding adhesive. *Am. J. Orthod. Dentofac. Orthop.* **1998**, *114*, 80–87. [CrossRef]
27. Cook, P.A.; Youngson, C.C. An in vitro Study of the Bond Strength of a Glass Ionomer Cement in the Direct Bonding of Orthodontic Brackets. *Br. J. Orthod.* **1988**, *15*, 247–253. [CrossRef]
28. Toledano, M.; Osorio, R.; Osorio, E.; Romeo, A.; De La Higuera, B.; García-Godoy, F. Bond strength of orthodontic brackets using different light and self-curing cements. *Angle Orthod.* **2003**, *73*, 56–63. [CrossRef]
29. Borges, M.A.P.; Matos, I.C.; Dias, K.R.H.C. Influence of two self-etching primer systems on enamel adhesion. *Braz. Dent. J.* **2007**, *18*, 113–118. [CrossRef]
30. Komori, A.; Ishikawa, H. Evaluation of a resin-reinforced glass ionomer cement for use as an orthodontic bonding agent. *Angle Orthod.* **1997**, *67*, 189–196. [CrossRef]
31. Cacciafesta, V.; Jost-Brinkmann, P.-G.; Süßenberger, U.; Miethke, R.-R. Effects of saliva and water contamination on the enamel shear bond strength of a light-cured glass ionomer cement. *Am. J. Orthod. Dentofac. Orthop.* **1998**, *113*, 402–407. [CrossRef]
32. Reddy, L.; Marker, V.A.; Ellis, E. Bond strength for orthodontic brackets contaminated by blood: Composite versus resin-modified glass ionomer cements. *J. Oral Maxillofac. Surg.* **2003**, *61*, 206–213. [CrossRef] [PubMed]
33. Yassaei, S.; Davari, A.; Moghadam, M.G.; Kamaei, A. Comparison of shear bond strength of RMGI and composite resin for orthodontic bracket bonding. *J. Dent.* **2014**, *11*, 282–289.
34. Rix, D.; Foley, T.F.; Mamandras, A. Comparison of bond strength of three adhesives: Composite resin, hybrid GIC, and glass-filled GIC. *Am. J. Orthod. Dentofac. Orthop.* **2001**, *119*, 36–42. [CrossRef] [PubMed]
35. Martha, K.; Ogodescu, A.; Zetu, I.; Ogodescu, E.; Gyergyay, R.; Pacurar, M. Comparative in vitro Study of the Tensile Bond Strength of Three Orthodontic Bonding Materials. *Mater. Plast.* **2013**, *50*, 208–211.

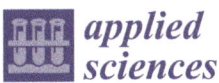

Article

Octacalcium Phosphate Bone Substitute (Bontree®): From Basic Research to Clinical Case Study

Joo-Seong Kim [1,†], Tae-Sik Jang [2,†], Suk-Young Kim [3] and Won-Pyo Lee [4,*]

1. Department of Biomedical Engineering, Yeungnam University, Daegu 42415, Korea; joorpediem@gmail.com
2. Department of Materials Science and Engineering, Chosun University, Gwangju 61452, Korea; tsjang@chosun.ac.kr
3. School of Materials Science and Engineering, Yeungnam University, Gyeongsan 38541, Korea; sykim@ynu.ac.kr
4. Department of Periodontology, School of Dentistry, Chosun University, Gwangju 61452, Korea
* Correspondence: wplee8@chosun.ac.kr; Tel.: +82-62-220-3850
† J.-S.K. and T.-S.J. are co-first authors and contributed equally to this work.

Featured Application: If a two-stage procedure comprising ridge or sinus augmentation using Bontree® followed by implant placement is planned, it is generally recommended that implants should be placed approximately 6 months after the healing period. However, as with other types of bone substitute materials, the implantation time can be decided on the basis of the surgeon's clinical experience and patient's condition.

Abstract: Bone grafts used in alveolar bone regeneration can be categorized into autografts, allografts, xenografts, and synthetic bones, depending on their origin. The purpose of this study was to evaluate the effect of a commercialized octacalcium phosphate (OCP)-based synthetic bone substitute material (Bontree®) in vitro, in vivo, and in clinical cases. Material characterization of Bontree® granules (0.5 mm and 1.0 mm) using scanning electron microscopy and X-ray diffraction showed that both 0.5 mm and 1.0 mm Bontree® granules were uniformly composed mainly of OCP. The receptor activator of NF-κB ligand (RANKL) and alkaline phosphatase (ALP) activities of MG63 cells were assessed and used to compare Bontree® with a commercial biphasic calcium phosphate ceramic (MBCP+™). Compared with MBCP+™, Bontree® suppressed RANKL and increased ALP activity. A rabbit tibia model used to examine the effects of granule size of Bontree® grafts showed that 1.0 mm Bontree® granules had a higher new bone formation ability than 0.5 mm Bontree® granules. Three clinical cases using Bontree® for ridge or sinus augmentation are described. All eight implants in the three patients showed a 100% success rate after 1 year of functional loading. This basic research and clinical application demonstrated the safety and efficacy of Bontree® for bone regeneration.

Keywords: biomaterial; bone regeneration; bone substitute; dental implant; octacalcium phosphate

1. Introduction

When teeth are lost, irreversible and gradual resorption of the alveolar bone occurs [1]. The loss of alveolar bone is one of the factors that makes it difficult prosthetically, esthetically, and functionally to restore lost teeth [2]. A sufficiently healthy alveolar bone is one of the main prerequisites for successful dental implant treatment [3]. Therefore, several studies have evaluated the concurrent use of a barrier membrane and graft materials for bone regeneration, which is commonly used to reconstruct resorbed alveolar bone [4].

Currently, bone graft materials used for bone regeneration are divided into autogenous bone grafts, allografts, xenografts, and synthetic bone grafts, depending on their origin. Autografts enable rapid healing without immunity-related problems and infection, and they contain growth factors that can facilitate new bone formation. However, the amount of bone that can be harvested is limited, and some limitations may lead to secondary bony defects at the donor site [5]. Allografts do not require surgery at the donor site and have osteoinduction and osteoconduction capabilities, but antigenicity- and infection-related problems may arise. In addition, new bone formation depends on the condition of the donor, which is a disadvantage [6]. Deproteinized bovine bone mineral (DBBM) is the most commonly used xenograft material in clinical practice. It has a calcium/phosphorus ratio similar to that of human bone, and its excellent osteoconductivity has been proven. However, xenografts have only osteoconductive ability and high absorption resistance; therefore, new bone formation is slower than that associated with autografts [7]. Synthetic bone graft materials can be mass-produced, their properties can be controlled, and there is no risk of cross-infection, although there are limitations such as low biodegradability depending on the material. Ceramics, tricalcium phosphate (TCP), and hydroxyapatite (HA) are used as synthetic bone materials. Several studies have been conducted on HA and β-TCP, which are calcium phosphate-based biomaterials [8].

Recently, octacalcium phosphate (OCP, $Ca_8H_2[PO_4]_6 \cdot 5H_2O$) was developed as a new synthetic bone substitute [9]. OCP is irreversibly converted to sustainable biological apatite under physiological conditions because OCP is a direct precursor of biological apatite [10]. OCP has been proven to be effective for new bone formation because of its high osteogenic capability and rapid bioabsorbability [11]. However, the sintering process changes the original crystal structure of OCP, and it cannot be formed into larger solid masses by sintering. In other words, OCP is generally fragile and difficult to develop as a synthetic bone substitute [12]. Due to these limitations, studies aimed at the commercialization of OCP-based bone substitutes have focused on coating OCP on DBBM [13] or mixing it with collagen [9,12,14]. However, a new synthesis method that does not require sintering was recently developed to mass-produce high-purity OCP with improved physical properties. This made it possible to commercialize an OCP-based synthetic bone substitute material (Bontree®, HudensBio Co., Gwangju, Korea), which is fully composed of apatite compounds with 80 wt.% OCP and 20 wt.% HA, with improved clinical handling while maintaining the inherent bone regeneration ability of OCP. In this article, we present the in vitro and in vivo evaluations of Bontree®. Its clinical use in three different surgical implant reconstructive procedures is also described.

2. Materials and Methods

2.1. Basic Research

2.1.1. Material Characterization

We purchased 0.5 mm and 1.0 mm diameter granules of the commercial OCP synthetic bone substitute material Bontree® (Bontree® 0.5-granule and Bontree® 1.0-granule, respectively, HudensBio Co., Gwangju, Korea) containing OCP and HA mixed at a weight ratio of 80:20 for experimental evaluation. A commercial biphasic calcium phosphate (BCP) synthetic bone substitute material (MBCP+™, composed of β-TCP and HA in a 80:20 weight ratio, Biomatlante Sarl, Vigneux de Bretagne, France) was also used for in vitro assays. Surface morphology was observed using field-emission scanning electron microscopy (FE-SEM, S-4700 Hitachi, Tokyo, Japan). Phase analysis was conducted using X-ray diffraction (XRD; X'Pert PRO MPD, Malvern Panalytical, Malvern, UK) with a Cu-Kα radiation source at a scan speed of 1.0°/min and a step size of 0.026°.

2.1.2. In Vitro Study

The biological properties of each sample were examined using a human osteoblast MG63 cell line (CTL-1427; ATCC, Manassas, VA, USA). MG63 cells were cultured in Dulbecco's modified Eagle's medium (DMEM; GIBCO Inc., Grand Island, NY, USA) supplemented with 10% fetal bovine serum (FBS; GIBCO Inc., Grand Island, NY, USA), 100 U/mL penicillin, and 100 μg/mL streptomycin (Gibco Inc., Grand Island, NY, USA). Prior to in vitro testing, Bontree® granules were compressed into 15 mm flat-faced tablets using a uniaxial press (Carver Inc., Chicago, IL, USA) for 30 s at a constant pressure of 55 MPa. The cells were incubated in a humidified incubator with 5% CO_2 at 37 °C. MG63 cells were seeded on each surface of the samples at a density of 1×10^4 cells/mL and cultured on the samples for 7 or 14 days. All the samples were sterilized with 70% ethanol solution for 30 min, followed by exposure under UV light for 12 h before MG63 cell seeding.

First, the content of the receptor activator of NF-κB ligand (RANKL) in the samples was determined using a commercial enzyme-linked immunosorbent assay (ELISA) kit. After a predetermined culturing time, the cells on the samples were detached using 0.25% trypsin-EDTA for 4 min at 37 °C, and the suspension containing the detached cells was vortexed and centrifuged at 13,000 rpm for 10 min. Standards and samples (100 µL) were added to the wells and incubated for 150 min at 25 °C. The wells were washed four times with a diluted wash solution. Next, 100 µL of biotinylated RANKL detection antibody diluted 80 times was added to each well and shaken gently for 1 h at 25 °C. Then, the wells were washed again with a wash solution diluted 20 times. Next, 100 µL of streptavidin–HRP conjugate solution diluted 200 times was added to each well, followed by shaking for 45 min at 25 °C, and washing with wash solution diluted 20 times. The wells were incubated with 100 µL of tetramethylbenzidine (TMB) for 30 min at 25 °C. The reaction was stopped by the addition of 50 µL of stop solution, and the color developed was measured at 450 nm.

Second, the differentiation of MG63 cells into osteoblasts was examined by an alkaline phosphatase (ALP) activity assay, which measured the transformation of *p*-nitrophenyl phosphate (*p*NPP, Sigma-Aldrich, Irvine, UK) into *p*-nitrophenol (*p*NP). After a predetermined culturing time, the cells were lysed in 0.2% Triton X-100 and incubated at 37 °C for 1 h after mixing with 50 µL of *p*NPP. The reaction was stopped by the addition of 50 µL of stop solution, and the color developed was measured at 405 nm.

2.1.3. In Vivo Study

All in vivo animal procedures, including surgical and sacrificial methods, were approved by the Ethics Committee on Animal Experimentation of the Institutional Animal Care and Use Committee of CRONEX (CRONEX-IACUC 201908004). The in vivo bone formation around the bone grafts was examined using a rabbit tibial defect model in 8 week old male New Zealand white rabbits (body weight 2–3 kg, KOSA Bio Inc., Seongnam, Korea). The rabbits were anesthetized using a mixture of xylaine, tiletamine, and a local anesthetic (lidocaine). In each proximal tibia, cylindrical defects of 3×6 mm were created using a hand drill. Two types of bone grafts, Bontree® 0.5-granule and Bontree® 1.0-granule, were placed in each tibial defect, and the soft tissue and skin were sutured carefully. Nongrafted tibial defects were also included as controls. The rabbits were sacrificed after 4 and 12 weeks of implantation.

Tibia extracted with implanted bone grafts were fixed in 10% formaldehyde solution and embedded in resin. The resin blocks were sectioned and stained with hematoxylin and eosin. Microscopic images of the stained sections were obtained using a polarized light Axioskop microscope (Olympus BX51, Olympus, Tokyo, Japan). The bone volume and remaining volume of implanted grafts were measured using ImageJ software (ImageJ version 1.50i, National Institutes of Health, Bethesda, MD, USA).

2.1.4. Statistical Analysis

The data were statistically analyzed using the Statistical Package for the Social Sciences (SPSS 23, SPSS Inc., Chicago, IL, USA). Data are presented as the mean ± standard deviation. For RANKL and ALP activities, Student's *t*-test was used to evaluate the differences. One-way analysis of variance was performed on the in vivo results of new bone and remaining graft volumes, followed by least significant difference post hoc tests. Statistical significance was set at $p < 0.05$.

2.2. Clinical Case Study

Patient Selection

Among the patients who visited the periodontal department of Chosun University Dental Hospital for implant surgery, we selected those who underwent sinus or alveolar ridge augmentation with Bontree® 1.0-granule with at least 1 year of functional loading. Patients were excluded if they (i) were not followed up, and (ii) did not have radiographs for evaluation. Three male patients were selected, and their ages ranged from 63 to 77 years (Table 1). This study was approved by the Institutional Review Board (IRB) of Chosun University Dental Hospital in Gwangju, Korea (CUDHIRB-2103-008). All treatment plans and procedures were explained to the patients, and they provided consent for surgery.

Table 1. Characteristics of the patients.

Case	Age	Sex	PMH	Procedure	Position of Implant Placement	ISQ (B/L)	Implant Prognosis
1	77	Male	HTN	Bone augmentation of peri-implant defects	#44i	78/84	Success
					#45i	80/79	Success
					#46i	85/85	Success
2	69	Male	HTNCVD	Vertical ridge augmentation	#24i	75/76	Success
					#26i	71/71	Success
					#27i	75/73	Success
3	63	Male	HTNDM	Sinus and ridge augmentation	#16i	62/75	Success
					#17i	61/71	Success

PMH, past medical history; ISQ (B/L), implant stability quotient (buccal/lingual); HTN, hypertension; CVD, cardiovascular disease; DM, diabetes mellitus.

3. Results

3.1. Basic Research

3.1.1. Material Characterization

Figure 1A shows the FE-SEM micrographs of two different granule sizes of Bontree®. At low magnification, both Bontree® granules had irregular shapes with clean and rough surface morphologies, and no cracks or defects were found on any Bontree® granule surface. High-magnification FE-SEM images clearly showed that micron-sized crystals uniformly covered the surface of the Bontree® granules. There were no significant differences between the surface qualities and morphologies of the two Bontree® granules.

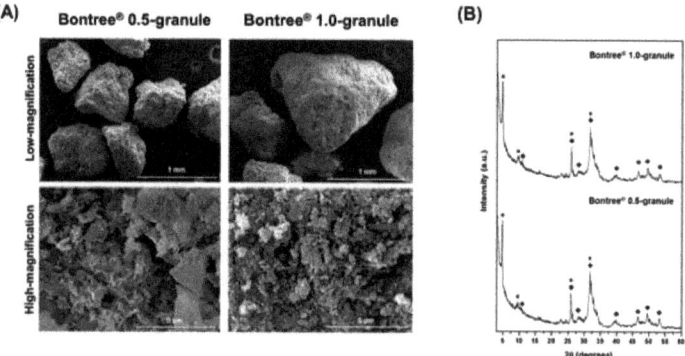

Figure 1. (A) Representative low- and high-magnification FE-SEM images of the Bontree® granules: Bontree® 0.5-granule and Bontree® 1.0-granule refer to Bontree® granules with diameters of 0.5 mm and 1.0 mm, respectively. (B) The XRD spectra of the Bontree® 0.5-granule and Bontree® 1.0-granule. The OCP and HA peaks are indicated by * and ♦, respectively. FE-SEM, field-emission scanning electron microscopy; XRD, X-ray diffraction; OCP, octacalcium phosphate; HA, hydroxyapatite.

Figure 1B shows the XRD patterns of Bontree® 0.5-granule and Bontree® 1.0-granule. XRD was conducted to examine the presence of OCP and HA in Bontree® grafts. The presence of diffraction peaks at 2θ = 10.8°, 26.3°, 31.8°, 32.2°, 32.9°, 39.8°, 46.6°, 49.3°, and 53.2° indicated the formation of apatite (HA), while the strongest intensity of the OCP diffraction peak (100) was observed at 4.7° in both samples [15,16]. Phase analysis using XRD showed that OCP is the main constituent of Bontree®, regardless of size.

3.1.2. In Vitro Study

The RANKL and ALP activities of the MG63 cells were assessed using ELISA to assess the role of Bontree® in bone formation and remodeling (Figure 2A,B). For comparison, a commercial biphasic calcium phosphate ceramic (MBCP+™) was also assessed as a reference [17]. Prior to in vitro testing, each specimen was compressed into tablets. Bontree® refers to both Bontree® 0.5-granule and Bontree® 1.0-granule samples.

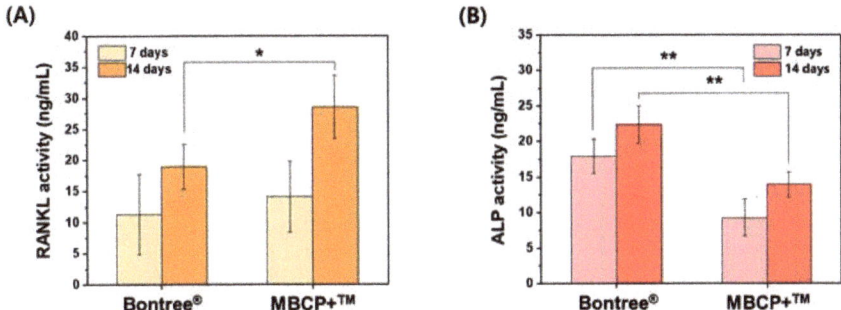

Figure 2. (**A**) RANKL activity and (**B**) ALP activity of MG63 cells in Bontree® and MBCP+™ cultures after 7 and 14 days of culture. Statistical significance was set at * $p < 0.05$ and ** $p < 0.01$, respectively. RANKL, receptor activator of NF-κB ligand; ALP, alkaline phosphatase.

The level of RANKL, an osteoclast differentiation factor [18], was lower in cultures with Bontree® than in those with MBCP+™ during both culturing periods; it was 11.3 ng/mL and 19.0 ng/mL for Bontree® and 14.1 ng/mL and 28.6 ng/mL for MBCP+™ after 7 and 14 days, respectively. In contrast, the activity of ALP, an osteoblast differentiation marker [19], was significantly elevated in cultures with Bontree® (17.9 ng/mL and 22.4 ng/mL at 7 and 14 days, respectively), showing 1.9- and 1.6-fold higher values than in cultures with MBCP+™ (9.2 ng/mL and 13.9 ng/mL at 7 and 14 days, respectively).

3.1.3. In Vivo Study

On the basis of the results of in vitro testing, Bontree® 0.5-granule and Bontree® 1.0-granule were selected for further evaluation of new bone formation in vivo. Figure 3A shows low- and high-magnification histological images of transverse cross-sections stained using hematoxylin and eosin; the cortical bone tissue stained light red or pink, and collagen fibers stained pale pink; the black areas represent the implanted Bontree® grafts [20]. To examine the size effect of bone grafts, two Bontree® grafts (Bontree® 0.5-granule and Bontree® 1.0-granule) were assessed in this in vivo study. At both 4 and 12 weeks after surgery, bone regeneration was observed in the histological images without any sign of local inflammation or rejection of the bone graft. In the control group (i.e., nongrafted defect), a small amount of new bone tissue was formed only at the edge of the tibial defect, and fibrous connective tissue and bone marrow nearly filled the entire tibial defect after 4 weeks of surgery. In contrast, defects filled with the Bontree® 0.5-granule and Bontree® 1.0-granule showed a significant amount of newly formed bone tissues that were uniformly distributed over the entire tibial defect and even in the bone marrow cavity. Notably, in the case of the Bontree® 1.0-granules, thick and dense new bone tissues were consistently generated between the graft granules, while relatively thin and less dense new bone tissues were formed with Bontree® 0.5-granules. Quantitative analysis of the new bone region (Figure 3B) showed 21.6% ± 5.3% and 26.0% ± 8.2% of new bone volumes after 4 weeks of grafting Bontree® 0.5- and 1.0-granules, respectively, which were significantly higher than that of the control (11.2% ± 2.9%) ($p < 0.01$).

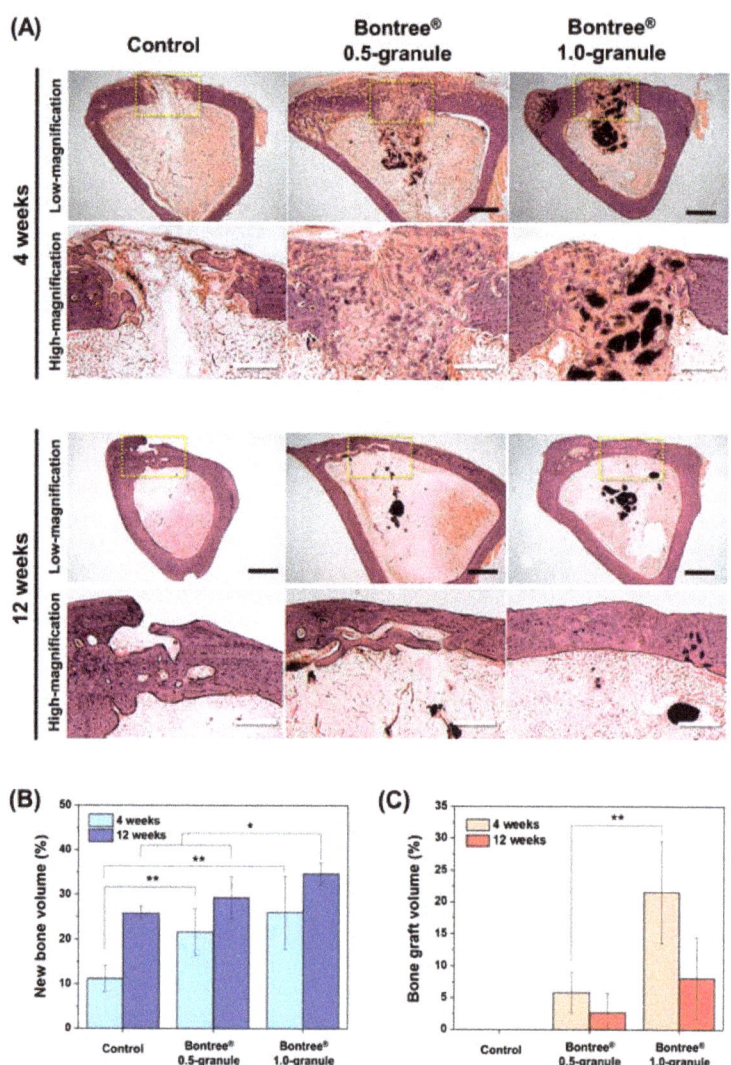

Figure 3. (**A**) Representative histological images with low- and high-magnifications of the bone graft implantation regions in a rabbit tibia 4 and 12 weeks after surgery. Magnified regions are marked with yellow rectangles in the low magnification images. Black and white bars indicate 2 mm and 1 mm, respectively. Percentages of (**B**) new bone and (**C**) bone graft volumes compared with the tibial defect volume at 4 and 12 weeks after surgery. Statistical significance was set at * $p < 0.05$ and ** $p < 0.01$, respectively.

The histological differences between the samples decreased with increasing implantation time. Twelve weeks after surgery (Figure 3A), all samples exhibited complete sealing of the bone defects; the tibial defects were fully filled with newly formed compact bone, and there was no open gap at the side of the cortical bone defect regions. However, in the control and Bontree® 0.5-granule groups, regenerated bone tissues were not fully dense, and they showed macroscopic inner pores within the bone structures. In contrast, tibias grafted with Bontree® 1.0-granule showed a fully dense regenerated bone structure at the wound site, and they showed good histomorphological continuity with adjacent old bone tissues. From the quantitative results (Figure 3B), the Bontree® 1.0-granule group showed significantly higher new bone volumes (34.5% ± 2.5%) than the control (25.8% ± 1.5%) and Bontree® 0.5-granule (29.2% ± 4.8%) groups ($p < 0.05$).

Regarding bone graft degradation, Bontree® 0.5-granule and Bontree® 1.0-granule showed apparent degradation over 12 weeks (Figure 3C). Four weeks after surgery, large amounts of bone graft remained inside the tibial defects in both groups, and the retention rates were 5.8% ± 3.2% and 21.5% ± 8.0% for the Bontree® 0.5-granule and Bontree® 1.0-granule groups, respectively. In contrast, at the end of the in vivo test (week 12), the bone grafts were significantly degraded, showing only several coarse remnants in the marrow cavities in both groups. The retention rates were 2.7% ± 3.0% and 8.1% ± 6.4%, respectively, which were 2.2 and 2.7 times lower than those at week 4, respectively.

3.2. Clinical Case Study

3.2.1. Description of Three Cases

All surgical procedures were performed by a single skilled periodontologist (W.-P.L.). Gargling was performed for 1 min using a 0.12% chlorhexidine solution before each surgery. After local anesthesia with 2% lidocaine containing epinephrine (1:100,000), bone was exposed by elevating a full-thickness flap after an alveolar ridge incision and a vertical incision with a #15 surgical blade. After curettage of the inflamed tissue, decortication was performed using a #330 carbide burr for bleeding. To facilitate the sticky bone substitute material condition, Bontree® and the entire blood harvested from the surgical site were mixed.

After each surgery, antibiotics (Augmentin 625 mg, Ilsung Pharm. Co., Seoul, Korea) and analgesics (aceclofenac 100 mg, Dona-A ST, Seoul, Korea) were administered orally for 7 days. In addition, the patients were advised to rinse the oral cavity with 0.12% chlorhexidine twice a day for 2 weeks. Complete stitch-out was performed 2 weeks after surgery. The implant stability quotient (ISQ) of each implant was measured at the second stage of implant surgery approximately 4 months after implantation.

The characteristic surgical procedure for each case is described below.

Case 1

A 77 year old man visited the clinic for implant placement in the 44–46 region. After local anesthesia, when implants (TS III SA®, Osstem, Seoul, Korea) were inserted, one implant thread was partially exposed buccally. Therefore, the guided bone regeneration (GBR) procedure was performed on the peri-implant dehiscence defect using a mixture of Bontree® and whole blood, followed by adaptation of a collagen barrier membrane (Ossix Plus®, Datum Dental Biotech, Lod, Israel). During the second-stage implant surgery performed 4 months after implantation, sufficient horizontal bone augmentation was observed around the implants. The final prosthesis was inserted approximately 6 months after implantation (Figure 4).

Case 2

A 69 year old man visited the clinic for bone augmentation and implant placement in the 24–27 region. As a severely atrophic alveolar ridge was expected, vertical ridge augmentation was performed first using Bontree® mixed with whole blood and a titanium mesh (Jeil Medical, Seoul, Korea) prefabricated on a 3D-printed model. The first stage of implant surgery for 24, 26, and 27 was performed 6 months after ridge augmentation. High primary stability was achieved at the time of implant (Luna®, Shinhung Co., Seoul,

Korea) placement, and sufficient buccal and lingual marginal bone width was confirmed. Four months after implantation, vestibular loss and a lack of buccal attached mucosa were observed with vertical bone loss. Therefore, an apically positioned flap was performed simultaneously with the second-stage implant surgery, followed by the application of an absorbable periodontal dressing (Reso-Pac®, Hager & Werken GmbH & Co., KG, Germany). The final prosthesis was provided approximately 6 months after implantation (Figure 5).

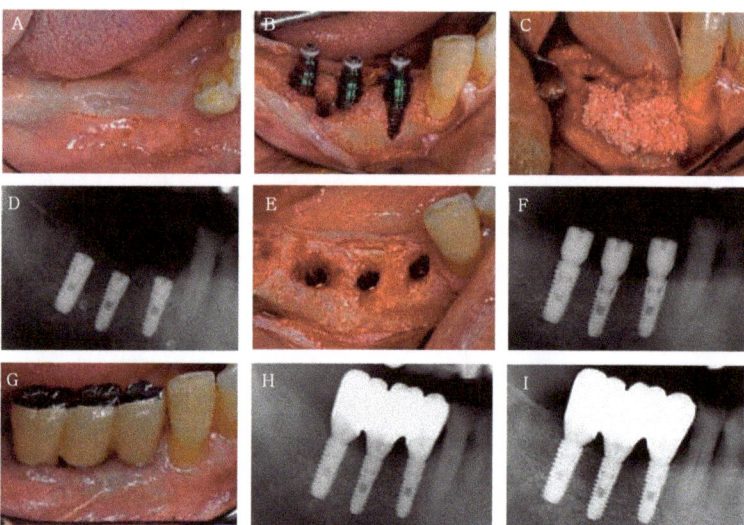

Figure 4. Clinical case 1. (**A**) Clinical view before bone augmentation and implantation of 44, 45, and 46. (**B**) Peri-implant dehiscence defects at 44 and 45. (**C**) Bone augmentation at 44 and 45 using Bontree® and collagen barrier membrane. (**D**) Radiograph after bone augmentation and implantation. (**E**) Clinical view after flap elevation during the second-stage implant surgery 4 months after implantation. (**F**) Radiograph after the second-stage implant surgery. (**G,H**) Clinical and radiographic views of the final prosthesis 6 months after implantation. (**I**) Radiograph at 1 year after loading.

Case 3

A 63 year old man visited the clinic for sinus augmentation and implant placement in the 16–17 region. Because oroantral communication (OAC) was expected on radiographic evaluation, vertical ridge augmentation with simultaneous sinus floor elevation was planned. After a piezoelectric lateral bony window osteotomy and sinus membrane elevation, sinus grafting was performed with a mixture of Bontree® and whole blood, followed by bony window replacement. Next, vertical ridge augmentation was performed with Bontree® mixed with whole blood and a titanium-reinforced d-PTFE membrane (Cytoplast® Ti-250, Osteogenics Biomedical, Lubbock, TX, USA). A single-stage implant surgery for 16 and 17 was planned 6 months postoperatively, because the radiograph showed sufficient hard tissue volume in the 16–17 region, indicating the resolution of OAC. A core biopsy was conducted before drilling at site 16 for implant placement. The biopsy was harvested through the alveolar process at a depth of 10 mm using a trephine bur with an inner diameter of 2 mm. High primary stability was obtained when the implants (Superline®, Dentium Co. Ltd., Seoul, Korea) for 16 and 17 were placed, and sufficient buccal and lingual marginal bone width was also confirmed. The harvested specimens were fixed using paraformaldehyde in 4% buffered saline, followed by demineralization. The specimens were processed into paraffin blocks, and a microtome was used for microsectioning. Next, hematoxylin and eosin staining was performed. Four months after implantation, modified periosteal fenestration [21–23], which we first suggested as a free gingival graft alternative, followed by the application of an absorbable periodontal dressing, was performed because of the loss of attached mucosa buccally. The final prosthesis was inserted 6 months after the single-stage implant surgery (Figure 6).

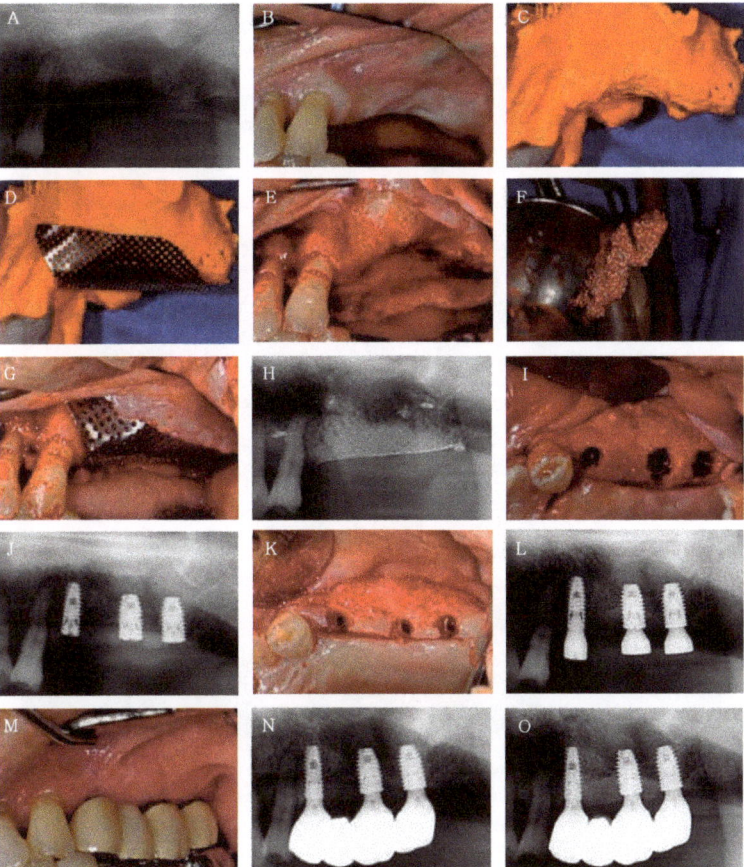

Figure 5. Clinical case 2. (**A,B**) Clinical and radiographic views before vertical ridge augmentation in the 24, 26, and 27 regions. (**C**) Three-dimensional printed model of the severely atrophic posterior maxilla. (**D**) A prefabricated titanium mesh on the 3D-printed model before clinical application. (**E**) Buccal view after flap elevation. (**F**) Bontree® mixed with whole blood. A sticky bone graft with good manipulability is observed. (**G**) Buccal view of vertical ridge augmentation using Bontree® and a titanium mesh. (**H**) Radiograph after vertical ridge augmentation. (**I**) Occlusal view of 24, 26, and 27 implants placed 6 months after vertical ridge augmentation. (**J**) Radiograph after the first-stage implant surgery. (**K**) Occlusal view of the second-stage implant surgery using apically positioned flap and punching technique 4 months after implantation. (**L**) Radiograph after the second-stage implant surgery. (**M,N**) Clinical and radiographic views of the final prosthesis 6 months after implantation. (**O**) Radiograph at 1 year after loading.

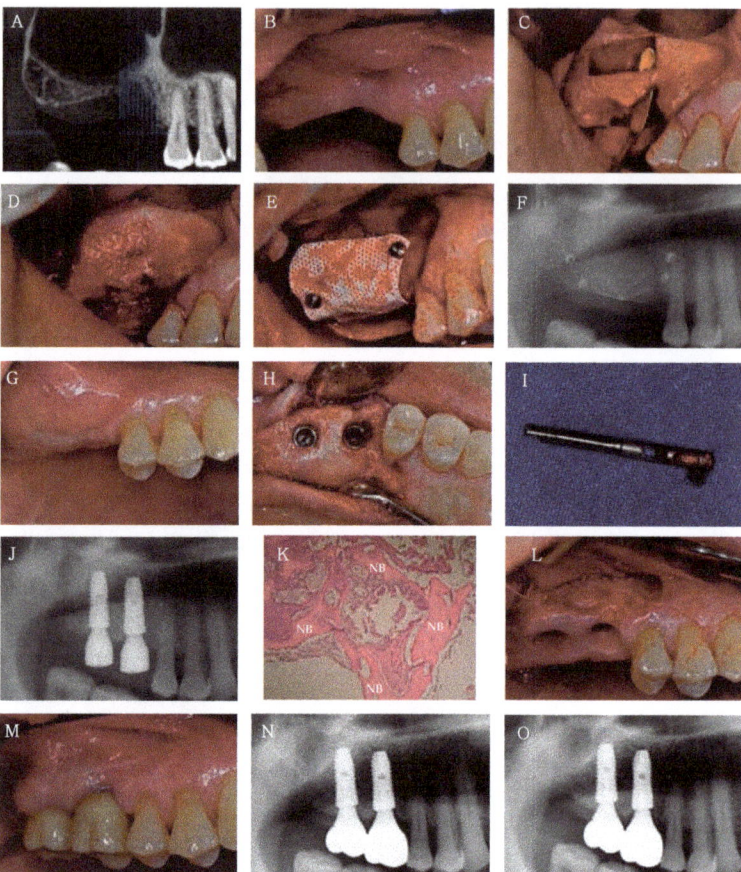

Figure 6. Clinical case 3. (**A,B**) Clinical and radiographic views before alveolar ridge and sinus augmentation in the 16 and 17 regions. (**C**) Buccal view after a piezoelectric bony window osteotomy and sinus membrane elevation. An oroantral communication is seen. (**D**) Sinus graft with Bontree®. (**E**) Vertical ridge augmentation with Bontree® and titanium-reinforced d-PTFE membrane after the replacement of the bony window. (**F**) Radiograph after sinus and ridge augmentation. (**G**) Buccal view before placement of implants 16 and 17, 6 months after sinus and ridge augmentation. A coronally positioned mucogingival junction line is observed. (**H**) Occlusal view of implants 16 and 17 immediately after placement. (**I**) The core biopsy in the 16 region using a trephine bur. (**J**) Radiograph after the single-stage implant surgery. (**K**) Histological examination. New bone formation (NB) is observed with no inflammatory tissue (H&E-stained; original magnification × 100). (**L**) Buccal view after performing a modified periosteal fenestration 4 months after the single-stage implant surgery. (**M,N**) Clinical and radiographic views of the final prosthesis 6 months after the single-stage implant surgery. (**O**) Radiograph at 1 year after loading.

3.2.2. Clinical and Radiological Findings

A total of eight implants were placed in three patients who underwent sinus or alveolar ridge bone grafting with Bontree®. None of the patients had postoperative complications other than slight swelling at the surgical site. At 4 months after implantation, the ISQ values were >60 for all implants, indicating good implant stability (Table 1). All eight implants in all three patients were followed up for at least 12 months after functional loading, and the success rate, which was evaluated on the basis of the International

Congress of Oral Implantologists Pisa Consensus implant health scale [24], was 100% (Table 1). The radiograph at the 1 year follow-up showed integration of the implant with the regenerated bone and no bone loss or peri-implant radiolucency. No decrease in graft height was observed on any radiograph, and healthy peri-implant mucosa was established around all implants during the 1 year loading period.

3.2.3. Histological Findings

Histological analysis at the site of 16 in case 3, where sinus and ridge grafting was performed with Bontree®, revealed the deposition of newly formed bone around the residual synthetic bone graft and satisfactory incorporation of the newly formed bone with the residual synthetic bone graft. No foreign body reactions or inflammatory signs were detected (Figure 6K).

4. Discussion

In this study, the safety and efficacy of Bontree® for bone regeneration were demonstrated using in vitro and in vivo experiments. In addition, in patients with bony defects in the alveolar ridge or maxillary sinus, oral rehabilitation using dental implants was possible after ridge or sinus augmentation using Bontree®.

Although OCP is a promising bone graft material with excellent biological properties, there are only a few commercially available OCP-based products, such as Ti-Oss® (Chiyewon, Guri, Korea) or Bonarc™ (Toyobo Co. Ltd., Osaka, Japan) bone grafts. However, even these products are not fully composed of Ca- and P-containing apatites; rather, they consist of a combination of OCP with naturally occurring bovine bone materials or collagens. In contrast, the recently introduced OCP bone graft, Bontree®, is fully composed of apatite compounds with 80 wt.% OCP and 20 wt.% HA, and it exhibits a commercially acceptable quality, defect-free homogeneous surface morphology, and relatively uniform size distribution (Figure 1A). In addition, numerous micron-scale crystals covering the entire surface of Bontree® granules are beneficial for increasing the rate of dissolution and resorption of Ca and P ions under physiological conditions, thereby enabling active mineralization on their surfaces.

Short-term in vitro and long-term in vivo studies were performed to investigate the bone formation ability of Bontree®. In the in vitro experiments, RANKL and ALP were used as key markers for bone formation. RANKL is a transmembrane protein that controls the differentiation, maturation, and activation of osteoclasts, which results in bone resorption during remodeling, whereas ALP is an enzyme secreted by osteoblasts and is involved in the mineralization and calcification of newly formed bone tissues. Therefore, the suppressed RANKL activity of MG63 cells is closely associated with reduced osteoclastic differentiation and bone resorption, while the improved ALP activity indicates better osteoblastic differentiation and new bone formation on the bone grafts [19,25,26]. If the bone graft material has insufficient ability to regenerate bone tissues, pores between the bone grafts allow infiltration of soft tissues that hinder the formation of new bone [27,28]. Moreover, the soft tissue is unable to provide sufficient mechanical support to the host bone and prevents the escape of bone grafts from the implanted site [29]. As shown in Figure 2A,B, Bontree® exhibited significantly higher values of ALP activity than MBCP+™ at 12 days of MG63 cell culturing, and a significant amount of newly formed bone tissues appeared uniformly distributed over the entire region of the Bontree® 0.5-granule- and Bontree® 1.0-granule-grafted tibial defects at 4 weeks after surgery. In previous studies, OCP showed outstanding osteoconductive and osteoinductive properties owing to its unique physicochemical properties [30]. When degraded and converted to HA, it releases numerous inorganic PO_4^{3-} and Ca^{2+} ions, which are known to promote osteoblastic differentiation and maturation better than HA, as evidenced by the increased ALP activity (Figure 2B) [31]. In addition, OCP is beneficial for the adsorption of bone-forming molecules and proteins, which could further increase the osteogenic differentiation of cells and initiate bone regeneration [32].

In terms of the size effect of bone grafts on bone regeneration, macroscopic bone grafts generally provide more free space than their microscopic counterparts for cells to move into and attach to, thereby promoting vascularization and ingrowth of newly formed bone tissue into the bone grafts [33]. As shown in Figure 3A,B, Bontree® 1.0-granule was associated with greater amounts of newly formed bone tissues than the Bontree® 0.5-granule at both 4 and 12 weeks. According to the results of in vitro and in vivo experiments, the Bontree® 1.0-granule has a high potential as a commercially applicable novel bone graft material, and it was selected for the evaluation of clinical significance.

On the basis of the results of this basic research, we attempted to perform alveolar ridge or sinus augmentation using Bontree® 1.0-granule during dental implant surgery. Eight implants in three patients showed a 100% success rate after 1 year of functional loading. During the surgical procedure, clinical and systemic complications, such as pain, severe inflammation, or significant infection, were not observed. In Case 1, GBR was performed on the peri-implant dehiscence bony defects using Bontree® and an absorbable collagen barrier membrane, and clinically successful horizontal hard tissue gain was observed after 4 months. In Cases 2 and 3, vertical ridge or sinus augmentation with Bontree® was performed 6 months before implant placement, sufficient horizontal/vertical bone width and height were obtained clinically, and sufficient implant primary stability ≥ 40 N was achieved. All ISQ values measured approximately 4 months after implant placement were >60, indicating successful secondary implant stability. In addition, no characteristic marginal bone loss around the implant was observed on radiographs for up to 1 year after loading. The clinically and radiographically successful bone regeneration with Bontree® can be attributed to the excellent new bone formation ability unique to OCP. In other words, OCP seems to provide a nucleus for promoting osteogenesis and creates numerous starting points for ossification, unlike HA and β-TCP [34]. In addition, Kawai et al. [14] reported that OCP-based bone grafts achieved comparable osseointegration to autologous bone grafts in a study of the mandible in a canine model. However, due to the limitations inherent to retrospective studies, the number of samples was too small, and we cannot confirm the clinical characteristics of Bontree® only on the basis of the three cases included in this study. In addition, the follow-up period of approximately 1 year may be too short to evaluate the success rate of the implants. Therefore, as a follow-up study, comparative studies with other bone substitute materials, long-term studies, and prospective studies using Bontree® in a much larger number of cases are needed.

5. Conclusions

According to our basic research and clinical applications, Bontree® showed significantly higher ALP activity than a commercial biphasic calcium phosphate ceramic (MBCP+™). Although both Bontree® 0.5-granule and Bontree® 1.0-granule are mainly composed of OCP distributed uniformly regardless of size, the Bontree® 1.0-granule has a higher potential for new bone formation. The clinical cases had predictable and successful outcomes, which demonstrated the safety and efficacy of Bontree® in alveolar ridge or sinus augmentation.

Author Contributions: Conceptualization, W.-P.L.; methodology, T.-S.J. and W.-P.L.; validation, S.-Y.K.; formal analysis, T.-S.J. and W.-P.L.; investigation, J.-S.K.; resources, J.-S.K. and W.-P.L.; data curation, T.-S.J. and J.-S.K.; writing—original draft preparation, J.-S.K., T.-S.J. and W.-P.L.; writing—review and editing, S.-Y.K. and W.-P.L.; visualization, T.-S.J. and W.-P.L.; supervision, S.-Y.K.; project administration, W.-P.L. All authors have read and agreed to the published version of the manuscript.

Funding: This research received no external funding.

Institutional Review Board Statement: This study was conducted in accordance with the guidelines of the Declaration of Helsinki and approved by the Institutional Review Board of the Dental Hospital of Chosun University in Gwangju, Korea (CUDHIRB-2103-008).

Informed Consent statement: Informed consent was obtained from all patients involved in the study.

Data Availability Statement: The datasets generated or analyzed during the current study are available from the corresponding author upon reasonable request.

Conflicts of Interest: The authors declare no conflict of interest.

References

1. Couso-Queiruga, E.; Stuhr, S.; Tattan, M.; Chambrone, L.; Avila-Ortiz, G. Post-extraction dimensional changes: A systematic review and meta-analysis. *J. Clin. Periodontol.* **2021**, *48*, 127–145. [CrossRef]
2. Jambhekar, S.; Kernen, F.; Bidra, A.S. Clinical and histologic outcomes of socket grafting after flapless tooth extraction: A systematic review of randomized controlled clinical trials. *J. Prosthet. Dent.* **2015**, *113*, 371–382. [CrossRef] [PubMed]
3. Breine, U.; Brånemark, P.-I. Reconstruction of alveolar jaw bone. *Scand. J. Plast. Reconstr. Surg.* **1980**, *14*, 23–48. [CrossRef] [PubMed]
4. Venugopalan, V.; Vamsi, A.R.; Shenoy, S.; Ashok, K.; Thomas, B. Guided Bone Regeneration-A Comprehensive Review. *J. Clin. Diagn. Res.* **2021**, *15*, 1–4.
5. Springfield, D. Autograft reconstructions. *Orthop. Clin. N. Am.* **1996**, *27*, 483–492. [CrossRef]
6. Betz, R.R. Limitations of autograft and allograft: New synthetic solutions. *Orthopedics* **2002**, *25*, S561–S570. [CrossRef]
7. Dos Santos Canellas, J.V.; Drugos, L.; Ritto, F.G.; Fischer, R.G.; Medeiros, P.J.D.A. Xenograft materials in maxillary sinus floor elevation surgery: A systematic review with network meta-analyses. *Br. J. Oral Maxillofac. Surg.* **2021**, *59*, 742–751. [CrossRef]
8. Lu, J.; Descamps, M.; Dejou, J.; Koubi, G.; Hardouin, P.; Lemaitre, J.; Proust, J.P. The biodegradation mechanism of calcium phosphate biomaterials in bone. *J. Biomed. Mater. Res.* **2002**, *63*, 408–412. [CrossRef]
9. Kawai, T.; Tanuma, Y.; Matsui, K.; Suzuki, O.; Takahashi, T.; Kamakura, S. Clinical safety and efficacy of implantation of octacalcium phosphate collagen composites in tooth extraction sockets and cyst holes. *J. Tissue Eng.* **2016**, *7*, 2041731416670770. [CrossRef]
10. Brown, W.E.; Smith, J.P.; Lehr, J.R.; Frazier, A.W. Octacalcium phosphate and hydroxyapatite: Crystallographic and chemical relations between octacalcium phosphate and hydroxyapatite. *Nature* **1962**, *196*, 1050–1055. [CrossRef]
11. Kamakura, S.; Sasano, Y.; Shimizu, T.; Hatori, K.; Suzuki, O.; Kagayama, M.; Motegi, K. Implanted octacalcium phosphate is more resorbable than β-tricalcium phosphate and hydroxyapatite. *J. Biomed. Mater. Res.* **2002**, *59*, 29–34. [CrossRef]
12. Kamakura, S.; Sasaki, K.; Homma, T.; Honda, Y.; Anada, T.; Echigo, S.; Suzuki, O. The primacy of octacalcium phosphate collagen composites in bone regeneration. *J. Biomed. Mater. Res. Part A* **2007**, *83*, 725–733. [CrossRef]
13. Jung, Y.; Kim, W.-H.; Lee, S.-H.; Ju, K.W.; Jang, E.-H.; Kim, S.-O.; Kim, B.; Lee, J.-H. Evaluation of New Octacalcium Phosphate-Coated Xenograft in Rats Calvarial Defect Model on Bone Regeneration. *Materials* **2020**, *13*, 4391. [CrossRef]
14. Kawai, T.; Matsui, K.; Ezoe, Y.; Kajii, F.; Suzuki, O.; Takahashi, T.; Kamakura, S. Efficacy of octacalcium phosphate collagen composite for titanium dental implants in dogs. *Materials* **2018**, *11*, 229. [CrossRef] [PubMed]
15. Robin, M.; Von Euw, S.; Renaudin, G.; Gomes, S.; Krafft, J.-M.; Nassif, N.; Azaïs, T.; Costentin, G. Insights into OCP identification and quantification in the context of apatite biomineralization. *CrystEngComm* **2020**, *22*, 2728–2742. [CrossRef]
16. Marycz, K.; Smieszek, A.; Trynda, J.; Sobierajska, P.; Targonska, S.; Grosman, L.; Wiglusz, R.J. Nanocrystalline hydroxyapatite loaded with resveratrol in colloidal suspension improves viability, metabolic activity and mitochondrial potential in human adipose-derived mesenchymal stromal stem cells (hASCs). *Polymers* **2019**, *11*, 92. [CrossRef] [PubMed]
17. Toker, H.; Ozdemir, H.; Ozer, H.; Eren, K. A comparative evaluation of the systemic and local alendronate treatment in synthetic bone graft: A histologic and histomorphometric study in a rat calvarial defect model. *Oral Surg. Oral Med. Oral Pathol. Oral Radiol.* **2012**, *114*, S146–S152. [CrossRef]
18. Ling, L.; Murali, S.; Stein, G.S.; Van Wijnen, A.J.; Cool, S.M. Glycosaminoglycans modulate RANKL-induced osteoclastogenesis. *J. Cell. Biochem.* **2010**, *109*, 1222–1231. [CrossRef]
19. Yeo, M.; Jung, W.-K.; Kim, G. Fabrication, characterisation and biological activity of phlorotannin-conjugated PCL/β-TCP composite scaffolds for bone tissue regeneration. *J. Mater. Chem.* **2012**, *22*, 3568–3577. [CrossRef]
20. Xie, L.; Liu, N.; Xiao, Y.; Liu, Y.; Yan, C.; Wang, G.; Jing, X. In vitro and in vivo osteogenesis induced by icariin and bone morphogenetic protein-2: A dynamic observation. *Front. Pharmacol.* **2020**, *11*, 1058. [CrossRef]
21. Park, D.Y.; Lee, W.P. Vestibuloplasty around teeth and dental implants using simplified periosteal fenestration (sPF): Case Reports. *J. Korean Dent. Assoc.* **2020**, *59*, 20–27.
22. Lee, W.P.; Kwon, Y.S. Vestibuloplasty around Dental Implants Using Modified Periosteal Fenestration (mPF): Case Series. *Implantology* **2020**, *24*, 22–30. [CrossRef]
23. Baek, J.-H.; Kim, B.-O.; Lee, W.-P. Implant Placement after Closure of Oroantral Communication by Sinus Bone Graft Using a Collagen Barrier Membrane in the Shape of a Pouch: A Case Report and Review of the Literature. *Medicina* **2021**, *57*, 626. [CrossRef] [PubMed]
24. Misch, C.E.; Perel, M.L.; Wang, H.-L.; Sammartino, G.; Galindo-Moreno, P.; Trisi, P.; Steigmann, M.; Rebaudi, A.; Palti, A.; Pikos, M.A. Implant success, survival, and failure: The International Congress of Oral Implantologists (ICOI) pisa consensus conference. *Implant Dent.* **2008**, *17*, 5–15. [CrossRef] [PubMed]
25. Marahleh, A.; Kitaura, H.; Ohori, F.; Kishikawa, A.; Ogawa, S.; Shen, W.-R.; Qi, J.; Noguchi, T.; Nara, Y.; Mizoguchi, I. TNF-α directly enhances osteocyte RANKL expression and promotes osteoclast formation. *Front. Immunol.* **2019**, *10*, 2925. [CrossRef] [PubMed]

26. Lee, M.-K.; Lee, H.; Kim, H.-E.; Lee, E.-J.; Jang, T.-S.; Jung, H.-D. Nano-Topographical Control of Ti-Nb-Zr Alloy Surfaces for Enhanced Osteoblastic Response. *Nanomaterials* **2021**, *11*, 1507. [CrossRef]
27. Chou, Y.-C.; Lee, D.; Chang, T.-M.; Hsu, Y.-H.; Yu, Y.-H.; Liu, S.-J.; Ueng, S.W.-N. Development of a three-dimensional (3D) printed biodegradable cage to convert morselized corticocancellous bone chips into a structured cortical bone graft. *Int. J. Mol. Sci.* **2016**, *17*, 595. [CrossRef] [PubMed]
28. Otero-Pérez, R.; Permuy, M.; López-Senra, E.; López-Álvarez, M.; López-Peña, M.; Serra, J.; González-Cantalapiedra, A.; Muñoz, F.M.; González, P. Preclinical Evaluation of an Innovative Bone Graft of Marine Origin for the Treatment of Critical-Sized Bone Defects in an Animal Model. *Appl. Sci.* **2021**, *11*, 2116. [CrossRef]
29. Choi, S.W.; Bae, J.Y.; Shin, Y.H.; Song, J.H.; Kim, J.K. Treatment of forearm diaphyseal non-union: Autologous iliac corticocancellous bone graft and locking plate fixation. *Orthop. Traumatol. Surg. Res.* **2021**, 102833. [CrossRef]
30. Kikawa, T.; Kashimoto, O.; Imaizumi, H.; Kokubun, S.; Suzuki, O. Intramembranous bone tissue response to biodegradable octacalcium phosphate implant. *Acta Biomater.* **2009**, *5*, 1756–1766. [CrossRef]
31. Wang, Z.; Ma, K.; Jiang, X.; Xie, J.; Cai, P.; Li, F.; Liang, R.; Zhao, J.; Zheng, L. Electrospun poly (3-hydroxybutyrate-co-4-hydroxybutyrate)/octacalcium phosphate nanofibrous membranes for effective guided bone regeneration. *Mater. Sci. Eng. C* **2020**, *112*, 110763. [CrossRef] [PubMed]
32. Jiang, P.; Liang, J.; Song, R.; Zhang, Y.; Ren, L.; Zhang, L.; Tang, P.; Lin, C. Effect of octacalcium-phosphate-modified micro/nanostructured titania surfaces on osteoblast response. *ACS Appl. Mater. Interfaces* **2015**, *7*, 14384–14396. [CrossRef] [PubMed]
33. Xin, F.; Jian, C.; Jianming, R.; Zhongcheng, Z.; Jianpeng, Z. Synthesis and degradation properties of beta-TCP/BG porous composite materials. *Bull. Mater. Sci.* **2011**, *34*, 357–364. [CrossRef]
34. Sakai, S.; Anada, T.; Tsuchiya, K.; Yamazaki, H.; Margolis, H.C.; Suzuki, O. Comparative study on the resorbability and dissolution behavior of octacalcium phosphate, β-tricalcium phosphate, and hydroxyapatite under physiological conditions. *Dent. Mater. J.* **2016**, *35*, 216–224. [CrossRef] [PubMed]

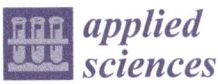

Article

Titanium Nitride Plating Reduces Nickel Ion Release from Orthodontic Wire

Arata Ito, Hideki Kitaura *, Haruki Sugisawa, Takahiro Noguchi, Fumitoshi Ohori and Itaru Mizoguchi

Division of Orthodontics and Dentofacial Orthopedics, Graduate School of Dentistry, Tohoku University, 4-1 Seiryo-machi, Aoba-ku, Sendai 980-8575, Japan; arata.ito.c7@tohoku.ac.jp (A.I.); mythread.and.bluesun71@gmail.com (H.S.); takahiro.noguchi.d4@tohoku.ac.jp (T.N.); fumitoshi.ohori.b4@tohoku.ac.jp (F.O.); itaru.mizoguchi.c3@tohoku.ac.jp (I.M.)
* Correspondence: hideki.kitaura.b4@tohoku.ac.jp; Tel.: +81-22-717-8374

Abstract: The leaching of metal ions from orthodontic appliances is a problem for their use in patients with metal allergies. Despite the development of a number of non-metal orthodontic appliances, including brackets, non-metal wires are not yet available. Therefore, it is necessary to modify the surfaces of orthodontic wires to prevent the leaching of metal ions into the oral environment for use in such patients. This study was performed to examine whether plating of orthodontic wire with titanium nitride (TiN), which does not impair its mechanical properties, could prevent the leaching of metal ions from the wire on immersion in acid. To investigate the acid corrosion resistance of the wire, the amount of metal ions eluted from the wire immersed in acid was measured by using inductively coupled plasma mass spectrometry (ICP-MS) and the dimethylglyoxime (DMG) test, the properties of the wire surface were examined by stereomicroscopy and scanning electron microscopy, and the surface roughness was measured using a surface roughness tester. The results indicated that TiN plating of orthodontic wire significantly suppressed the elution of metal ions on immersion in acid.

Keywords: TiN ion plating; metal allergy; orthodontic wire

Citation: Ito, A.; Kitaura, H.; Sugisawa, H.; Noguchi, T.; Ohori, F.; Mizoguchi, I. Titanium Nitride Plating Reduces Nickel Ion Release from Orthodontic Wire. *Appl. Sci.* 2021, *11*, 9745. https://doi.org/10.3390/app11209745

Academic Editor: Vittorio Checchi

Received: 6 September 2021
Accepted: 14 October 2021
Published: 19 October 2021

Publisher's Note: MDPI stays neutral with regard to jurisdictional claims in published maps and institutional affiliations.

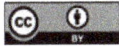

Copyright: © 2021 by the authors. Licensee MDPI, Basel, Switzerland. This article is an open access article distributed under the terms and conditions of the Creative Commons Attribution (CC BY) license (https://creativecommons.org/licenses/by/4.0/).

1. Introduction

The number of patients with metal allergies has increased in recent years [1,2]. The metals used in dentistry are considered to be among the factors responsible for metal allergies. Many orthodontic materials also contain such metals associated with allergic reactions, and therefore care is required in the orthodontic treatment of patients with metal allergies [3–5]. Some metals commonly used in dental practice, including nickel (Ni), cobalt (Co), and chromium (Cr), are known allergens for patients with metal-allergic disease [6,7]. These metals are also present in various orthodontic materials [8]. Several studies have shown that Ni is the most common allergen associated with metal-allergic disease [2,9,10]. Previously, we evaluated the surface elements of orthodontic materials by X-ray fluorescence spectroscopy, and found that Ni was present in almost all the orthodontic metal materials [8]. Metal ions can be eluted from orthodontic materials due to the electrochemical corrosion caused by saliva, electrolytes in food debris, and acids produced by bacteria [11]. Therefore, orthodontic patients can be exposed to Ni from orthodontic appliances. In fact, Fors et al. [12] reported significantly elevated Ni levels in the dental plaque of patients with orthodontic appliances than in that of non-orthodontic patients.

Despite the development of many non-metal orthodontic appliances, including brackets, non-metal wires are still not available [5]. Therefore, it is necessary to improve orthodontic wires to achieve high corrosion resistance. Plating can be used to provide increased surface hardness, wear resistance, corrosion resistance, low friction, and improved esthetics, as well as to improve interactions with biological and material substrates [13]. Physical vapor deposition (PVD) ion plating is a particularly suitable plating method to produce thin films on substrates. TiN layers fabricated by ion plating have demonstrated favorable characteristics in terms of corrosion resistance [14], wear resistance [15], hardness [16], and low friction [17], and may therefore be useful for the modification of the surfaces of orthodontic wires.

We described the mechanical and frictional properties of TiN-coated wires previously [17], but the details of corrosion resistance have yet to be elucidated. We focused on two acids as potential sources of metal ion leaching from orthodontic wires in the oral cavity. First, as fixed orthodontic appliances induce the retention of bacterial plaque, leading to an increase in levels of caries-inducing bacteria in the oral cavity, such as *Lactobacillus* spp. and *Streptococcus mutans* [18], and bacteria corrode orthodontic appliances [19], we focused on lactic acid, which is the main metabolite that causes low pH [20]. We also focused on gastric acid, mainly hydrochloric acid (HCl), which enters the oral cavity due to gastroesophageal reflux disease (GERD), which has a high incidence, of 10–20%, in adults [21]. In addition to acid erosion of teeth and dissolution of dental restorations [22], gastric acid has been reported to be involved in the elution of metal ions from orthodontic wires [23].

In the present study, we evaluated the corrosion resistance of TiN-plated stainless steel (SS) and nickel titanium (NiTi) orthodontic arch wire immersed in acids by measuring the concentrations of released metal ions, by stereomicroscopic and scanning electron microscopic observation of the wire surface, and by surface roughness measurement.

2. Materials and Methods

2.1. TiN Ion Plating

SS wire and NiTi wire (0.016 × 0.022 inches) (American Orthodontics, Sheboygan, WI, USA) were plated with TiN using the hollow cathode discharge method, as described previously [17]. Briefly, a 180-mm length of wire was wiped clean with ethanol and coated using an ion plating system (HCD Ion Plating System X-27; Tigold Co., Ltd., Chiba, Japan) with 1.49 Pa argon (Ar) gas, 1.69 Pa nitrogen (N_2) gas, and a bias voltage of −20 V. The temperature of the substrate was kept at approximately 220 °C for 7 min, and after the wire was completely covered with the TiN layer, except at the two ends, it was slowly cooled under vacuum for 60 min. The coating thickness was set to 0.3 µm. The thickness of the TiN coating was measured as described previously [17].

2.2. Metal Ion Release Testing

Orthodontic wire samples consisting of uncoated SS wire, TiN-coated SS wire, uncoated NiTi wire, and TiN-coated NiTi wire were separately immersed in plastic dishes (untreated 60 × 15 mm dishes; Falcon, Tewksbury, MA, USA) containing 10 mL of physiological saline, sterile water, 35% HCl (pH −1.1) (Wako Pure Chemical Industries, Ltd., Osaka, Japan), and 88% lactic acid (pH 1.2) (Wako Pure Chemical Industries, Ltd., Osaka, Japan). The dishes were placed in an incubator at 37 °C for 30 min, and the concentrations of Cr, manganese (Mn), iron (Fe), and Ni ions released from the SS wires and of the Ni and Ti ions released from the Ni-Ti wires into the solutions were measured by triple quadrupole inductively coupled plasma mass spectrometry (ICP-MS) (ICP-QQQ-Agilent 8800; Agilent Technologies, Santa Clara, CA, USA). The concentrations of metal ions are shown as the mean ± SD of four replicates for each sample.

2.3. DMG Tests

The dimethylglyoxime (DMG) test was performed to detect the leaching of Ni from the surface of orthodontic wires immersed in physiological saline, sterile water, 35% HCl, and 88% lactic acid at 37 °C for 30 min. As described previously [24], two drops of 1% DMG in absolute ethanol and two drops of 10% ammonium hydroxide were added to a cotton swab, which was then rubbed on the sample for 30 s. The strength of the color reaction on the cotton swab was then evaluated visually; the development of a red color was considered a positive reaction, indicating the release of Ni from the wire surface. For positive reactions, points were allocated according to the following criteria: dark red, 3 points; red, 2 points; pink, 1 point; and colorless, 0 points. All the tests were performed in triplicate by the same operator. The values for all the tests are shown as the mean ± SD of three replicates for each sample.

2.4. Observation of the Wire Surface

The wire surface was then observed and photographed under a stereomicroscope (M165FC; Leica, Wetzlar, Germany) and by scanning electron microscopy (SEM) (VE-7800; Keyence, Osaka, Japan) at a magnification of 200× and 1000× with an acceleration voltage of 15 kV.

2.5. Measurement of Surface Roughness

Surface roughness was assessed using a surface roughness tester (Surftest SJ-210; Mitutoyo Corporation, Tokyo, Japan), according to ISO 1997, with a diamond tip radius of 5 µm, a measurement force of 4.0 mN, a scanning speed of 0.5 mm/s, a cut-off length of 0.8 mm, and a Gaussian filter. The samples were each fixed under the stylus of the tester, and the mean surface roughness values (Ra, µm) were determined. The values for each sample are shown as the mean ± SD of three replicates for each sample.

2.6. Statistics

Statistical analyses were performed with JMP® Pro software (version 16.0.0, SAS Institute Inc., Cary, NC, USA). The data obtained from the DMG test and the surface roughness test were analyzed using the Tukey–Kramer HSD test. The Shapiro–Wilk test for normality indicated that the ICP-MS data had a non-parametric distribution, so the concentrations of the eluted metal ions were analyzed using non-parametric comparisons for each pair with Wilcoxon's method. In all the analyses, $p < 0.05$ was taken to indicate statistical significance.

3. Results

3.1. TiN Coating of Orthodontic Wires Suppresses the Elution of Metal Ions from the Wire Surface

The amount of metal ions released from the TiN-coated and uncoated wires after immersion in sterile water, physiological saline, HCl, or lactic acid for 30 min, are shown in Tables 1 and 2. All the data are shown as the mean ± SD of four replicates.

Following immersion in HCl for 30 min, the TiN-coated SS wire showed significantly reduced Cr, Mn, Fe, and Ni ion concentrations compared to the uncoated SS wire and the HCl-only immersion solution, which was used as a control (Figure 1a). On the other hand, following the immersion of the NiTi wire in HCl for 30 min, the concentrations of Ni and Ti ions were significantly reduced in the TiN-coated wire sample compared to the uncoated NiTi wire sample and the HCl-immersion-solution-only control (Figure 1b). Furthermore, the leaching of Ni ions from the uncoated SS and NiTi wire immersed in lactic acid for 30 min was significantly increased compared to the lactic-acid-only immersion solution control (Figure 1c,d). There were no significant differences in the amounts of metal ions released when the wires were immersed in sterile water or physiological saline for 30 min between the TiN-coated wire, the uncoated wire, and the immersion-solution-only control.

Table 1. Metal ion release from SS wire (μg/L).

Wire	Solution	Immersion Time (min)	Cr Mean	Cr SD	Mn Mean	Mn SD	Fe Mean	Fe SD	Ni Mean	Ni SD
TiN-coated SS wire	Sterile water	0	4.78	6.83	0.76	0.54	49.26	52.90	0.43	0.28
		30	3.08	2.85	0.51	0.31	22.07	17.00	0.48	0.26
	Physiological saline	0	2.38	2.48	1.01	0.31	16.61	12.25	1.06	0.87
		30	2.21	0.38	2.54	1.67	19.33	15.39	11.82	12.23
	Hydrochloric acid	0	5.22	1.32	1.08	0.35	70.09	30.67	8.03	11.02
		30	24,625.05	7557.31	2070.16	725.35	81,189.98	25,124.15	15,839.44	5752.39
	Lactic acid	0	32.15	0.48	0.83	0.32	71.60	1.29	1.34	0.07
		30	31.74	0.51	0.64	0.10	77.52	4.71	1.55	0.10
Uncoated SS wire	Sterile water	0	4.78	6.83	0.76	0.54	49.26	52.90	0.43	0.28
		30	3.29	2.27	0.86	0.40	33.03	14.57	2.25	1.72
	Physiological saline	0	2.38	2.48	1.01	0.31	16.61	12.25	1.06	0.87
		30	3.89	2.72	1.52	0.24	22.22	11.94	17.36	22.61
	Hydrochloric acid	0	5.22	1.32	1.08	0.35	70.09	30.67	8.03	11.02
		30	171,051.75	41,866.15	15,044.11	2118.26	653,585.22	116,232.28	82,007.05	15,393.43
	Lactic acid	0	32.15	0.48	0.83	0.32	71.60	1.29	1.34	0.07
		30	32.33	0.58	0.77	0.20	81.63	2.24	4.14	3.49

Table 2. Metal ion release from NiTi wire (µg/L).

Wire	Solution	Immersion Time (min)	Ni		Ti	
			Mean	SD	Mean	SD
TiN-coated SS wire	Sterile water	0	0.43	0.28	1.82	0.99
		30	1.35	0.95	2.57	2.11
	Physiological saline	0	1.06	0.87	1.76	0.77
		30	4.16	2.05	7.29	10.30
	Hydrochloric acid	0	8.03	11.02	13.01	10.59
		30	13,536.28	10,012.85	12,005.95	9871.59
	Lactic acid	0	1.34	0.07	24.19	0.27
		30	1.44	0.03	24.56	0.33
Uncoated SS wire	Sterile water	0	0.43	0.28	1.82	0.99
		30	2.38	1.47	2.18	2.43
	Physiological saline	0	1.06	0.87	1.76	0.77
		30	3.37	0.91	1.17	0.29
	Hydrochloric acid	0	8.03	11.02	13.01	10.59
		30	215,499.84	64,463.60	173,761.82	73,627.09
	Lactic acid	0	1.34	0.07	24.19	0.27
		30	2.29	0.19	25.37	0.36

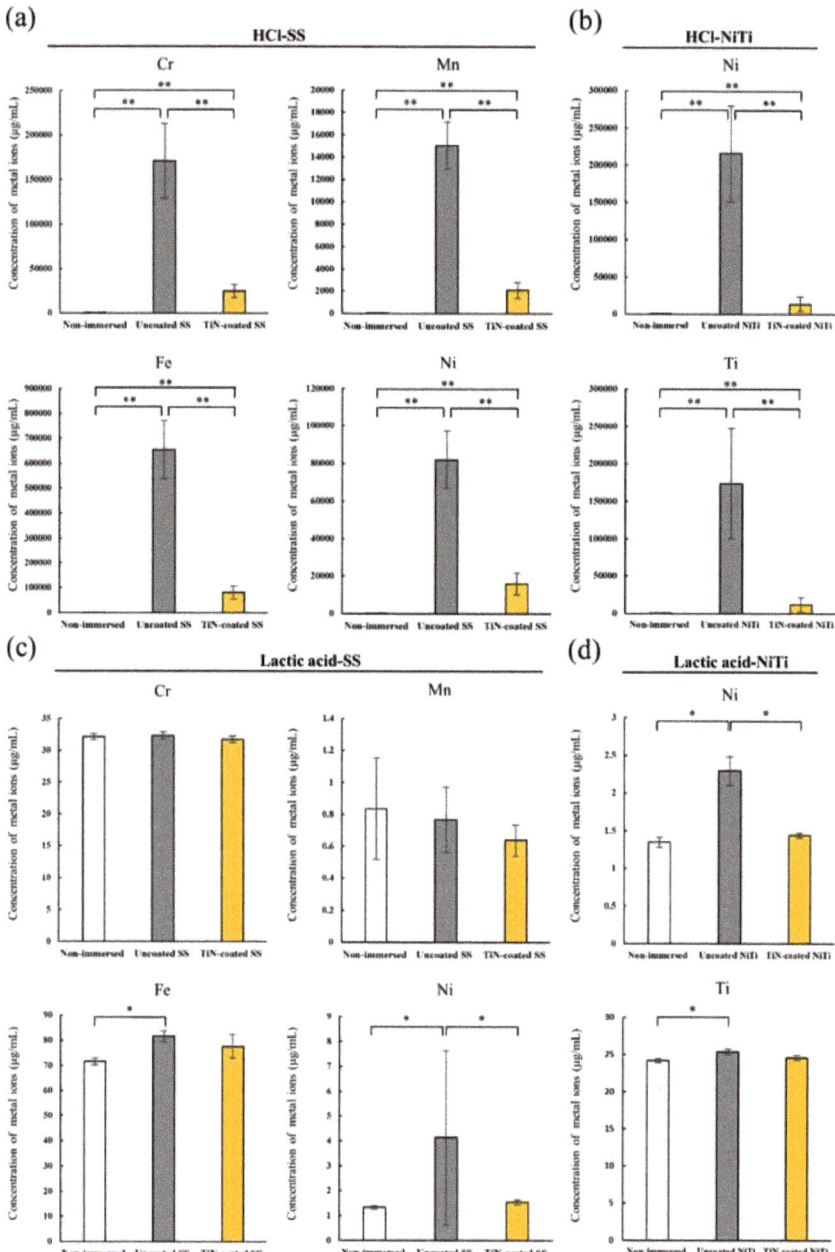

Figure 1. Metal ions released from orthodontic arch wire immersed in different solutions. After immersion in HCl or lactic acid solution for 30 min, the amount of metal ions eluted from the wire was determined by ICP-MS. The concentrations of the eluted metal ions from TiN-coated SS wire and uncoated SS wire were: (**a**) SS immersed in HCl; (**b**) NiTi immersed in HCl; (**c**) SS immersed in lactic acid; (**d**) NiTi immersed in lactic acid. The statistical significance of differences was determined by the Shapiro-Wilk (* $p < 0.05$, ** $p < 0.01$).

3.2. DMG Test

The results of the DMG test were scored according to the degree of red color development as an indicator of the strength of the positive response, as shown in Figure 2a. The DMG test results for Ni release are shown in Tables 3 and 4. The TiN-coated and uncoated SS and NiTi wire immersed in HCl for 30 min showed positive reactions on the DMG test, while negative reactions were observed for the other conditions. Following immersion in HCl for 30 min, the scores for the TiN-coated and uncoated SS wire were 1.0 ± 0.0 and 2.67 ± 0.58, respectively (Figure 2b, Table 3), and those for the TiN-coated and uncoated NiTi wire were 1.0 ± 0.0 and 2.67 ± 0.58, respectively (Figure 2c, Table 4).

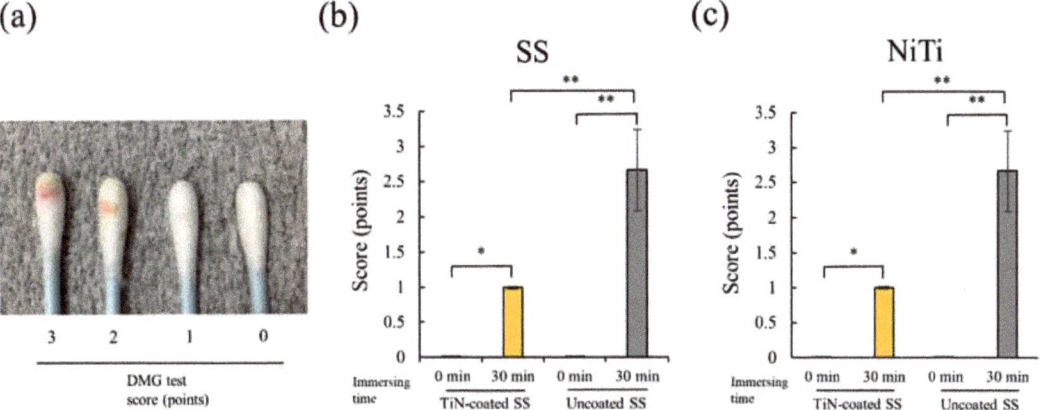

Figure 2. DMG test: (**a**) Positive reactions were scored; (**b**) SS wire immersed in HCl; (**c**) NiTi wire immersed in HCl. The statistical significance of differences was determined by the Tukey-Kramer HSD test. (* $p < 0.05$, ** $p < 0.01$).

Table 3. DMG test results for SS wire.

Wire	Solution	Immersion Time (min)	Mean	SD
TiN-coated SS wire	Sterile water	0	0.00	0.00
		30	0.00	0.00
	Physiological saline	0	0.00	0.00
		30	0.00	0.00
	Hydrochloric acid	0	0.00	0.00
		30	1.00	0.00
	Lactic acid	0	0.00	0.00
		30	0.00	0.00
Uncoated SS wire	Sterile water	0	0.00	0.00
		30	0.00	0.00
	Physiological saline	0	0.00	0.00
		30	0.00	0.00
	Hydrochloric acid	0	0.00	0.00
		30	2.67	0.47
	Lactic acid	0	0.00	0.00
		30	0.00	0.00

Table 4. DMG test results for NiTi wire.

Wire	Solution	Immersion Time (min)	Mean	SD
TiN-coated NiTi wire	Sterile water	0	0.00	0.00
		30	0.00	0.00
	Physiological saline	0	0.00	0.00
		30	0.00	0.00
	Hydrochloric acid	0	0.00	0.00
		30	1.00	0.00
	Lactic acid	0	0.00	0.00
		30	0.00	0.00
Uncoated NiTi wire	Sterile water	0	0.00	0.00
		30	0.00	0.00
	Physiological saline	0	0.00	0.00
		30	0.00	0.00
	Hydrochloric acid	0	0.00	0.00
		30	2.67	0.47
	Lactic acid	0	0.00	0.00
		30	0.00	0.00

3.3. Observation of the Wire Surface

Figure 3 shows stereomicrographs of the surfaces of the wire samples. Corrosion of the surface was found on both the TiN-coated and uncoated SS and NiTi wire after immersion in HCl for 30 min. There were no differences between the non-immersed wire and wire immersed in lactic acid for 30 min.

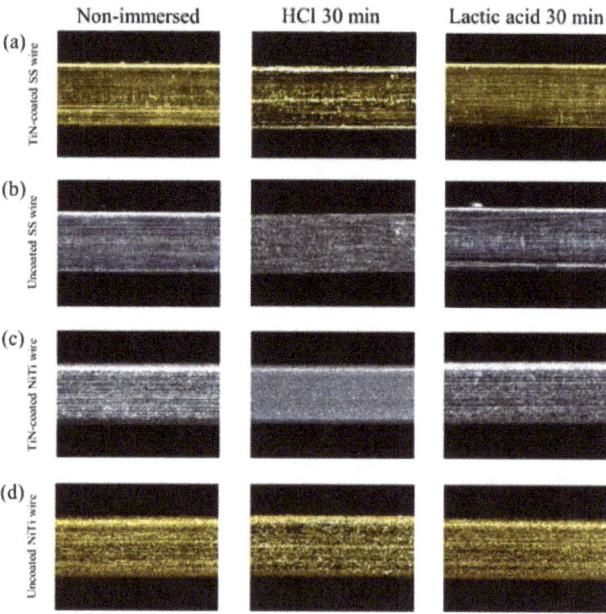

Figure 3. Stereomicrographs of orthodontic wire immersed in HCl or lactic acid for 30 min: (**a**) TiN-coated SS wire; (**b**) Uncoated SS wire; (**c**) TiN-coated NiTi wire; (**d**) Uncoated NiTi wire.

SEM images of the wire surface are shown in Figure 4. At a magnification of 200×, corrosion was found on both the TiN-coated and uncoated SS and NiTi wires after immersion in HCl for 30 min. At a magnification of 1000×, the TiN-coated SS and NiTi wires demonstrated pitting corrosion, while the uncoated SS and NiTi wires showed uniform corrosion. There were no differences in surfaces between non-immersed wires or TiN-coated and uncoated wire immersed in lactic acid for 30 min.

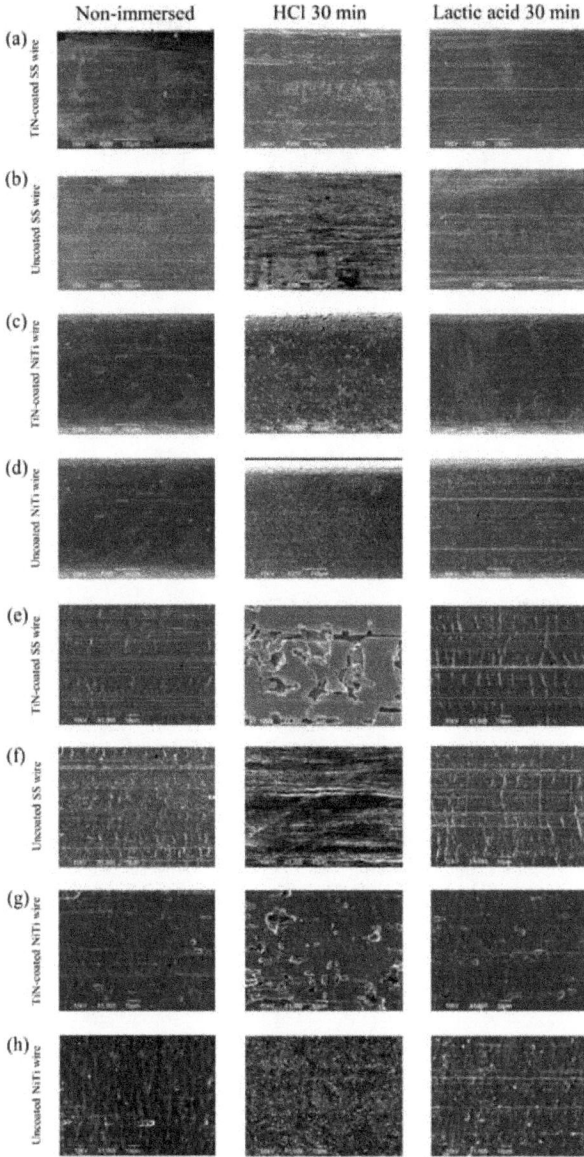

Figure 4. Scanning electron micrographs of orthodontic arch wire immersed in HCl or lactic acid for 30 min. (×200): (**a**) TiN-coated SS wire; (**b**) Uncoated SS wire; (**c**) TiN-coated NiTi wire; (**d**) Uncoated NiTi wire. (×1000): (**e**) TiN-coated SS wire; (**f**) Uncoated SS wire; (**g**) TiN-coated NiTi wire; (**h**) Uncoated NiTi wire.

3.4. Surface Roughness

Both the uncoated and the TiN-coated SS and NiTi wires immersed in HCl for 30 min showed significantly increased surface roughness compared to the non-immersed wire (Figure 5). On the other hand, immersion in lactic acid for 30 min was associated with significantly increased surface roughness compared to non-immersed wire only for the uncoated SS and NiTi specimens.

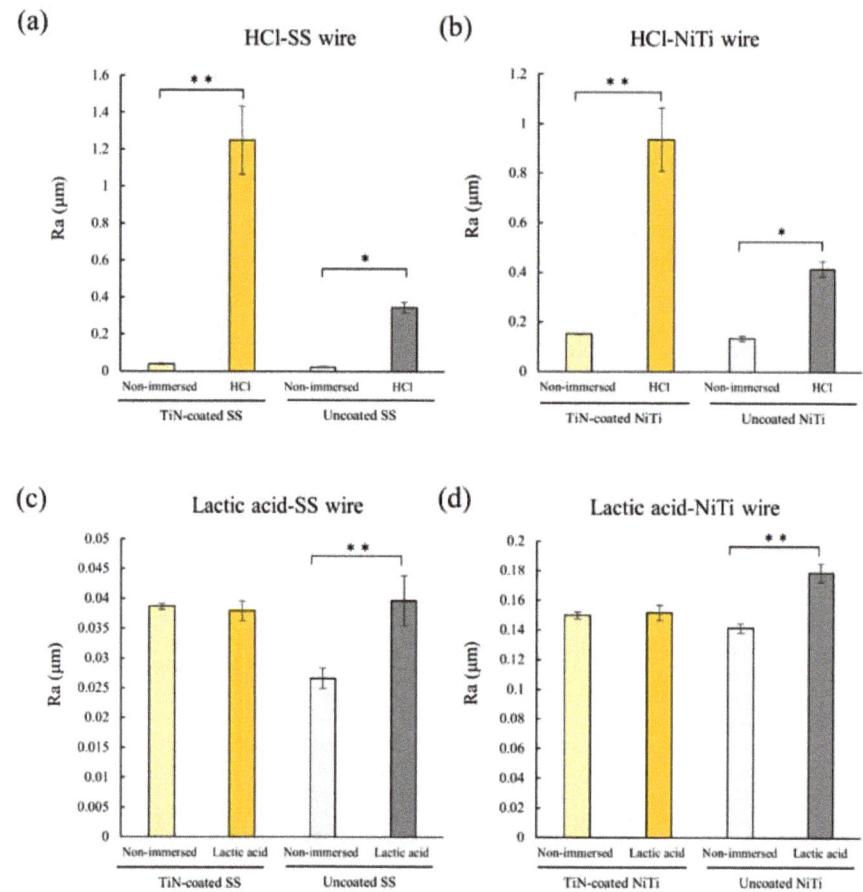

Figure 5. Comparison of surface roughness of orthodontic arch wires after immersion in HCl or lactic acid. After immersion in HCl or lactic acid for 30 min, the surface roughness (Ra) of orthodontic arch wires was assessed using a surface roughness tester: (**a**) SS wire immersed in HCl; (**b**) NiTi wire immersed in HCl; (**c**) SS wire immersed in lactic acid; (**d**) NiTi immersed in lactic acid. The statistical of differences was determined by the Tukey-Kramer HSD test. (* $p < 0.05$, ** $p < 0.01$).

4. Discussion

As the release of metal ions from orthodontic materials in the oral environment is closely related to their corrosion, metal surfaces are coated to improve corrosion resistance [13]. A number of plating techniques and materials are available for coating such metal components, and TiN ion plating was used in this study. The Ti of TiN components forms a passivation film, which improves the surface properties of the substrate material [25,26]. TiN ion plating results in little degradation of the mechanical properties of the substrate material because it is performed at low temperatures. Previously, we reported that TiN-coated orthodontic wire has a reduced friction coefficient, and the mechanical properties of the base material are maintained [17]. This study was performed to investigate whether the elution of metal ions can be suppressed by coating orthodontic wires with TiN film.

The ICP-MS data showed that the elution of metal ions was significantly suppressed in the TiN-coated wire compared to the uncoated wire after immersion in HCl for 30 min. Similarly, the DMG test confirmed that that the amount of Ni leached from both the SS and the NiTi wire after immersion in HCl were significantly lower for the TiN-coated than for the uncoated wire. The leaching of metal ions by HCl was suppressed by TiN coating. On the other hand, with immersion in lactic acid, Ni ions were leached from the uncoated but not the TiN-coated SS and NiTi wire, suggesting that the TiN-coated SS and NiTi wire was resistant to corrosion by lactic acid. Wire immersed in lactic acid showed no positive reaction on the DMG test, which may have been because the concentration of Ni was below the limit of detection of the test (10 µg/mL, 10 ppm) [27]. ICP-MS also showed that the amount of Ni ions eluted from the wire immersed in lactic acid was < 10 µg/mL, suggesting that it would be difficult to detect Ni elution associated with immersion in lactic acid on the DMG test. The amount of metal ions eluted from the TiN-coated SS and NiTi wire and the variations in the data were considered to be greater because of the high concentration of HCl used in this experiment. As the HCl derived from GERD has a lower concentration than that used in this study [23] and the immersion time in GERD-derived HCl is likely to be < 30 min in the oral cavity, the amount of elution is expected to be much smaller than in this experiment. However, as the threshold for Ni allergies is 1.5 µg [28], and there is a risk of onset of metal allergy when exposed to very small amounts of the metal, further experiments are required to examine the use of HCl at a concentration closer to that likely to be present in the oral cavity. Furthermore, the amount of Ni ion elution from uncoated SS wire immersed in lactic acid showed a high standard deviation. The immersion time of 30 min in lactic acid is considered to be the starting point of erosion for the SS wire used in this experiment. In some samples, the amount of Ni ion elution was small because dissolution had only just begun, and this may have resulted in the high degree of variation in the data.

The stereomicroscopy and SEM analyses showed the corrosion of all the wires following immersion in HCl, but the types of corrosion differed between the TiN-coated and uncoated wires. That is, pitting corrosion occurred in the TiN-coated SS and NiTi wire, while the uncoated SS and NiTi wire showed uniform corrosion. Such uniform corrosion is known to occur when metal is immersed in HCl [29], and this was confirmed in the present study. Pitting corrosion tends to occur in TiN with a coating thickness <6 µm [30]. In the present study, the TiN coating was 0.3 µm thick, which was intended to be used for orthodontic treatment, so the pitting corrosion may have occurred easily. Preliminary experiments showed that the peeling of TiN coating gradually became noticeable under the stereomicroscope when immersed in HCl for more than 30 min, so the immersion time was set to 30 min in this study.

The surface roughness of both the uncoated and the TiN-coated wire immersed in HCl was increased significantly compared to that of the non-immersed samples, suggesting that the wire surface was corroded by HCl, confirming the results of the microscopic analyses. Furthermore, the surface roughness of the TiN-coated wire was greater than that of the uncoated wire despite the reduced amount of metal ion elution. This may have been due to the difference in corrosion patterns between the TiN-coated and uncoated wires, as revealed by the stereomicroscopy and SEM analyses. The uniform corrosion of the uncoated wire was seen over its entire surface, but the pitting corrosion of TiN-coated wire induced by HCl in this study was randomly scattered, and the SEM images showed small fragments of coating material that seemed to have been peeled off around the pores, which may have caused an increase in the surface roughness. The surface roughness (Ra) measured in this study is a two-dimensional measurement, so a three-dimensional measurement of surface roughness (Sa) may be useful for further detailed analyses [31].

Microscopic examination indicated that the surface condition of the TiN-coated SS and NiTi wire was not altered by immersion in lactic acid and there was no change in the surface roughness, suggesting no corrosion by lactic acid. On the other hand, for the uncoated SS and NiTi wire, although microscopy revealed no changes in the surface condition, the surface roughness was increased by immersion in lactic acid, suggesting the possibility of corrosion by lactic acid.

Taken together, the results outlined above indicated that pitting corrosion occurred on the surface of TiN-coated SS and NiTi wire immersed in HCl, but that the corrosion did not spread over the entire surface of the wire, so the leaching of metal ions was significantly suppressed compared to the uncoated wire. The leaching of Ni ions from the TiN-coated SS and NiTi wire immersed in lactic acid was also shown to be significantly suppressed compared to the uncoated wire. These results indicated that TiN coating inhibits acid-induced corrosion and the elution of metal ions. GERD is associated with the regurgitation of gastric acid, mainly HCl, into the oral cavity. Thus, the results presented above suggest that the use of TiN-coated wires may be effective in preventing the leaching of metal ions from orthodontic appliances by HCl in gastric acid and reduce the rates of induction and exacerbation of metal allergy in patients with GERD. In addition, *Lactobacillus acidophilus* present in the oral cavity has been suggested to be related to the corrosion of metals mediated by lactic acid production [11]. The TiN-coated wire used in this study was resistant to corrosion by lactic acid, and is expected to be applicable to orthodontic treatment of patients with metal allergies.

We analyzed the acid corrosion resistance of TiN-coated wires in vitro. The following issues should be considered in future experiments. First, it is necessary to examine how long the TiN coating can be maintained in good condition in the oral cavity during orthodontic treatment. Second, the TiN coating is expensive, so cost reduction must be considered for clinical use. We plan to reduce the cost by coating as many wires as possible at once. Although TiN coating has excellent biocompatibility, as demonstrated previously in a device for atrial septal defect closure [14], it will be necessary to study its biocompatibility in the oral cavity, where it will be exposed to various chemical substances in food and drink, as well as saliva.

5. Conclusions

TiN plating of orthodontic wires can inhibit acid-mediated corrosion, and thus reduce the elution of Ni ions from the wire surface. These results suggest that TiN plating may be useful for the orthodontic treatment of patients with metal allergies. In addition, TiN plating has the potential for use in other dental applications, such as coating the metal parts of removable dentures and for wires to splint the teeth after orthodontic treatment.

Author Contributions: Conceptualization, A.I. and H.K.; methodology, A.I. and H.K.; validation, A.I. and H.K.; formal analysis, A.I.; investigation, A.I. and H.S.; resources, A.I. and H.K.; data curation, A.I.; writing—original draft preparation, A.I.; writing—review and editing, H.K.; visualization, A.I., T.N. and F.O.; supervision, H.K. and I.M.; project administration, H.K.; funding acquisition, A.I. All authors have read and agreed to the published version of the manuscript.

Funding: This work was supported in part by JSPS KAKENHI grants from the Japan Society for the Promotion of Science (No. K20K187740).

Informed Consent Statement: Not applicable.

Data Availability Statement: The data and analysis in this study are available on request from the corresponding author.

Conflicts of Interest: The authors declare there are no conflicts of interest.

Abbreviations

TiN	titanium nitride
ICP-MS	inductively coupled plasma mass spectrometry
DMG	dimethylglyoxime
Ni	nickel
Co	cobalt
Cr	chromium
PVD	physical vapor deposition
SS	stainless steel
NiTi	nickel titanium
Ar	argon
N_2	nitrogen
HCl	hydrochloric acid
Mn	manganese
Fe	iron
SEM	scanning electron microscopy
GERD	gastroesophageal reflux disease

References

1. Mortz, C.G.; Bindslev-Jensen, C.; Andersen, K.E. Prevalence, incidence rates and persistence of contact allergy and allergic contact dermatitis in The Odense Adolescent Cohort Study: A 15-year follow-up. *Br. J. Dermatol.* **2013**, *168*, 318–325. [CrossRef]
2. Thyssen, J.P.; Linneberg, A.; Menné, T.; Johansen, J.D. The epidemiology of contact allergy in the general population—Prevalence and main findings. *Contact Dermat.* **2007**, *57*, 287–299. [CrossRef]
3. Kitaura, H.; Fujimura, Y.; Nakao, N.; Eguchi, T.; Yoshida, N. Treatment of a patient with metal hypersensitivity after orthognathic surgery. *Angle Orthod.* **2007**, *77*, 923–930. [CrossRef]
4. Lindsten, R.; Kurol, J. Orthodontic appliances in relation to nickel hypersensitivity. A review. *J. Orofac. Orthop.* **1997**, *58*, 100–108. [PubMed]
5. Noble, J.; Ahing, S.I.; Karaiskos, N.E.; Wiltshire, W.A. Nickel allergy and orthodontics, a review and report of two cases. *Br. Dent. J.* **2008**, *204*, 297–300. [CrossRef] [PubMed]
6. Bajaj, A.K.; Saraswat, A.; Mukhija, G.; Rastogi, S.; Yadav, S. Patch testing experience with 1000 patients. *Indian J. Dermatol. Venereol. Leprol.* **2007**, *73*, 313–318. [CrossRef] [PubMed]
7. Dotterud, L.K.; Smith-Sivertsen, T. Allergic contact sensitization in the general adult population: A population-based study from Northern Norway. *Contact Dermat.* **2007**, *56*, 10–15. [CrossRef]
8. Adachi, N.; Kitaura, H.; Ikeda, M.; Kobayashi, K. Quantitative analysis of the surface elements of orthodontic metal materials using an X-ray fluorescence spectroscope. *Orthod. Waves* **2000**, *59*, 128–137.
9. Nielsen, N.H.; Linneberg, A.; Menné, T.; Madsen, F.; Frølund, L.; Dirksen, A.; Jørgensen, T. Allergic contact sensitization in an adult Danish population: Two cross-sectional surveys eight years apart (the Copenhagen Allergy Study). *Acta Derm. Venereol.* **2001**, *81*, 31–34. [CrossRef]
10. Dotterud, L.K. The prevalence of allergic contact sensitization in a general population in Tromsø, Norway. *Int. J. Circumpolar Health* **2007**, *66*, 328–334. [CrossRef]
11. Chaturvedi, T.P.; Upadhayay, S.N. An overview of orthodontic material degradation in oral cavity. *Indian J. Dent. Res.* **2010**, *21*, 275–284. [CrossRef]
12. Fors, R.; Persson, M. Nickel in dental plaque and saliva in patients with and without orthodontic appliances. *Eur. J. Orthod.* **2006**, *28*, 292–297. [CrossRef]
13. Jabbari, Y.S.A.; Fehrman, J.; Barnes, A.C.; Zapf, A.M.; Zinelis, S.; Berzins, D.W. Titanium nitride and nitrogen ion implanted coated dental materials. *Coatings* **2012**, *2*, 160–178. [CrossRef]
14. Zhang, Z.; Fu, B.; Zhang, D.Y.; Zhang, Z.; Cheng, Y.; Sheng, L.; Lai, C.; Xi, T. Safety and efficacy of nano lamellar TiN coatings on nitinol atrial septal defect occluders in vivo. *Mater. Sci. Eng. C Mater. Biol. Appl.* **2013**, *33*, 1355–1360. [CrossRef] [PubMed]
15. Kim, H.; Kim, C.Y.; Kim, D.W.; Lee, I.S.; Lee, G.H.; Park, J.C.; Lee, S.J.; Lee, K.Y. Wear performance of self-mating contact pairs of TiN and TiAlN coatings on orthopedic grade Ti-6Al-4V. *Biomed. Mater.* **2010**, *5*, 044108. [CrossRef]
16. Steele, J.G.; McCabe, J.F.; Barnes, I.E. Properties of a titanium nitride coating for dental instruments. *J. Dent.* **1991**, *19*, 226–229. [CrossRef]
17. Sugisawa, H.; Kitaura, H.; Ueda, K.; Kimura, K.; Ishida, M.; Ochi, Y.; Kishikawa, A.; Ogawa, S.; Takano-Yamamoto, T. Corrosion resistance and mechanical properties of titanium nitride plating on orthodontic wires. *Dent. Mater. J.* **2018**, *37*, 286–292. [CrossRef] [PubMed]
18. Smiech-Slomkowska, G.; Jablonska-Zrobek, J. The effect of oral health education on dental plaque development and the level of caries-related *Streptococcus* mutans and *Lactobacillus* spp. *Eur. J. Orthod.* **2007**, *29*, 157–160. [CrossRef]

19. Kameda, T.; Oda, H.; Ohkuma, K.; Sano, N.; Batbayar, N.; Terashima, Y.; Sato, S.; Terada, K. Microbiologically influenced corrosion of orthodontic metallic appliances. *Dent. Mater. J.* **2014**, *33*, 187–195. [CrossRef]
20. Dashper, S.G.; Reynolds, E.C. Lactic acid excretion by Streptococcus mutans. *Microbiology* **1996**, *142*, 33–39. [CrossRef] [PubMed]
21. Dent, J.; El-Serag, H.; Wallander, M.A.; Johansson, S. Epidemiology of gastro-oesophageal reflux disease: A systematic review. *Gut* **2005**, *54*, 710–717. [CrossRef]
22. Sulaiman, T.A.; Abdulmajeed, A.A.; Shahramian, K.; Hupa, L.; Donovan, T.E.; Vallittu, P.; Närhi, T.O. Impact of gastric acidic challenge on surface topography and optical properties of monolithic zirconia. *Dent. Mater.* **2015**, *31*, 1445–1452. [CrossRef] [PubMed]
23. Elsaka, S.; Hassan, A.; Elnaghy, A. Effect of gastric acids on surface topography and bending properties of esthetic coated nickel-titanium orthodontic archwires. *Clin. Oral Investig.* **2021**, *25*, 1319–1326. [CrossRef] [PubMed]
24. Nakao, N.; Kitaura, H.; Yoshida, N. Analysis of the release of nickel from orthodontic wires using the dimethylglyoxime spot test: In vitro and in vivo study. *Orthod. Waves* **2002**, *61*, 478–481.
25. Iijima, M.; Endo, K.; Ohno, H.; Yonekura, Y.; Mizoguchi, I. Corrosion behavior and surface structure of orthodontic Ni-Ti alloy wires. *Dent. Mater. J.* **2001**, *20*, 103–113. [CrossRef] [PubMed]
26. Lee, T.H.; Huang, T.K.; Lin, S.Y.; Chen, L.K.; Chou, M.Y.; Huang, H.H. Corrosion resistance of different nickel-titanium archwires in acidic fluoride-containing artificial saliva. *Angle Orthod.* **2010**, *80*, 547–553. [CrossRef] [PubMed]
27. Rycroft, R.J.; Menné, T.; Frosch, P.J.; Lepoittevin, J.-P. *Textbook of Contact Dermatitis*; Springer: Berlin/Heidelberg, Germany, 2013.
28. Emmett, E.A.; Risby, T.H.; Jiang, L.; Ng, S.K.; Feinman, S. Allergic contact dermatitis to nickel: Bioavailability from consumer products and provocation threshold. *J. Am. Acad. Dermatol.* **1988**, *19*, 314–322. [CrossRef]
29. Tjahjanti, P.; Kurniawan, M.; Firdaus, R.; Iswanto, A. *Experimental Study of Corrosion Rate on st60 Steel as a Result of Immersion in HCl, NaOH, and NaCl Solutions*; IOP Conference Series: Materials Science and Engineering; IOP Publishing: Bristol, UK, 2020; p. 012038.
30. Lang, F.; Yu, Z. The corrosion resistance and wear resistance of thick TiN coatings deposited by arc ion plating. *Surf. Coat. Technol.* **2001**, *145*, 80–87. [CrossRef]
31. Ardila-Rodríguez, L.A.; Rans, C.; Poulis, J.A. Effect of surface morphology on the Ti-Ti adhesive bond performance of Ti6Al4V parts fabricated by selective laser melting. *Int. J. Adhes. Adhes.* **2021**, *110*, 102918. [CrossRef]

Article

Influence of Selected Restorative Materials on the Environmental pH: In Vitro Comparative Study

Anna Lehmann [1,†], Kacper Nijakowski [1,*,†], Michalina Nowakowska [2], Patryk Woś [2], Maria Misiaszek [2] and Anna Surdacka [1]

1. Department of Conservative Dentistry and Endodontics, Poznan University of Medical Sciences, 60-812 Poznan, Poland; annalehmann@ump.edu.pl (A.L.); annasurd@ump.edu.pl (A.S.)
2. Student's Scientific Group, Department of Conservative Dentistry and Endodontics, Poznan University of Medical Sciences, 60-812 Poznan, Poland; michalina1n@gmail.com (M.N.); patrykwos4@gmail.com (P.W.); mariamisiaszek1@gmail.com (M.M.)
* Correspondence: kacpernijakowski@ump.edu.pl
† These authors contributed equally to this work.

Abstract: In dental caries treatment, it is worth using such restorative materials that may limit plaque accumulation. The pH of the filling seems to be an important factor affecting the potential bacterial colonisation. Our study aimed to assess how selected restorative materials influence the environmental pH. A total of 150 specimens (30 of each: Ketac Molar, Riva LC, Riva SC, Filtek Bulk Fill, and Evetric) were placed in 100 sterile hermetic polyethene containers with saline and stored in 37 °C. The pH of each sample was measured using the electrode Halo HI13302 (Hanna Instruments, Poland) at specific points in time for 15 days. The initial pH levels were significantly lower for glass ionomer cements (3.9–4.7) compared to composites (5.9–6.0). With time, the pH increased for samples with glass ionomer cements (by nearly 1.5), whereas it decreased for samples with composites (maximally by 0.8). In the end, all materials were in the pH range between 5.3 and 6.0. The highest final pH was obtained with Ketac Molar at about 5.9. Double samples had lower pH values than single samples, irrespective of the type of material. In conclusion, immediately after application, restorative materials decreased the environmental pH, especially light-cured glass ionomer cements. For glass ionomers, within two weeks, the pH increased to levels comparable with composites.

Keywords: dental material; restorative material; composite; glass ionomer; resin-modified glass ionomer; pH; acidity; oral environment; dental filling; dental restoration

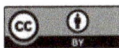

1. Introduction

Acid demineralisation of enamel due to the metabolic activity of bacterial plaque is the first stage of the caries process, leading to the formation of a cavity [1–3]. The destructed dental tissues are restored with various materials; however, on the contact surface of the tooth and the filling, there is usually a niche that favours the plaque accumulation and may increase the risk of secondary caries. Therefore, it is worth using such restorative materials that may prevent bacterial adhesion or limit the development of bacterial plaque. The pH of the filling seems to be an essential factor influencing the potential bacterial colonisation [4]. Numerous in vitro studies show that at acidic pH, the surface of the composite material is more stable than the surface of glass ionomer cement [4–6]. Thus far, few researchers have analysed the potential effect of the filling materials on the environmental pH. However, conventional glass ionomer cements (GICs) can buffer lactic acid and release fluoride, which appears to be very beneficial in a clinical approach [7–9].

It is believed that there are no clear limits to the number of fillings a dentist can perform in one visit. If necessary, it is recommended to perform several fillings in the same area within the conduction anaesthesia. However, other factors can affect the amount of time a patient spends in the dental chair. Most often, apart from the time limitations of the doctor and the patient, the general health condition and ailments related to the temporomandibular joint can pose a limitation. After two hours with an open mouth, it is recognised that there may be irreversible changes in the joint [10]. There are no previous articles on how the pH in the oral cavity changes after tooth restoration depending on the number of fillings.

The literature reports the hydrolysis process of fillings under low and high pH conditions in vitro. The carious bacteria fermentation and gastric acid attack are most often simulated by lactic acid and hydrochloric acid, respectively [11,12]. Both composite materials and glass ionomer cements undergo hydrolysis at acidic pH [4,13,14]. However, GICs seem to exhibit more favourable properties than resin-based materials, among others: chemical adhesion to enamel and dentin in the presence of moisture, resistance to microleakage, good marginal integrity, dimensional stability at high humidity, coefficient of thermal expansion like tooth structure, biocompatibility, fluoride release, rechargeability with fluoride, and less shrinkage than resins upon setting with no free monomer being released [15]. In the case of composite materials, the key is proper preparation of the cavity edge, gradual material application, and a meticulous polishing procedure [1,16]. However, even in vitro, a microleakage can be observed in the most carefully placed composite [17]. Certain limitations can also be seen in the bonding systems. All adhesive systems are somehow unstable and susceptible to hydrolytic degradation, which may be responsible for the partial failure of the material adhesion to the tooth, leading to marginal leakage [18,19]. The literature shows that resin restoration degradation is a complex process involving the hydrolysis of the resin and the dentin collagen fibril phases within the hybrid layer. Inhibition of the collagenolytic activity, as well as the use of cross-linking agents, are the two main strategies to increase the resistance of the hybrid layer to enzymatic degradation [20,21]. There is still no answer as to whether the effect of the restorations' pH on the oral environment could be a helpful factor in reducing secondary caries. It is known that despite the continuous modernising of the filling materials, the enamel still has a more significant buffer capacity than the composite or glass ionomer cement [22,23].

Our study aimed to analyse the potential pH effect of the most used dental materials, i.e., composites and glass ionomers, on the oral environment modelled in vitro. We tried to answer the following questions:

1. How do restorative materials influence the environmental pH within the first two weeks after their application?
2. Can a larger number of one-time fillings affect the surrounding pH more?
3. Which filling materials are more stable in terms of pH?

2. Materials and Methods
2.1. Materials Used in the Study

In this in vitro study, we used five dental restorative materials. Detailed characteristics of the materials are presented in Table 1.

Table 1. Detailed characteristics of the dental restorative materials used in the study.

Material	Material Group	Manufacturer	Acronym	Composition	Lot Number
Filtek Bulk Fill, Shade A3	composite	3M/ESPE, Seefeld, Germany	FBF	Organic matrix: AUDMA, UDMA, 1,12-dodecane-DMA 20 nm silica; Filler fraction (wt%/vol%) 76.5/58.4, Fillers: 4–11 nm zirconia, ytterbium trifluoride filler consisting of agglomerate 100 nm particles	N867070

Table 1. Cont.

Material	Material Group	Manufacturer	Acronym	Composition	Lot Number
Evetric, Shade A3	composite	Ivoclar Vivadent, Schaan, Liechtenstein	ER	Organic matrix: Bis-GMA, Bis-EMA, UDMA; Filler fraction (wt%/vol%) 80–81/55–57, Fillers: barium glass, ytterbium trifluoride, mixed oxide, copolymers (size 40–3000 nm)	Y20235
Ketac Molar Easymix, Shade A3	glass-ionomer cement	3M/ESPE, Seefeld, Germany	KM	Liquid: polyacrylic acid 20–30%, tartaric acid 10–15%, water Powder: fluoroaluminosilicate glass 90–95%, polyacrylic acid 5–10%	7870998
Riva SC, Shade A3	glass-ionomer cement	SDI Limited, Victoria, Australia	RSC	Liquid: polyacrylic acid 20–30%, tartaric acid 10–15%, water Powder: fluoroaluminosilicate glass 90–95%, polyacrylic acid 5–10%	B1912041
Riva LC, Shade A3	resin-modified glass ionomer cement	SDI Limited, Victoria, Australia	RLC	Liquid: polyacrylic acid 20–30%, tartaric acid 5–10%, HEMA 20–25%, dimethacrylate cross linker 10–25%, acid monomer 10–20% Powder: fluoroaminosilicate powder 95–100%	J2011171

2.2. Specimen Preparation

All specimen preparation was completed by one operator to reduce variability. A total of 150 specimens (30 from one material) were prepared using metal moulds with 6 mm diameter and 2 mm thickness. All materials were inserted into the mould and intentionally overfilled. Then, the mould was sandwiched between transparent Mylar strips to expel excess material. The uncured resin-modified glass ionomer and composites were light-cured for 40 s, according to the manufacturer's instructions (light intensity of 1200 mW/cm^2, Translux Wave, Kulzer GmbH, Hanau, Germany). Conventional glass ionomer cement (CGIC) was prepared according to the powder-liquid mixing ratio indicated by the manufacturers. After 30 min, the CGIC specimens were removed from the moulds.

2.3. Specimen Storage and pH Evaluation

The samples were placed in 100 sterile hermetic polyethene containers (ApteoCare, Sanmed, Bydgoszcz, Poland; lot: 06/KS/2021/S) and incubated in 37 °C. Each type of material was divided into 20 containers. In the first 10, there was one sample of the filling material and in the next 10, two samples. To each container, 5 mL of saline (Polpharma, Stargard Gdanski, Poland; lot: 1280620) was added.

The pH of each sample was measured using the electrode Halo HI13302 (Hanna Instruments, Olsztyn, Poland) by immersing it into the central part of the solution. Between procedures, the electrode was cleaned and recalibrated. All measurements were made in duplicate and then averaged. The pH evaluation was performed at the following time points: after 1, 6, 12 and 24 h and after 3, 6, 9, 12 and 15 days from the specimen preparation.

2.4. Statistical Analysis

The determined pH values were analysed using a two-way repeated-measures analysis of variance (in the model with the interaction). The pH changes were compared separately at specific points in time depending on the kind of used dental restorative material and the number of the incubated samples. The significance level was defined as $\alpha = 0.05$. The statistical analysis was performed using Statistica 13.3 (Statsoft, Cracow, Poland).

3. Results

For a better interpretation, all results are presented in the form of graphs. Figures 1–3 show the differences in pH changes over time depending on the dental materials used.

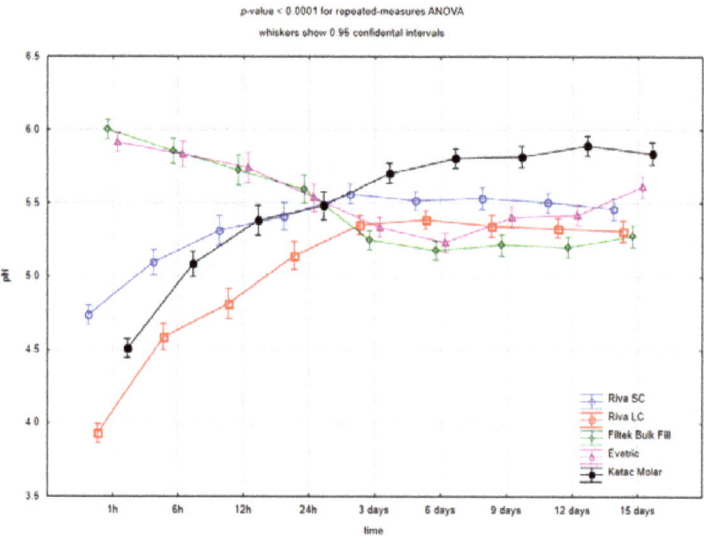

Figure 1. Repeated-measures analysis of variance for pH values in the individual time points depending on the dental restorative material (without subdividing by number of samples).

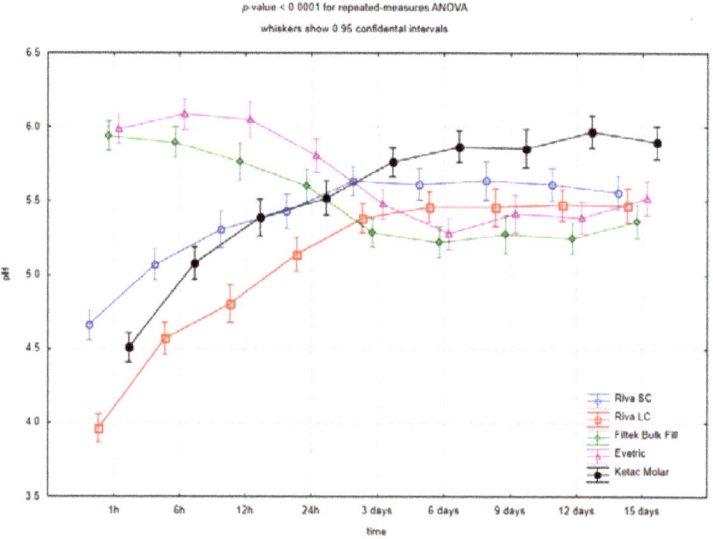

Figure 2. Repeated-measures analysis of variance for pH values in the individual time points depending on the dental restorative material for the one sample.

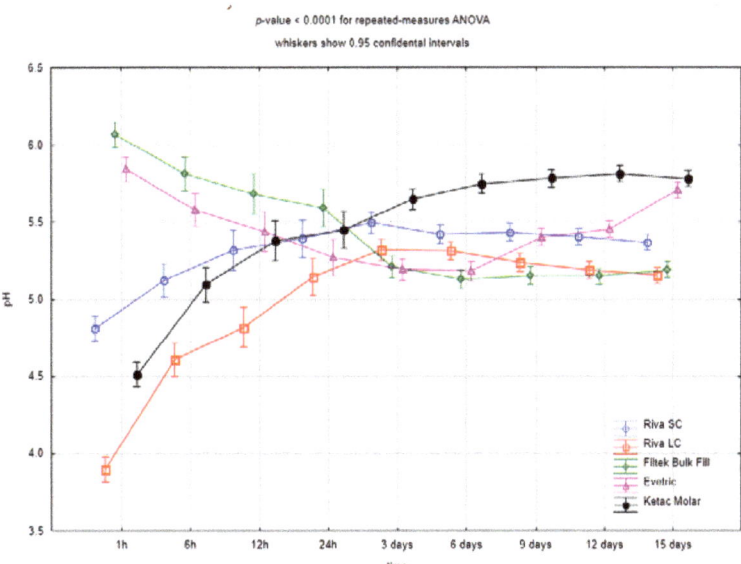

Figure 3. Repeated-measures analysis of variance for pH values in the individual time points depending on the dental restorative material for the two samples.

In general, all materials of a given group showed similar trends in pH change over time, regardless of the number of samples. Glass ionomer materials showed a significant increase in initial pH level from acidic to more neutral. The lowest initial pH level was found for the light-cured glass ionomer. However, for this material, the final pH level was higher by nearly 1.5. A similar increase was found for Ketac Molar. In contrast, for composite materials, a decrease in pH level by less than 1 was observed. At the endpoint, all materials had pH levels close to each other between 5 and 6, with Ketac Molar having the highest value. Moreover, after about a week, this material had a significantly higher environmental pH than all the others.

The changes in pH over time for individual materials depending on the number of the samples are presented in Figures 4–8.

For glass ionomer materials, already after three days, significant differences between pH levels can be seen depending on the number of samples. In the case of dual samples, lower values were obtained. In contrast, for Evetric composite material, significant differences were observed in pH level depending on the number of samples during the first three days. Additionally, the two samples showed significantly lower values, although higher variability was determined for the measurements of composite materials. On the other hand, Filtek Bulk Fill was the only material without pH variation depending on the number of samples, although there were changes in pH over time.

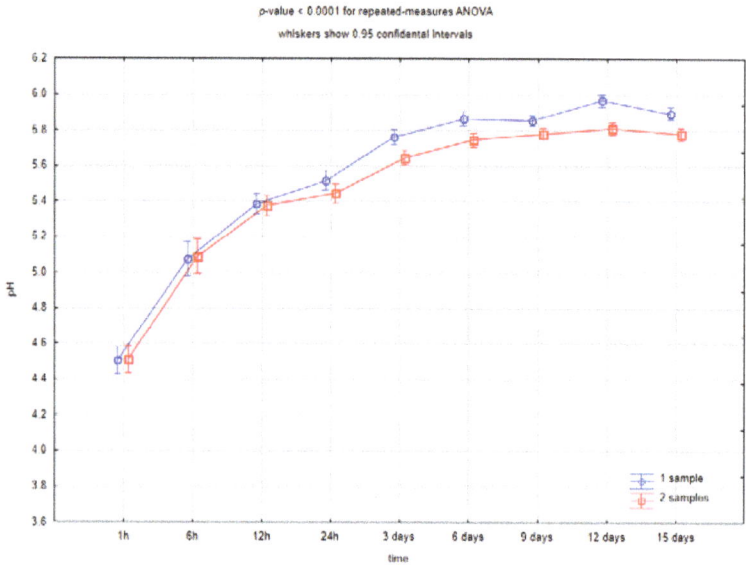

Figure 4. Repeated-measures analysis of variance for pH values in the individual time points depending on the number of the samples for Ketac Molar Easymix.

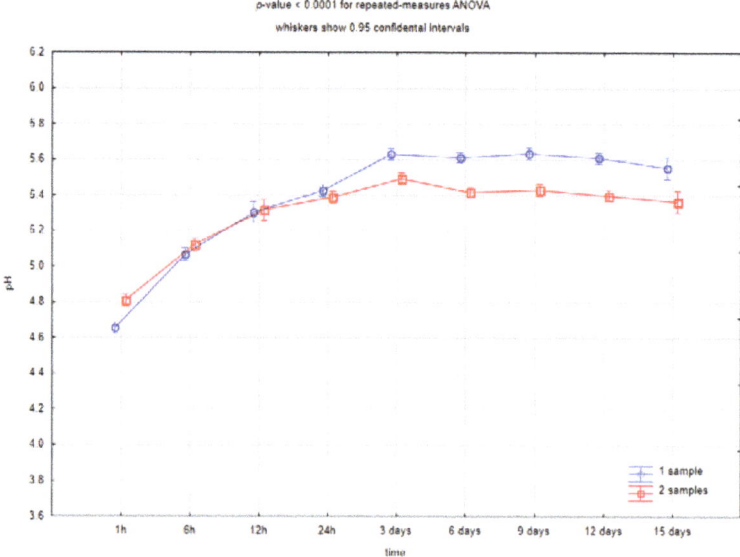

Figure 5. Repeated-measures analysis of variance for pH values in the individual time-points depending on the number of the samples for RIVA SC.

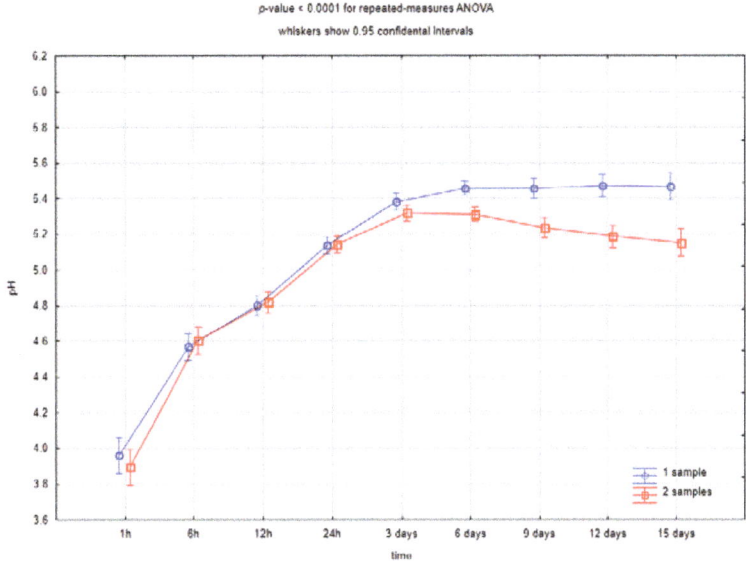

Figure 6. Repeated-measures analysis of variance for pH values in the individual time points depending on the number of the samples for RIVA LC.

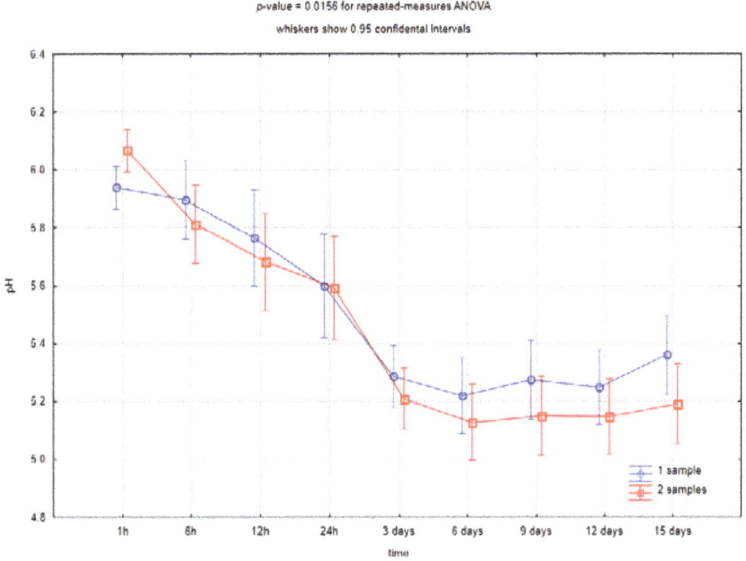

Figure 7. Repeated-measures analysis of variance for pH values in the individual time points depending on the number of the samples for Filtek Bulk Fill.

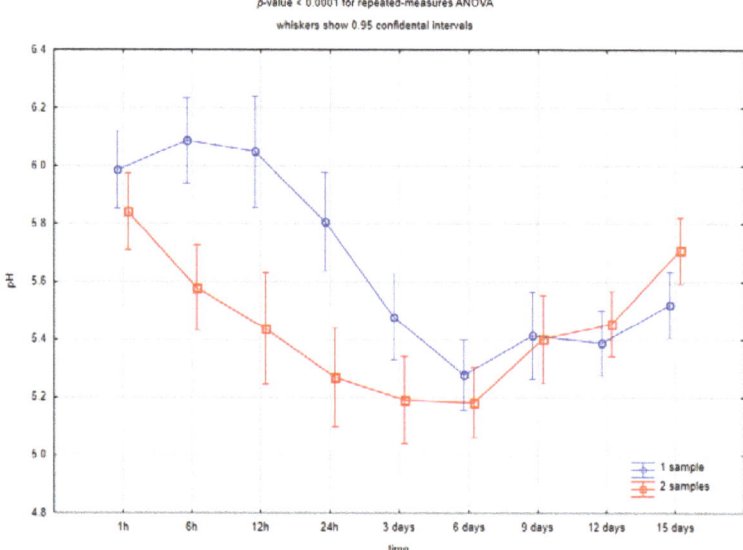

Figure 8. Repeated-measures analysis of variance for pH values in the individual time points depending on the number of the samples for Evetric.

4. Discussion

Unlike many researchers, we have chosen saline as a research medium to create an oral environment [13,18,24]. It should be noted that the use of distilled water, even at human body temperature, does not reflect oral conditions [25]. Several authors have already used saline with interesting findings [26–28]. Researchers also use artificial saliva to determine the pH of dental materials [29,30]. However, its composition is very variable; the search for the best composition is still ongoing [31]. Apart from the eating situation, the oral cavity contains maximally about 1.1 mL of saliva as this amount forces the swallowing reflex [32]. For our analysis, we used 5 mL of saline so that the pH electrode was completely immersed in the solution.

In our study, we found significant differences in the effects of different materials on the environmental pH. After 15 days, all tested materials reached a pH between 5 and 6 on the pH scale. It seems that this fact may have some clinical implications.

It is well known that glass ionomer cements in the initial setting phase are characterised by a low pH that can irritate the pulp [13,15]. Therefore, it was surprising that they finally reached a pH higher than composites. Interestingly, conventional glass ionomers acidified the environment to a lesser extent than those modified with resin during the entire 15-day observation period. It is believed that this is a consequence of the lack of any buffering capacity of composite materials [4,33]. Many researchers indicate this fact as the main cause of secondary caries in materials based on synthetic resin [34,35]. We also observed that a single sample of the GIC lowered the environmental pH less than dual samples. The highest final pH about 5.9 was achieved by Ketac Molar. According to other researchers, it may even reach a pH close to 7 [13]. The first three days of material maturation seem to be crucial, when the pH increase was faster. The pH variation of Riva SC was similar but with a lower amplitude of the pH value at about 0.8 (compared to 1.4). This behaviour can be explained by releasing unreacted acrylic (or another organic acid) and its calcium salt, a weak acid, and conjugate base, which constitute a typical chemical buffer [35]. Some researchers state that it may result from the acid groups being bound to polymer molecules with limited diffusivity [2]. The most acidifying material was Riva LC which had the lowest initial pH of below 4.0 (below the critical point for enamel). In the case of two samples, it was also the most acidic material after 15 days with a pH of about 5.2. It is commonly believed that RMGICs are more composites than glass ionomers [36,37], which was confirmed by the findings of our experiment.

The research methodology on composite materials focuses largely on subjecting them to cyclical changes in pH [38,39]. However, there is no clear answer as to whether these materials are chemically stable at a neutral pH. Despite the daily and routine placement of composite restorations, dentists' knowledge about the composite properties and the main factors of the polymerisation process is not adequate. It can lead to incorrect curing protocol, resulting in the incomplete polymerisation as well as relying on residual monomers and pH changes [40,41]. Moreover, chemical degradation of composite resin results in the release of final products, such as methacrylic acid which could acidify the environment [42,43].

Contrary to other studies [35,44], composite materials used in our research (Filtek Bulk Fill and Evetric) acidified the environment. Despite the initially relatively high pH of about 6, we observed a significant decrease to about 5.3 during the next 3 days of measurements. Around day 6, the pH started to rise slightly, and on day 15, it reached about 5.5. The Evetric composite, containing the Bis-EMA resin, turned out to be less acidifying in our study. Some researchers suggest that Bis-EMA, due to its hydrophobicity and high conversion character, is characterised by lower water sorption and lower solubility [45]. Another theory claims that UDMA composites are less hydrophilic than Bis-GMA-based composites. Also, it is suggested that the main difference between UDMA and Bis-GMA is their flexibility. Therefore, systems containing carboxylic or phosphate groups as functional monomers are more hydrophilic than the resins containing the Bis-GMA/TEGDMA monomer system [41,46]. It is believed that differences in the water absorption of the polymer network can be observed depending on the type of monomer. TEGDMA, Bis-GMA and UDMA seem to be the most hydrophilic [41].

Our study showed that medium-sized fillings are capable of inducing pH changes in the aquatic environment. Interestingly, the acidifying effect was visible in the case of resin-based materials, and two fillings lowered the environmental pH more than one. The literature shows that the lower the cross-linking of the composite, the higher the water absorption. It follows that the polymerisation quality of the composite may affect the pH stability [46]. In clinical practice, the irradiation of a portion of the material is not always optimal—a lower degree of conversion may adversely affect the quality of the filling and its subsequent durability [47]. We are planning further analyses to assess the possibility of changes in acidification by modifying the exposure time of the samples, the distance from the polymerisation lamp, and the diameter of the lamp optical fibre. The soaking of the filling materials in saline would also affect the dimensional, mechanical, and chemical properties. Therefore, it would also be advisable to evaluate the surface roughness of the samples or the release of chemicals such as residual monomers and metal ions.

5. Conclusions

Restorative materials lowered the environmental pH immediately after application, especially light-cured glass ionomer cements. Within two weeks, the pH level for glass ionomers rose to values comparable to composite materials. Moreover, dual samples reached lower pH levels than single samples. Self-cured materials showed larger amplitudes of pH changes than light-cured ones.

Author Contributions: Conceptualisation, A.L.; methodology, A.L. and K.N.; formal analysis, K.N. and A.L.; investigation and resources, A.L., K.N., M.N., P.W. and M.M.; writing—original draft preparation, A.L., K.N., and M.N.; writing—review and editing, K.N., A.L. and A.S.; visualisation, K.N.; supervision, A.S. All authors have read and agreed to the published version of the manuscript.

Funding: This research received no external funding.

Institutional Review Board Statement: Not applicable.

Informed Consent Statement: Not applicable.

Data Availability Statement: Data are available on request from the corresponding author.

Acknowledgments: The project was implemented with the use of funds for science, awarded by the Poznan University of Medical Sciences.

Conflicts of Interest: The authors declare no conflict of interest.

References

1. Cavallari, T.; Arima, L.Y.; Ferrasa, A.; Moysés, S.J.; Moysés, S.T.; Herai, R.H.; Werneck, R.I. Dental Caries: Genetic and Protein Interactions. *Arch. Oral Biol.* **2019**, *108*, 104522. [CrossRef]
2. Nedeljkovic, I.; De Munck, J.; Vanloy, A.; Declerck, D.; Lambrechts, P.; Peumans, M.; Teughels, W.; Van Meerbeek, B.; Van Landuyt, K.L. Secondary Caries: Prevalence, Characteristics, and Approach. *Clin. Oral Investig.* **2020**, *24*, 683–691. [CrossRef]
3. Schwendicke, F.; Lamont, T.; Innes, N. Removing or Controlling? How Caries Management Impacts on the Lifetime of Teeth. *Monogr. Oral Sci.* **2018**, *27*, 32–41. [CrossRef] [PubMed]
4. Fuss, M.; Wicht, M.J.; Attin, T.; Derman, S.H.M.; Noack, M.J. Protective Buffering Capacity of Restorative Dental Materials in vitro. *J. Adhes. Dent.* **2017**, *19*, 177–183. [CrossRef]
5. Mohamed-Tahir, M.A.; Yap, A.U.J. Effects of PH on the Surface Texture of Glass Ionomer Based/Containing Restorative Materials. *Oper. Dent.* **2004**, *29*, 586–591. [PubMed]
6. Xavier, A.M.; Sunny, S.M.; Rai, K.; Hegde, A.M. Repeated Exposure of Acidic Beverages on Esthetic Restorative Materials: An in-vitro Surface Microhardness Study. *J. Clin. Exp. Dent.* **2016**, *8*, e312–e317. [CrossRef]
7. Czarnecka, B.; Limanowska-Shaw, H.; Nicholson, J.W. Buffering and Ion-Release by a Glass-Ionomer Cement under near-Neutral and Acidic Conditions. *Biomaterials* **2002**, *23*, 2783–2788. [CrossRef]
8. Nicholson, J.W.; Aggarwal, A.; Czarnecka, B.; Limanowska-Shaw, H. The Rate of Change of PH of Lactic Acid Exposed to Glass-Ionomer Dental Cements. *Biomaterials* **2000**, *21*, 1989–1993. [CrossRef]
9. Nicholson, J.W.; Czarnecka, B.; Limanowska-Shaw, H. A Preliminary Study of the Effect of Glass-Ionomer and Related Dental Cements on the PH of Lactic Acid Storage Solutions. *Biomaterials* **1999**, *20*, 155–158. [CrossRef]
10. Sahebi, S.; Moazami, F.; Afsa, M.; Zade, M.R.N. Effect of Lengthy Root Canal Therapy Sessions on Temporomandibular Joint and Masticatory Muscles. *J. Dent. Res. Dent. Clin. Dent. Prospect.* **2010**, *4*, 95–97. [CrossRef]
11. Wang, L.; Cefaly, D.F.G.; dos Santos, J.L.; dos Santos, J.R.; Lauris, J.R.P.; Mondelli, R.F.L.; Atta, M.T. In Vitro Interactions between Lactic Acid Solution and Art Glass-Ionomer Cements. *J. Appl. Oral Sci.* **2009**, *17*, 274–279. [CrossRef] [PubMed]
12. Turssi, C.P.; Amaral, F.L.B.; França, F.M.G.; Basting, R.T.; Hara, A.T. Effect of Sucralfate against Hydrochloric Acid-Induced Dental Erosion. *Clin. Oral Investig.* **2019**, *23*, 2365–2370. [CrossRef] [PubMed]
13. Cardoso, A.M.R.; de Sousa Leitão, A.; Neto, J.C.L.; de Almeida, T.L.M.; Lima, D.M.B.; Brandt, L.M.T.; de Castro, R.D.; Cavalcanti, A.L. Evaluation of Fluoride Release, PH and Microhardness of Glass Ionomer Cements. *Pesqui. Bras. Odontopediatria Clín. Integr.* **2015**, *15*, 23–29. [CrossRef]
14. Gupta, N.; Jaiswal, S.; Nikhil, V.; Gupta, S.; Jha, P.; Bansal, P. Comparison of Fluoride Ion Release and Alkalizing Potential of a New Bulk-Fill Alkasite. *J. Conserv. Dent.* **2019**, *22*, 296–299. [CrossRef]
15. Almuhaiza, M. Glass-Ionomer Cements in Restorative Dentistry: A Critical Appraisal. *J. Contemp. Dent. Pract.* **2016**, *17*, 331–336. [CrossRef]
16. Lehmann, A.; Nijakowski, K.; Potempa, N.; Sieradzki, P.; Król, M.; Czyż, O.; Radziszewska, A.; Surdacka, A. Press-On Force Effect on the Efficiency of Composite Restorations Final Polishing—Preliminary In Vitro Study. *Coatings* **2021**, *11*, 705. [CrossRef]
17. Chisnoiu, A.M.; Moldovan, M.; Sarosi, C.; Chisnoiu, R.M.; Rotaru, D.I.; Delean, A.G.; Pastrav, O.; Muntean, A.; Petean, I.; Tudoran, L.B.; et al. Marginal Adaptation Assessment for Two Composite Layering Techniques Using Dye Penetration, AFM, SEM and FTIR: An In-Vitro Comparative Study. *Appl. Sci.* **2021**, *11*, 5657. [CrossRef]
18. Bucur, S.M.; Bud, A.; Gligor, A.; Vlasa, A.; Cocoş, D.I.; Bud, E.S. Observational Study Regarding Two Bonding Systems and the Challenges of Their Use in Orthodontics: An In Vitro Evaluation. *Appl. Sci.* **2021**, *11*, 7091. [CrossRef]
19. Cadenaro, M.; Maravic, T.; Comba, A.; Mazzoni, A.; Fanfoni, L.; Hilton, T.; Ferracane, J.; Breschi, L. The Role of Polymerization in Adhesive Dentistry. *Dent. Mater.* **2019**, *35*, e1–e22. [CrossRef]
20. Frassetto, A.; Breschi, L.; Turco, G.; Marchesi, G.; Di Lenarda, R.; Tay, F.R.; Pashley, D.H.; Cadenaro, M. Mechanisms of Degradation of the Hybrid Layer in Adhesive Dentistry and Therapeutic Agents to Improve Bond Durability—A Literature Review. *Dent. Mater.* **2016**, *32*, e41–e53. [CrossRef]
21. Breschi, L.; Maravic, T.; Cunha, S.R.; Comba, A.; Cadenaro, M.; Tjäderhane, L.; Pashley, D.H.; Tay, F.R.; Mazzoni, A. Dentin Bonding Systems: From Dentin Collagen Structure to Bond Preservation and Clinical Applications. *Dent. Mater.* **2018**, *34*, 78–96. [CrossRef]
22. Kasraei, S.; Haghi, S.; Valizadeh, S.; Panahandeh, N.; Nejadkarimi, S. Phosphate Ion Release and Alkalizing Potential of Three Bioactive Dental Materials in Comparison with Composite Resin. *Int. J. Dent.* **2021**, *2021*, e5572569. [CrossRef]
23. Kaga, N.; Nagano-Takebe, F.; Nezu, T.; Matsuura, T.; Endo, K.; Kaga, M. Protective Effects of GIC and S-PRG Filler Restoratives on Demineralization of Bovine Enamel in Lactic Acid Solution. *Materials* **2020**, *13*, 2140. [CrossRef] [PubMed]
24. Ben-Amar, A.; Liberman, R.; Apatowsky, U.; Pilo, R. PH Changes of Glass-Ionomer Lining Materials at Various Time Intervals. *J. Oral Rehabil.* **1999**, *26*, 847–852. [CrossRef] [PubMed]

25. Herman, K.; Wujczyk, M.; Dobrzynski, M.; Diakowska, D.; Wiglusz, K.; Wiglusz, R.J. In Vitro Assessment of Long-Term Fluoride Ion Release from Nanofluorapatite. *Materials* **2021**, *14*, 3747. [CrossRef] [PubMed]
26. Lucchetti, M.C.; Fratto, G.; Valeriani, F.; De Vittori, E.; Giampaoli, S.; Papetti, P.; Spica, V.R.; Manzon, L. Cobalt-Chromium Alloys in Dentistry: An Evaluation of Metal Ion Release. *J. Prosthet. Dent.* **2015**, *114*, 602–608. [CrossRef] [PubMed]
27. Briddell, J.W.; Riexinger, L.E.; Graham, J.; Ebenstein, D.M. Comparison of Artificial Saliva vs. Saline Solution on Rate of Suture Degradation in Oropharyngeal Surgery. *JAMA Otolaryngol.—Head Neck Surg.* **2018**, *144*, 824–830. [CrossRef]
28. Jayaprakash, K.; Shetty, K.H.K.; Shetty, A.N.; Nandish, B.T. Effect of Recasting on Element Release from Base Metal Dental Casting Alloys in Artificial Saliva and Saline Solution. *J. Conserv. Dent.* **2017**, *20*, 199–203. [CrossRef]
29. Viana, Í.; Alania, Y.; Feitosa, S.; Borges, A.B.; Braga, R.R.; Scaramucci, T. Bioactive Materials Subjected to Erosion/Abrasion and Their Influence on Dental Tissues. *Oper. Dent.* **2020**, *45*, E114–E123. [CrossRef]
30. Akay, C.; Tanış, M.Ç.; Sevim, H. Effect of Artificial Saliva with Different PH Levels on the Cytotoxicity of Soft Denture Lining Materials. *Int. J. Artif. Organs* **2017**, *40*, 581–588. [CrossRef] [PubMed]
31. Łysik, D.; Niemirowicz-Laskowska, K.; Bucki, R.; Tokajuk, G.; Mystkowska, J. Artificial Saliva: Challenges and Future Perspectives for the Treatment of Xerostomia. *Int. J. Mol. Sci.* **2019**, *20*, 3199. [CrossRef] [PubMed]
32. Iorgulescu, G. Saliva between Normal and Pathological. Important Factors in Determining Systemic and Oral Health. *J. Med. Life* **2009**, *2*, 303–307. [PubMed]
33. Odermatt, R.; Par, M.; Mohn, D.; Wiedemeier, D.B.; Attin, T.; Tauböck, T.T. Bioactivity and Physico-Chemical Properties of Dental Composites Functionalized with Nano- vs. Micro-Sized Bioactive Glass. *J. Clin. Med.* **2020**, *9*, 772. [CrossRef] [PubMed]
34. Thomas, R.Z.; van der Mei, H.C.; van der Veen, M.H.; de Soet, J.J.; Huysmans, M.C.D.N.J.M. Bacterial Composition and Red Fluorescence of Plaque in Relation to Primary and Secondary Caries next to Composite: An in Situ Study. *Oral Microbiol. Immunol.* **2008**, *23*, 7–13. [CrossRef] [PubMed]
35. Nedeljkovic, I.; De Munck, J.; Slomka, V.; Van Meerbeek, B.; Teughels, W.; Van Landuyt, K.L. Lack of Buffering by Composites Promotes Shift to More Cariogenic Bacteria. *J. Dent. Res.* **2016**, *95*, 875–881. [CrossRef] [PubMed]
36. Boing, T.F.; de Geus, J.L.; Wambier, L.M.; Loguercio, A.D.; Reis, A.; Gomes, O.M.M. Are Glass-Ionomer Cement Restorations in Cervical Lesions More Long-Lasting than Resin-Based Composite Resins? A Systematic Review and Meta-Analysis. *J. Adhes. Dent.* **2018**, *20*, 435–452. [CrossRef]
37. Hussainy, S.N.; Nasim, I.; Thomas, T.; Ranjan, M. Clinical Performance of Resin-Modified Glass Ionomer Cement, Flowable Composite, and Polyacid-Modified Resin Composite in Noncarious Cervical Lesions: One-Year Follow-Up. *J. Conserv. Dent.* **2018**, *21*, 510–515. [CrossRef]
38. Somacal, D.C.; Manfroi, F.B.; Monteiro, M.; Oliveira, S.D.; Bittencourt, H.R.; Borges, G.A.; Spohr, A.M. Effect of PH Cycling Followed by Simulated Toothbrushing on the Surface Roughness and Bacterial Adhesion of Bulk-Fill Composite Resins. *Oper. Dent.* **2020**, *45*, 209–218. [CrossRef]
39. Moon, J.-D.; Seon, E.-M.; Son, S.-A.; Jung, K.-H.; Kwon, Y.-H.; Park, J.-K. Effect of Immersion into Solutions at Various PH on the Color Stability of Composite Resins with Different Shades. *Restor. Dent. Endod.* **2015**, *40*, 270–276. [CrossRef]
40. Dikova, T.; Maximov, J.; Todorov, V.; Georgiev, G.; Panov, V. Optimization of Photopolymerization Process of Dental Composites. *Processes* **2021**, *9*, 779. [CrossRef]
41. Bociong, K.; Szczesio, A.; Sokolowski, K.; Domarecka, M.; Sokolowski, J.; Krasowski, M.; Lukomska-Szymanska, M. The Influence of Water Sorption of Dental Light-Cured Composites on Shrinkage Stress. *Materials* **2017**, *10*, 1142. [CrossRef] [PubMed]
42. Szczesio-Wlodarczyk, A.; Sokolowski, J.; Kleczewska, J.; Bociong, K. Ageing of Dental Composites Based on Methacrylate Resins—A Critical Review of the Causes and Method of Assessment. *Polymers* **2020**, *12*, 882. [CrossRef]
43. Yap, A.U.; Lee, H.K.; Sabapathy, R. Release of Methacrylic Acid from Dental Composites. *Dent. Mater.* **2000**, *16*, 172–179. [CrossRef]
44. Degradation of Glass Filler in Experimental Composites—PubMed. Available online: https://pubmed.ncbi.nlm.nih.gov/6457066/ (accessed on 12 November 2021).
45. Prado, V.; Santos, K.; Fontenele, R.; Soares, J.; Vale, G. Effect of over the Counter Mouthwashes with and without Alcohol on Sorption and Solubility of Bulk Fill Resins. *J. Clin. Exp. Dent.* **2020**, *12*, e1150–e1156. [CrossRef] [PubMed]
46. Craciun, A.; Prodan, D.; Constantiniuc, M.; Ispas, A.; Filip, M.; Moldovan, M.; Badea, M.; Ioan, P.; Crişan, M. Stability of Dental Composites in Water and Artificial Saliva. *Mater. Plast.* **2019**, *57*, 57–66. [CrossRef]
47. Palin, W.M.; Fleming, G.J.P.; Burke, F.J.T.; Marquis, P.M.; Randall, R.C. The Influence of Short and Medium-Term Water Immersion on the Hydrolytic Stability of Novel Low-Shrink Dental Composites. *Dent. Mater.* **2005**, *21*, 852–863. [CrossRef] [PubMed]

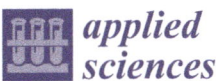

Article

SEM and FT-MIR Analysis of Human Demineralized Dentin Matrix: An In Vitro Study

Lucia Memè [1,*], Enrico M. Strappa [2], Riccardo Monterubbianesi [1], Fabrizio Bambini [1] and Stefano Mummolo [3]

[1] Department of Clinical Sciences and Stomatology, Polytechnic University of Marche, 60126 Ancona, Italy; r.monterubbianesi@pm.univpm.it (R.M.); f.bambini@staff.univpm.it (F.B.)
[2] IRCCS Istituto Ortopedico Galeazzi, University of Milan, 20161 Milan, Italy; estrappa@yahoo.it
[3] Department of Life, Health and Environmental Sciences, University of L'Aquila, 67100 L'Aquila, Italy; stefano.mummolo@univaq.it
* Correspondence: l.meme@staff.univpm.it

Abstract: Recently, the demineralized dentin matrix has been suggested as an alternative material to autologous bone grafts and xenografts for clinical purposes. The aim of this study was to investigate the effect of different times of demineralization on the chemical composition and the surface morphology of dentinal particles. Extracted teeth were ground and divided into 5 groups based on demineralization time (T0 = 0 min, T2 = 2 min, T5 = 5 min, T10 = 10 min, and T60 = 60 min) with 12% EDTA. The analysis was performed using Fourier-Transform Mid-Infrared spectroscopy (FT-MIR) and Scanning Electron Microscopy (SEM) ($p < 0.05$). The FT-MIR analysis showed a progressive reduction of the concentration of both PO_4^{3-} and CO_3^{2-} in the specimens (T0 > T2 > T5 > T10 > T60). On the contrary, the organic (protein) component did not undergo any change. The SEM examination showed that increasing the times of demineralization resulted in a smoother surface of the dentin particles and a higher number of dentinal tubules.

Keywords: demineralized dentin matrix; human demineralized dentin matrix; human; bone graft; FT-MIR; SEM

1. Introduction

After tooth extraction, hard and soft tissue withstand remodeling processes. Alveolar ridge undergoes resorption, mostly in the horizontal but also in the vertical dimension [1]. Several studies analyzed the changes after tooth extraction [2]. The majority of horizontal and vertical changes take place during the first 3–6 months after tooth extraction and continue through the first year [3]. In fact, the horizontal bone loss is higher on the buccal side of the alveolar ridge than on the lingual/palatal side. On the other hand, the vertical resorption is minor and mainly on the buccal aspect of the alveolar ridge. This volumetric contraction of the alveolar ridge may jeopardize an appropriate implant-supported prosthetic rehabilitation.

Several surgical techniques have been developed to reduce or, at least, minimize the changes of soft and hard tissue following tooth loss. The main alveolar ridge preservation techniques concern on soft-tissue preservation, hard-tissue preservation (guided bone regeneration) and the combination of soft tissue and hard tissue preservation (socket seal technique) [4]. Moreover, different regenerative techniques have been tested: the use of bone grafts alone; barrier membranes alone, either resorbable or not; the combination of barrier membranes and bone graft. Metanalyses have shown that alveolar ridge preservation techniques are effective in significantly reducing vertical and horizontal alveolar ridge contraction [5,6]. Also Troiano et al. [7] reported positive results in the use of bone grafting and resorbable membrane compared with spontaneous healing. Autologous bone represents the ideal graft material due to its osteoinductive and osteoconductive properties [8]. Nevertheless, its limits are the small amount of bone graft available, the morbidity

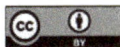

of the donor area, and the risk of resorption of the bone graft itself. The research has led to developing alternatives, such as allogenic grafts, alloplastic grafts, and xenogenic grafts [9].

In the past decades, the use of demineralized dentin matrix (DDM) as a potential bone substitute has been proposed. Dentin consists of (i) 70% inorganic component (hydroxyapatite, tricalcium phosphate, octacalcium phosphate, and amorphous calcium phosphate); (ii) 20% organic component (collagen I 90%, collagen III and V in small quantities, and non-collagenic proteins); (iii) 10% water [10]. Its composition is, therefore, similar to that of bone tissue. Dentin also contains various growth factors, such as Fibroblast Growth Factors -2 (FGF-2), transforming growth factors-β1 (TGF-β1), insulin growth factor-1 (IGF-1) and, above all, bone morphogenetic proteins (BMPs) involved in the osteogenesis process [10].

Through demineralization, dentin can release the growth factors [11] and consequently express its osteoinductive and osteoconductive properties [12]. Thereby acting as a scaffold, dentin promotes the formation of bone tissue (osteoconduction), but at the same time, it releases the growth factors that promote the formation of bone (osteoinduction). Moreover, different in vivo studies have reported encouraging results [13–15] that led to this material being considered as a possible alternative to autologous bone grafts [16].

It has been shown that the preparation procedure, the shape, and the size of the dentin particles can influence dentin's osteoconductive and osteoinductive properties [17]. Excessive demineralization can damage the structure of the dentin and negatively affect the composition and function of growth factors; on the other hand, a reduced demineralization produces a scaffold with osteoconductive and osteoinductive properties [18].

The aims of this study were: (i) to examine the changes in the chemical composition of dentin particles using Fourier-transform mid-infrared spectroscopy (FT-MIR) analysis after different exposure times to demineralizing agent; (ii) to evaluate the surface morphology of the dentin particles by Scanning Electron Microscopy (SEM) analysis after different exposure times to demineralizing agent.

2. Materials and Methods

2.1. Experimental Design and Specimen Preparation

For this study, we used extracted teeth with unfavorable prognoses with the consent of patients. The criteria for exclusion were: (i) teeth with carious lesions; (ii) teeth with root canal treatment. After extraction of the specimens, the enamel and root cementum were removed with a dental drill (Figure 1a). Next, each tooth was washed with physiological solution, rinsed with an air-spray tool, and stored at $-20\,^\circ$C. The teeth were placed in a sterile container (Figure 1b) and ground using a Smart Dentin Grinder (KometaBio Inc., Cresskill, NJ, USA) for 3 s (Figure 1c). Then, the dentinal powder was sieved to distinguish two specimens with different grain sizes: the first with granules of smaller sizes (<300 μm) (A); and the second with granules of sizes between 300 μm and 1200 μm (B). The specimens were collected in sterile containers (Figure 1d,e). In this study, we used only the second specimen (B), while the first was excluded (specimen A).

Following the instructions of the machine producer, the dentinal powder was immersed in basic alcohol for 10 min in a sterile glass container. The basic alcohol was composed of 0.5 M NaOH and 20% ethanol. Next, the dentinal powder was picked up and washed two times with sterile phosphate-buffered saline solution (3 min for each wash) (Figure 1f). The dentinal powder was washed with a physiological solution and rinsed as much as possible.

The dentinal powder was randomly divided into five groups (0.075 g of dentin each) based on the time of demineralization (Table 1): T2, 2 min; T5, 5 min; T10, 10 min; T60, 60 min. T0 was not-demineralized and was considered as the control group.

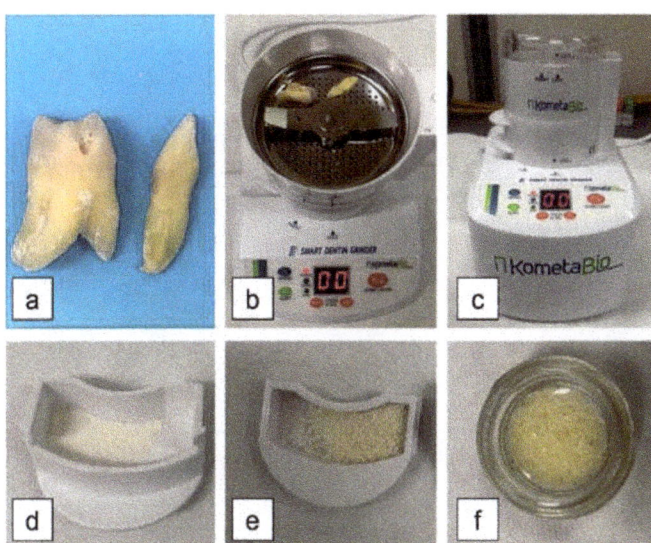

Figure 1. Specimen preparation: (**a**) Example of the final specimens after enamel and cementum removal with a dental drill; (**b**) specimens in the sterile trituration chamber; (**c**) detail of Smart Dentin Grinder machine (KometaBio Inc., Cresskill, NJ, USA); (**d**) ground dentin with particle size less than 300 µm; (**e**) ground dentin with particle size between 300 µm and 1200 µm; (**f**) dentin particulate immersed in a sterile container with sterile saline solution.

Table 1. Group nomenclature based on demineralization process.

Nomenclature	Demineralization Process
T0	not-demineralized
T2	2 min in 12% EDTA dentin particles
T5	5 min in 12% EDTA dentin particles
T10	10 min in 12% EDTA dentin particles
T60	60 min in 12% EDTA dentin particles

12 %EDTA was used to demineralize the dentin. Specifically, 1.7 g EDTA disodium salt was dissolved in 10mL distilled water at 25 °C. A saturated solution was obtained, from which only the supernatant was taken. Through this process, we obtained EDTA at 12%. The choice of this concentration was made according to previous articles published in the literature [12,17]. An amount of 1.1 mL EDTA was applied for the established time using a specific tool (Vortex). Once the process was completed, EDTA was removed, and the specimens were stored at −20 °C. Each specimen was washed two times with a physiologic solution (400 µL) to stop the demineralizing process. Next, the physiologic solution was aspirated.

The water had to be removed from the specimens to allow the spectrophotometry analysis. This process was completed by putting the specimens in a centrifuge (SpeedVac Concentrator, Savant SPD111V) (Figure 2a) for 30 min. The specimens were also weighed at different times: (i) ground and centrifuged dentin, before the demineralization process (D1); (ii) ground and demineralized dentin (D2); (iii) ground and centrifuged dentin after demineralization process (D3).

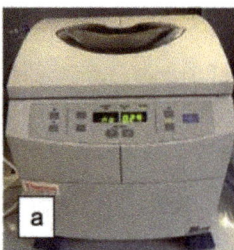
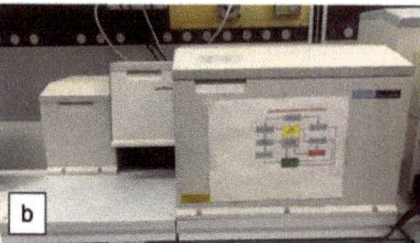
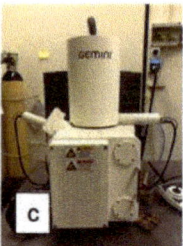

Figure 2. Instruments used in this study. (**a**) SpeedVac Concentrator, Savant SPD111V was used for the elimination of residual water; (**b**) FT-IR Perkin Elmer Spectrum One. Acquisition range 4000–450 cm^{-1}; (**c**) scanning electron microscope (Supra 40, Zeiss).

2.2. FT-MIR Analysis

FT-MIR analysis was carried out using the FT-IR Perkin Elmer Spectrum One (Figure 2b) (Department of Life and Environmental Sciences, Polytechnic University of Marche, Ancona, Italy). The analysis of all specimens was performed in reflection UATR mode (Attenuate Total Reflection) with a range between 4000–600 cm^{-1} (spectral resolution 4 cm^{-1}, 16 scans). The bands used for this study were: band 1021 cm^{-1}, which indicated the percentage of PO_4^{3-}; band 1649 cm^{-1}, which corresponded to the protein component and was performed to determine the percentage of mineralization of each specimen; and band 872 cm^{-1}, which reflected the CO_3^{2-} percentage.

2.3. SEM Analysis

The specimens were gold-coated and analyzed through SEM (Department of Materials, Environmental Science and Urban Planning, Polytechnic University of Marche, Ancona, Italy). The superficial morphology of each specimen was evaluated through detector SE2 (Figure 2c) at different magnifications: (i) 400×; (ii) 2000×; (iii) 8000×.

2.4. Statistical Analysis

Statistical analysis of data included analysis of variance (ANOVA) and Tukey's test ($p < 0.05$).

3. Results

3.1. Weight Analysis of the Specimens

Table 2 shows the average weight of D1, D2 and D3.

Table 2. The weights of the specimens (expressed in g) in D1 (triturated and centrifuged dentin), D2 (triturated and demineralized dentin), and D3 (triturated, demineralized, and centrifuged dentin).

Specimen	T2	T5	T10	T60
D1	0.075 g	0.075 g	0.075 g	0.075 g
D2	0.093 g	0.081 g	0.051 g	0.024 g
D3	0.061 g	0.057 g	0.034 g	0.014 g

3.2. FT-MIR

MIR spectra were acquired for each specimen in the 4000–600 cm^{-1} spectral range, and NIR in the 10000–4000 cm^{-1} range. The main MIR absorption bands considered in this study are shown in Figure 3, which shows the spectrum of the dentin not subjected to demineralization (T0). Based on previous studies [19–21], the main absorption bands analyzed in this study were: (i) ~1649 cm^{-1} band corresponding to the protein component of dentin (band A); (ii) ~1021 cm^{-1} band corresponding to the phosphate ion PO_4^{3-} (band B); (iii) ~872 cm^{-1} band corresponding to the stretching of the carbonate CO_3^{2-} (band C).

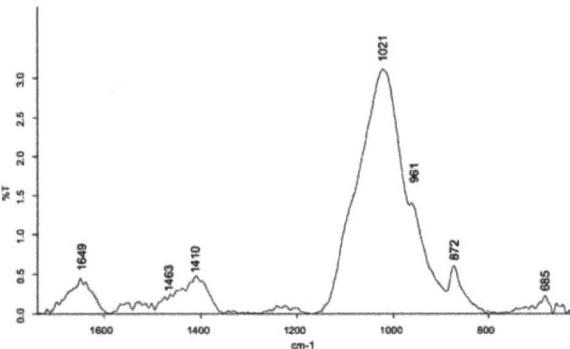

Figure 3. Spectrum acquired through FT-MIR analysis of dentin particles not subjected to demineralization with 12% EDTA.

The variations in the MIR spectral profiles of the analyzed specimens (T0, T2, T5, T10, T60) were acquired in the spectral range 4000–600 cm^{-1}. Then, the spectra were normalized compared to the 1649 cm^{-1} band, which corresponded to the protein component of dentin, and which remained constant even after the demineralization treatment. Through this procedure, it was possible to observe the trends of the PO_4^{3-} and CO_3^{2-} groups (Figure 4).

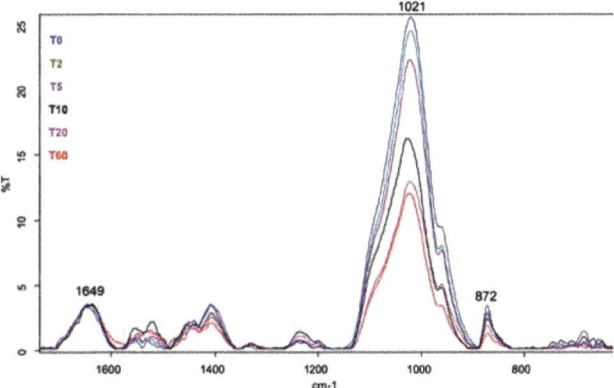

Figure 4. Spectra of the analyzed specimens normalized at the level of the 1649 cm^{-1} band, which corresponded to the protein component of dentin. Reductions were observed in the band at 1021 cm^{-1}, which resembled the phosphate group, and at 872 cm^{-1}, which corresponded to the carbonate group.

The concentrations of the inorganic components of dentin (PO_4^{3-} and CO_3^{2-} groups) decreased with increasing exposure time to the demineralizing agent. The amount of the mineralized component of the dentin was greater in T0, followed by T2, T5, T10. The T60 specimens were subject to the longest time of demineralization and showed the least amount of mineralized component.

The ratio between band B (1021 cm^{-1}), which described the percentage of PO_4^{3-}, and band A (1649 cm^{-1}), which corresponded to the protein component, was measured to determine the percentage of mineralization of each specimen (Figure 5a). Band C (872 cm^{-1}), which reflected the CO_3^{2-} percentage, was also compared with band A (1649 cm^{-1}), which corresponded to the protein component (Figure 5b).

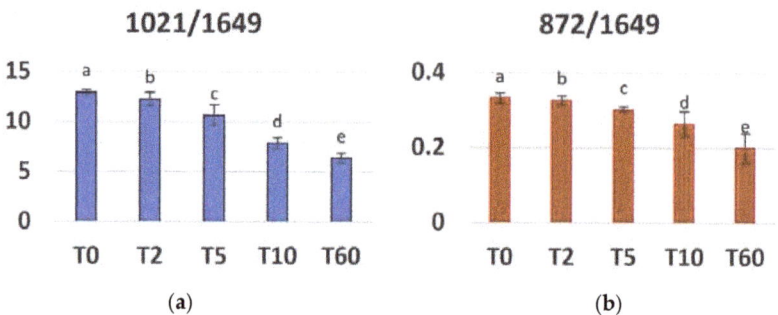

Figure 5. FT-MIR Analysis. (**a**) The ratio between band B (1021 cm^{-1}), which corresponded to the PO_4^{3-} group, and band A (1649 cm^{-1}), which reflected the protein component; (**b**) the ratio between band C (872 cm^{-1}), which represented the CO_3^{2-} group, and band A (1649 cm^{-1}), which corresponded to the protein component. Different letters represent statistically significant differences ($p < 0.05$).

At T0, dentin was not treated with 12% EDTA, so it was considered as the control group, assuming 100% mineralization. Next, we calculated the quantity of PO_4^{3-} and CO_3^{2-} as a percentage of each specimen (Figure 6).

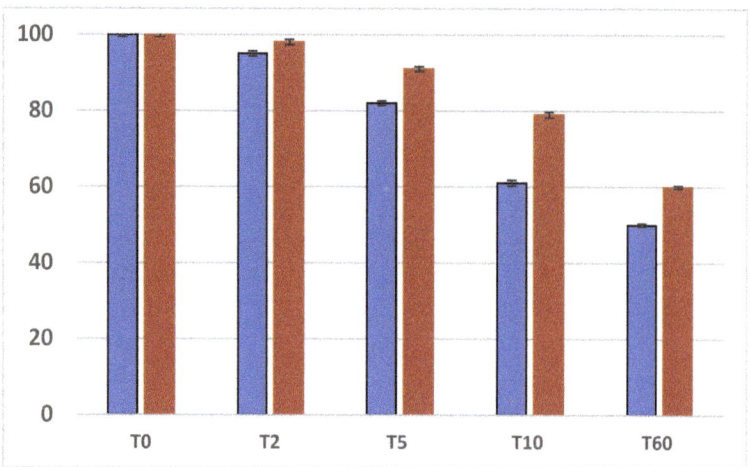

Figure 6. The graph represents the percentage of mineralization of the analyzed specimens after different exposure times. The blue expresses the quantity (%) of the PO_4^{3-} group; the orange describes the quantity (%) of the CO_3^{2-} group.

3.3. SEM

Finally, in this study, an SEM morphological evaluation of the specimens was performed (Figure 7). For each specimen, the obtained microanalysis was derived from the average of the results obtained on the most representative area. The voltage used was 25 kW, while the focal length was 15 mm.

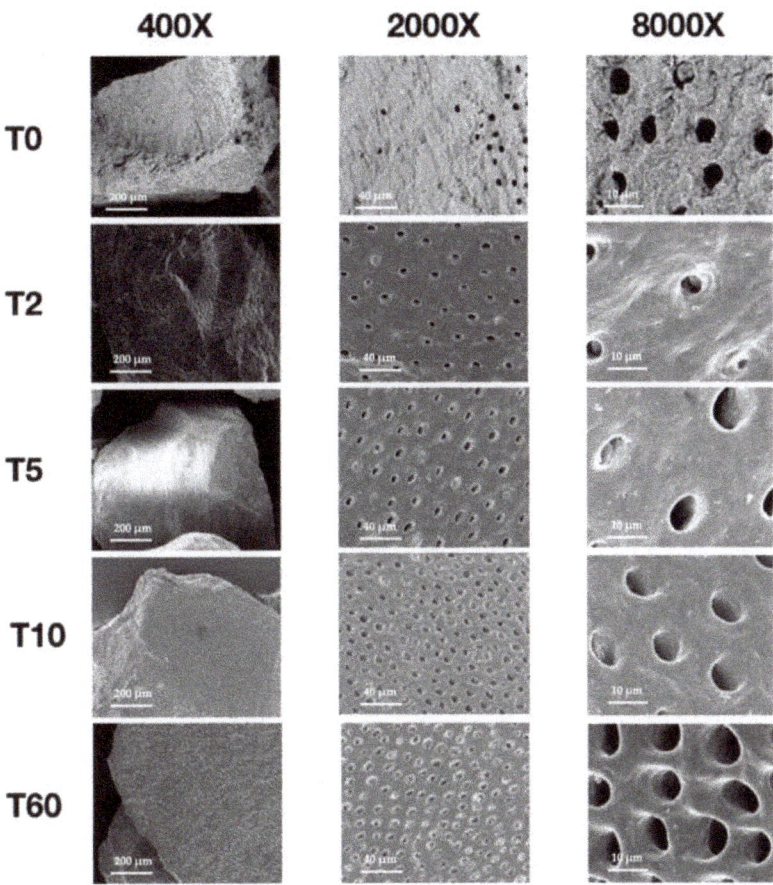

Figure 7. The acquired SEM images of the specimens T0, T2, T5, T10, T60 at different magnifications: 400×, 2000×, and 8000×.

The images were acquired at different magnifications (400×, 2000×, and 8000×). This analysis allowed us to investigate the form and number of dentinal tubules exposed on the surface of the specimen. At 2000× magnification, it was seen that the number of the dentinal tubules in the same surface area increased T0 < T2 < T5 < T10 < T60.

Comparing the image at 8000× magnification of T0 with the one of T60, we observed a difference at the surface of the specimens. In the T0 specimens, the surface of the dentin was rough and non-homogeneous, while the dentin surface of the T60 specimen was smoother and more homogeneous. According to these results, it was assumed that the surface roughness tended to decrease with longer exposure to the demineralizing agent.

4. Discussion

An ideal bone graft should be biocompatible, biomechanically stable, capable of degrading over a certain time, and exhibit osteoconductive, osteogenic, and osteoconductive properties [22]. Although the gold standard is exemplified by autologous bone, the limited amount of bone available, the morbidity of the donor site, and the high rate of resorption affect its use. Therefore, alternative materials for autologous bone grafts are required.

In recent years, it has been proposed that DDM be used as a potential bone graft. In Japan and Korea, this type of graft is widely used, as demonstrated by the number of scientific works published in the literature by scientific authors [23]. It has been shown that the preparation process, the size, and shape of the dentin particles seem to influence their osteoinductive and osteoconductive properties [17].

In summary, the concentration of the phosphate group (inorganic component of dentin, corresponding to the spectral peak at 1021 cm^{-1}) and the carbonate group (inorganic component of dentin, corresponding to the spectral peak at 872 cm^{-1}) decreased with increasing time of demineralization (T0 > T2 > T5 > T10 > T60). In addition, with increasing demineralization time, the number of exposed dentinal tubules in the same surface area increased, and the particles become more homogeneous and smoother.

In the present study, the enamel and the cementum were removed from the extracted teeth. In fact, the hydroxyapatite in the enamel is structured as highly crystalline calcium phosphate, while the dentin contains hydroxyapatite in low crystalline calcium phosphate form. In the first case, the high crystalline content is not easy to decompose by osteoclasts. Consequently, the resorption rate is slow, and the material's osteoconductivity is reduced. On the contrary, hydroxyapatite in dentin has a low crystalline structure, and this makes its resorption easier [11]. Bone tissues also contain low crystalline apatite. Recently, Elfana et al. [24] performed a randomized clinical trial comparing autologous whole tooth grafts and the autologous demineralized dentin grafts. The histological results showed a higher amount of newly formed bone and a smaller number of remnant grafts in the autologous demineralized dentin grafts group. The authors hypothesized that in the autologous demineralized dentin grafts group, the lower mineral content made particle degradation faster than that in the autologous whole tooth grafts group, and this allowed the release of growth factors earlier.

Regarding the size of the particles, a clear consensus has not yet been reached on which precise size is most suitable for bone grafts. Shapoff et al. [25] stated that the particle size of bone grafts should be between 100 μm and 300 μm. Nam et al. [26] conducted an in vivo study testing the new bone formation capabilities of DDM grafts with different densities and particle sizes. The histomorphometric analysis demonstrated the superiority of the specimens with grafting particles sized between 250 μm and 1000 μm and spaces of 200 μm between the particles compared to the results obtained with grafts with larger particles (1000–2000 μm). Koga et al. [12] reported better results in terms of new bone formation with particle sizes between 1200 μm and 800 μm compared to those obtained with smaller particle sizes. The authors also observed that the smaller particles underwent faster resorption than the larger ones. Therefore, it was suggested that the larger-sized particles (1200–800 μm) offer a greater surface area than those of smaller sizes (180–212 μm and 425–600 μm) for the adhesion of osteoprogenitor cells and osteoblasts. In addition, the adhesion of these cells could prevent the absorption of DDM particles and start the formation of new bone. For these reasons, in our study, demineralized dentin particles ranging in size from 300 μm to 1200 μm were used, excluding the smaller-sized particles (<300 μm).

Many studies have reported different tooth processing methods. Generally, there are four main categories [17]: (i) extraction of non-collagenic proteins from dentin; (ii) demineralization; (iii) elimination of the organic matrix (denaturation); (iv) use of tooth particles without modification. Denaturation is a little-used method because it eliminates the proteins in the matrix, including the growth factors responsible for the osteoinductive capacity of the dentin itself. Currently, the most used protocol is demineralization, as demonstrated by a large number of studies in the literature. The most used demineralizing agents are: (i) EDTA [17,24,27]; (ii) HNO$_3$ [12,27]; and (iii) HCl [28–30].

Demineralization does not affect the organic component of the dentin or damage the growth factors contained therein. This process increases the osteoinductivity of the dentin particles, since it promotes the release of growth factors [11], favors the adhesion of osteoblasts through the exposure of collagen fibers [12], and reduces dentin's antigenicity. Demineralization is necessary because crystalline hydroxyapatite inhibits the release of growth factors, such as BMPs [11]. It has been observed that the amount of time during which a demineralizing agent acts influences the characteristics of dentin. An excessive demineralization can damage the dentin structure and adversely affect the composition and function of odontogenic factors. On the other hand, a mild demineralization produces a scaffold with poor osteoinductive capabilities [18].

Tanoue et al. [27] performed an FIB/SEM analysis of the demineralized (HNO_3 2%) dentin matrix grafted in a rat calvaria bone defect model. This method allowed the 3D reconstruction of the interface between the implanted dentin particles and the surrounding bone. The diameters of the exposed dental tubules averaged 3 μm. Mesenchymal cells, such as osteoblasts and bone tissue cells, are between 10–20 μm in size, while osteoclasts are 20–100 μm. The results of this study showed that osteocytes surrounded the grafted dentin particles, forming a network on their surfaces. In addition, cytoplasmatic extensions of osteocytes were observed in the dentinal tubules contained within the dentin particles. The authors also hypothesized a possible biological sequence of events that occurs when demineralized dentin particles are grafted into the recipient site. The release of BMPs induces mesenchymal cells to differentiate into osteoblasts, as also shown by the immunohistochemical analysis of de Oliviera et al. [31]. These cells produce a matrix that undergoes mineralization and forms new bone. At this point, the osteoblasts differentiate into osteocytes, which adhere to the surface of the demineralized dentin particles, forming a network on their surface. Cytoplasmatic extensions from the network spread into the dentinal tubules contained within the dentin particles. Afterward, the dentin particles will be reabsorbed and replaced by new bone, as confirmed by Kim et al. [13].

BMPs belong to the large family of TGF-β. Urist [32] was the first to describe their biological activity. In the following years, considerable efforts were made to isolate these growth factors and study both their in vitro and in vivo features. The BMPs promote the differentiation of mesenchymal cells into osteoblasts and chondroblasts [33], participating in the development of bone and cartilage [34], rather than the formation of dental hard tissues [35]. Bessho et al. [36,37] showed that BMPs obtained from demineralized dentin have osteoinductive properties similar to those derived from bone tissue. The BMPs induced new bone formation through endochondral (indirect) and intramembranous (direct) ossification, as shown by the histological findings of Murata et al. [30].

In our study, the dentin particles underwent a demineralization process with 12% EDTA. This agent is widely used in endodontics as a chelating agent for the enlargement of the canals and the removal of the smear layer. The longer the EDTA works on dentin, the more evident its effects are on dentin, as demonstrated by the release of phosphorus [38]. The specimens in our study were divided based on the exposure time of EDTA (0 min; 2 min; 5 min; 10 min; 60 min). The effect of the demineralizing agent was demonstrated by the analysis of the weight of the specimens, the FT-MIR analysis, and also SEM.

The weight of each specimen was lower after the demineralization process. One of the most used methods to confirm demineralization is SEM [18]. The results of our SEM analysis showed that the longer the EDTA was allowed to work, the less rough, or smoother, the surfaces of the particles became. Furthermore, it was observed that the longer the duration of demineralization, the greater the number of dentinal tubules exposed on the same surface area of the particles.

Koga et al. [12] conducted an in vivo study comparing non-demineralized, partially demineralized, and completely demineralized dentin specimens. Similarly to our study, the SEM analysis showed that the surfaces of the demineralized dentin specimens were smoother while those of the non-demineralized dentin were rougher. Interestingly, the osteoblasts adhered only to the surfaces of demineralized dentin but not to those of non-demineralized dentin. The authors hypothesized that the exposure of collagen fibers following demineralization could promote the adhesion of osteoblasts. The specimens of partially and completely demineralized dentin matrix, above all, showed greater osteogenic power than the non-demineralized ones.

Similar SEM results were achieved by Tabatabei et al. [18] performed a SEM analysis of dentin particles, reaching results similar to those of our study. The specimens of demineralized dentin showed greater exposure of the dentinal tubules and smoother surfaces compared to the non-demineralized specimens. Furthermore, the surfaces of the demineralized dentin particles demonstrated better suitability for cell proliferation (human dental pulp stem cells) than the surfaces of the non-demineralized particles. The authors also reported that the surfaces of the demineralized dentin particles were less biocompatible than those of the deproteinized dentin particles. It was suggested that these results were due to the demineralization process, during which a certain amount of the proteins may have been denatured. The authors also assumed that if the release of proteins following the demineralization process exceeds a certain threshold, it could be unfavorable, resulting in lethality for the cells.

The FT-MIR analysis was performed to investigate the functional groups on the surfaces of dentin particles [18]. This analysis offered information regarding the degree of demineralization for each specimen. The results of our study showed that the inorganic mineral component (CO_3^{2-} and PO_4^{3-}) content decreased with increasing duration of exposure to 12% EDTA. In contrast, the protein component remained unchanged. The reference spectra values were considered on the basis of findings from previous investigations [19–21].

Clearly, demineralization is effective but within a certain range. If the dentin is poorly demineralized, it results in a poorly osteoinductive scaffold. Nevertheless, if the demineralization is excessive, the substrate becomes ineffective. Therefore, an appropriate balance must be achieved. The demineralized dentine particles have a porous structure due to the presence of the dentinal tubules. This means that the dentin particles may act as an osteoconductive scaffold, which allows cells proliferation. Literature on the effects of different demineralization agent exposure times on the biological properties of dentin particles is limited. In fact, most of the studies compare specimens of demineralized dentin, non-demineralized dentin, and deproteinized dentin. To the best of our knowledge, there are no in vitro or in vivo studies regarding the effect of different durations of demineralization on dentine particles. Although the present study has some limitations, as the limited demineralized substances used and the possibility of inaccurate removal of enamel and cementum from the specimens, it can be considered a pilot study for future in vivo studies to find the best degree of demineralization that can be used as a graft material for bone regeneration.

It seems that the use of DDM offers several advantages. Both dentin and alveolar bone tissue derive from the neural crest and also share similarities in composition. Dentin consists of (i) 70% inorganic components (hydroxyapatite, tricalcium phosphate, octacalcium phosphate, and amorphous calcium phosphate); (ii) 20% organic components (mainly collagen I; collagen III and V in small quantities; non-collagenic proteins); and (iii) 10% water [10]. Non-collagenous proteins of dentin are known to be involved in bone calcification [39]. Dentin has shown not only osteoconductive but also osteoinductive properties [11,13]. Clearly, DDM can be considered an autologous graft since it is obtained from the extracted tooth of the same patient. Therefore, there is no risk of a cross-infection or rejection reaction, as confirmed by retrospective clinical studies of Lee et al. [40] and Kim et al. [41]. Although the results of in vitro and in vivo studies suggested that DDM can be considered as an alternative to autologous bone grafts [42] and xenografts [15,43], the number of clinical studies is still limited. Hence, further studies are still needed to validate the performance of DDM for clinical purposes.

5. Conclusions

Demineralized dentin matrix could be considered as a suitable alternative to autologous bone grafts and xenografts. According to previous studies, an adequate balance should be achieved in the demineralization process of dentin particles. However, due to the lack of scientific data, this study described the chemical and surface characterization of DDM after different demineralization processes. The following can be concluded:

- there is a progressive reduction in the concentration of both PO_4^{3-} and CO_3^{2-} with increasing demineralization time;
- the organic (protein) component does not change during the demineralization process;
- increasing the duration of demineralization results in dentin particles with smoother surfaces and higher numbers of dentinal tubules.

Author Contributions: Conceptualization, F.B; methodology, L.M., E.M.S., F.B. and S.M.; software, S.M.; validation, L.M. and F.B.; formal analysis, E.M.S. and R.M.; investigation, E.M.S. and S.M.; resources, L.M. and F.B.; data curation, E.M.S. and F.B.; writing—original draft preparation, E.M.S. and F.B.; writing—review and editing, E.M.S. and R.M.; visualization, F.B.; supervision, L.M. and F.B.; project administration, L.M. and F.B.; funding acquisition, L.M. and F.B. All authors have read and agreed to the published version of the manuscript.

Funding: This research received no external funding.

Institutional Review Board Statement: Not applicable.

Informed Consent Statement: Not applicable.

Data Availability Statement: The data presented in this study are available on request from the corresponding author.

Conflicts of Interest: The authors declare no conflict of interest.

References

1. Tan, W.L.; Wong, T.L.T.; Wong, M.C.M.; Lang, N.P. A Systematic Review of Post-Extractional Alveolar Hard and Soft Tissue Dimensional Changes in Humans. *Clin. Oral Implants Res.* **2012**, *23* (Suppl. S5), 1–21. [CrossRef] [PubMed]
2. Hansson, S.; Halldin, A. Alveolar Ridge Resorption after Tooth Extraction: A Consequence of a Fundamental Principle of Bone Physiology. *J. Dent. Biomech.* **2012**, *3*, 1758736012456543. [CrossRef] [PubMed]
3. Schropp, L.; Wenzel, A.; Kostopoulos, L.; Karring, T. Bone Healing and Soft Tissue Contour Changes Following Single-Tooth Extraction: A Clinical and Radiographic 12-Month Prospective Study. *Int. J. Periodontics Restor. Dent.* **2003**, *23*, 313–323. [PubMed]
4. Jung, R.E.; Ioannidis, A.; Hämmerle, C.H.F.; Thoma, D.S. Alveolar Ridge Preservation in the Esthetic Zone. *Periodontology 2000* **2018**, *77*, 165–175. [CrossRef] [PubMed]
5. Vignoletti, F.; Matesanz, P.; Rodrigo, D.; Figuero, E.; Martin, C.; Sanz, M. Surgical Protocols for Ridge Preservation after Tooth Extraction. A Systematic Review. *Clin. Oral Implants Res.* **2012**, *23* (Suppl. S5), 22–38. [CrossRef]
6. Vittorini Orgeas, G.; Clementini, M.; De Risi, V.; de Sanctis, M. Surgical Techniques for Alveolar Socket Preservation: A Systematic Review. *Int. J. Oral Maxillofac. Implants* **2013**, *28*, 1049–1061. [CrossRef] [PubMed]
7. Troiano, G.; Zhurakivska, K.; Lo Muzio, L.; Laino, L.; Cicciù, M.; Lo Russo, L. Combination of Bone Graft and Resorbable Membrane for Alveolar Ridge Preservation: A Systematic Review, Meta-Analysis, and Trial Sequential Analysis. *J. Periodontol.* **2018**, *89*, 46–57. [CrossRef] [PubMed]
8. Miron, R.J.; Hedbom, E.; Saulacic, N.; Zhang, Y.; Sculean, A.; Bosshardt, D.D.; Buser, D. Osteogenic Potential of Autogenous Bone Grafts Harvested with Four Different Surgical Techniques. *J. Dent. Res.* **2011**, *90*, 1428–1433. [CrossRef]
9. Zizzari, V.L.; Zara, S.; Tetè, G.; Vinci, R.; Gherlone, E.; Cataldi, A. Biologic and Clinical Aspects of Integration of Different Bone Substitutes in Oral Surgery: A Literature Review. *Oral Surg. Oral Med. Oral Pathol. Oral Radiol.* **2016**, *122*, 392–402. [CrossRef]
10. Goldberg, M.; Kulkarni, A.B.; Young, M.; Boskey, A. Dentin: Structure, Composition and Mineralization. *Front. Biosci. Elite Ed.* **2011**, *3*, 711–735. [CrossRef]
11. Kim, Y.-K.; Lee, J.; Um, I.-W.; Kim, K.-W.; Murata, M.; Akazawa, T.; Mitsugi, M. Tooth-Derived Bone Graft Material. *J. Korean Assoc. Oral Maxillofac. Surg.* **2013**, *39*, 103–111. [CrossRef] [PubMed]
12. Koga, T.; Minamizato, T.; Kawai, Y.; Miura, K.I.T.; Nakatani, Y.; Sumita, Y.; Asahina, I. Bone Regeneration Using Dentin Matrix Depends on the Degree of Demineralization and Particle Size. *PLoS ONE* **2016**, *11*, e0147235. [CrossRef] [PubMed]
13. Kim, Y.-K.; Kim, S.-G.; Byeon, J.-H.; Lee, H.-J.; Um, I.-U.; Lim, S.-C.; Kim, S.-Y. Development of a Novel Bone Grafting Material Using Autogenous Teeth. *Oral Surg. Oral Med. Oral Pathol. Oral Radiol. Endod.* **2010**, *109*, 496–503. [CrossRef] [PubMed]
14. Kim, Y.-K.; Kim, S.-G.; Bae, J.-H.; Um, I.-W.; Oh, J.-S.; Jeong, K.-I. Guided Bone Regeneration Using Autogenous Tooth Bone Graft in Implant Therapy: Case Series. *Implant Dent.* **2014**, *23*, 138–143. [CrossRef]
15. Pang, K.-M.; Um, I.-W.; Kim, Y.-K.; Woo, J.-M.; Kim, S.-M.; Lee, J.-H. Autogenous Demineralized Dentin Matrix from Extracted Tooth for the Augmentation of Alveolar Bone Defect: A Prospective Randomized Clinical Trial in Comparison with Anorganic Bovine Bone. *Clin. Oral Implants Res.* **2017**, *28*, 809–815. [CrossRef]
16. Kim, Y.-K.; Kim, S.-G.; Yun, P.-Y.; Yeo, I.-S.; Jin, S.-C.; Oh, J.-S.; Kim, H.-J.; Yu, S.-K.; Lee, S.-Y.; Kim, J.-S.; et al. Autogenous Teeth Used for Bone Grafting: A Comparison with Traditional Grafting Materials. *Oral Surg. Oral Med. Oral Pathol. Oral Radiol.* **2014**, *117*, e39–e45. [CrossRef]

17. Tabatabaei, F.S.; Tatari, S.; Samadi, R.; Moharamzadeh, K. Different Methods of Dentin Processing for Application in Bone Tissue Engineering: A Systematic Review. *J. Biomed. Mater. Res. A* **2016**, *104*, 2616–2627. [CrossRef]
18. Tabatabaei, F.S.; Tatari, S.; Samadi, R.; Torshabi, M. Surface Characterization and Biological Properties of Regular Dentin, Demineralized Dentin, and Deproteinized Dentin. *J. Mater. Sci. Mater. Med.* **2016**, *27*, 164. [CrossRef]
19. Kolmas, J.; Kalinowski, E.; Wojtowicz, A.; Kolodziejski, W. Mid-Infrared Reflectance Microspectroscopy of Human Molars: Chemical Comparison of the Dentin–Enamel Junction with the Adjacent Tissues. *J. Mol. Struct.* **2010**, *966*, 113–121. [CrossRef]
20. Iafisco, M.; Palazzo, B.; Martra, G.; Margiotta, N.; Piccinonna, S.; Natile, G.; Gandin, V.; Marzano, C.; Roveri, N. Nanocrystalline Carbonate-Apatites: Role of Ca/P Ratio on the Upload and Release of Anticancer Platinum Bisphosphonates. *Nanoscale* **2011**, *4*, 206–217. [CrossRef]
21. Lopes, C. de C.A.; Limirio, P.H.J.O.; Novais, V.R.; Dechichi, P. Fourier Transform Infrared Spectroscopy (FTIR) Application Chemical Characterization of Enamel, Dentin and Bone. *Appl. Spectrosc. Rev.* **2018**, *53*, 747–769. [CrossRef]
22. Janicki, P.; Schmidmaier, G. What Should Be the Characteristics of the Ideal Bone Graft Substitute? Combining Scaffolds with Growth Factors and/or Stem Cells. *Injury* **2011**, *42* (Suppl. S2), S77–S81. [CrossRef] [PubMed]
23. Murata, M.; Akazawa, T.; Mitsugi, M.; Um, I.-W.; Kim, K.-W.; Kim, Y.-K. *Human Dentin as Novel Biomaterial for Bone Regeneration*; IntechOpen: London, UK, 2011; ISBN 978-953-307-418-4.
24. Elfana, A.; El-Kholy, S.; Saleh, H.A.; Fawzy El-Sayed, K. Alveolar Ridge Preservation Using Autogenous Whole-Tooth versus Demineralized Dentin Grafts: A Randomized Controlled Clinical Trial. *Clin. Oral Implants Res.* **2021**, *32*, 539–548. [CrossRef] [PubMed]
25. Shapoff, C.A.; Bowers, G.M.; Levy, B.; Mellonig, J.T.; Yukna, R.A. The Effect of Particle Size on the Osteogenic Activity of Composite Grafts of Allogeneic Freeze-Dried Bone and Autogenous Marrow. *J. Periodontol.* **1980**, *51*, 625–630. [CrossRef]
26. Nam, J.-W.; Kim, M.-Y.; Han, S.-J. Cranial Bone Regeneration According to Different Particle Sizes and Densities of Demineralized Dentin Matrix in the Rabbit Model. *Maxillofac. Plast. Reconstr. Surg.* **2016**, *38*, 27. [CrossRef]
27. de Oliveira, G.S.; Miziara, M.N.; da Silva, E.R.; Ferreira, E.L.; Biulchi, A.P.F.; Alves, J.B. Enhanced Bone Formation during Healing Process of Tooth Sockets Filled with Demineralized Human Dentine Matrix. *Aust. Dent. J.* **2013**, *58*, 326–332. [CrossRef]
28. Tanoue, R.; Ohta, K.; Miyazono, Y.; Iwanaga, J.; Koba, A.; Natori, T.; Iwamoto, O.; Nakamura, K.; Kusukawa, J. Three-Dimensional Ultrastructural Analysis of the Interface between an Implanted Demineralised Dentin Matrix and the Surrounding Newly Formed Bone. *Sci. Rep.* **2018**, *8*, 2858. [CrossRef]
29. Inoue, T.; Deporter, D.A.; Melcher, A.H. Induction of Cartilage and Bone by Dentin Demineralized in Citric Acid. *J. Periodontal Res.* **1986**, *21*, 243–255. [CrossRef]
30. Ike, M.; Urist, M.R. Recycled Dentin Root Matrix for a Carrier of Recombinant Human Bone Morphogenetic Protein. *J. Oral Implantol.* **1998**, *24*, 124–132. [CrossRef]
31. Murata, M.; Sato, D.; Hino, J.; Akazawa, T.; Tazaki, J.; Ito, K.; Arisue, M. Acid-Insoluble Human Dentin as Carrier Material for Recombinant Human BMP-2. *J. Biomed. Mater. Res. A* **2012**, *100*, 571–577. [CrossRef]
32. Urist, M.R. Bone: Formation by Autoinduction. *Science* **1965**, *150*, 893–899. [CrossRef] [PubMed]
33. Rosen, V.; Thies, R.S. The BMP Proteins in Bone Formation and Repair. *Trends Genet. TIG* **1992**, *8*, 97–102. [CrossRef]
34. Cao, X.; Chen, D. The BMP Signaling and in Vivo Bone Formation. *Gene* **2005**, *357*, 1–8. [CrossRef] [PubMed]
35. Kawai, T.; Urist, M.R. Bovine Tooth-Derived Bone Morphogenetic Protein. *J. Dent. Res.* **1989**, *68*, 1069–1074. [CrossRef] [PubMed]
36. Bessho, K.; Tagawa, T.; Murata, M. Purification of Rabbit Bone Morphogenetic Protein Derived from Bone, Dentin, and Wound Tissue after Tooth Extraction. *J. Oral Maxillofac. Surg. Off. J. Am. Assoc. Oral Maxillofac. Surg.* **1990**, *48*, 162–169. [CrossRef]
37. Bessho, K.; Tanaka, N.; Matsumoto, J.; Tagawa, T.; Murata, M. Human Dentin-Matrix-Derived Bone Morphogenetic Protein. *J. Dent. Res.* **1991**, *70*, 171–175. [CrossRef] [PubMed]
38. Serper, A.; Çalt, S. The Demineralizing Effects of EDTA at Different Concentrations and PH. *J. Endod.* **2002**, *28*, 501–502. [CrossRef] [PubMed]
39. Ritchie, H.H.; Ritchie, D.G.; Wang, L.H. Six Decades of Dentinogenesis Research. Historical and Prospective Views on Phosphophoryn and Dentin Sialoprotein. *Eur. J. Oral Sci.* **1998**, *106* (Suppl. S1), 211–220. [CrossRef]
40. Lee, J.-Y.; Kim, Y.-K. Retrospective Cohort Study of Autogenous Tooth Bone Graft. *Oral Biol. Res.* **2012**, *36*, 39–43.
41. Kim, Y.-K.; Bang, K.-M.; Murata, M.; Mitsugi, M.; Um, I.-W. Retrospective Clinical Study of Allogenic Demineralized Dentin Matrix for Alveolar Bone Repair. *J. Hard Tissue Biol.* **2017**, *26*, 95–102. [CrossRef]
42. Nampo, T.; Watahiki, J.; Enomoto, A.; Taguchi, T.; Ono, M.; Nakano, H.; Yamamoto, G.; Irie, T.; Tachikawa, T.; Maki, K. A New Method for Alveolar Bone Repair Using Extracted Teeth for the Graft Material. *J. Periodontol.* **2010**, *81*, 1264–1272. [CrossRef]
43. Santos, A.; Botelho, J.; Machado, V.; Borrecho, G.; Proença, L.; Mendes, J.J.; Mascarenhas, P.; Alcoforado, G. Autogenous Mineralized Dentin versus Xenograft Granules in Ridge Preservation for Delayed Implantation in Post-Extraction Sites: A Randomized Controlled Clinical Trial with an 18 Months Follow-Up. *Clin. Oral Implants Res.* **2021**, *32*, 905–915. [CrossRef]

Article

Prospective Pilot Study of Immediately Provisionalized Restorations of Trabecular Metal-Enhanced Titanium Dental Implants: A 5-Year Follow-Up Report

Peter van der Schoor [1,†], Markus Schlee [2,3] and Hai-Bo Wen [4,*]

1. Independent Researcher, 3886 LC Garderen, The Netherlands
2. Independent Researcher, 91301 Forchheim, Germany; markus.schlee@32schoenezaehne.de
3. Department of Oral Surgery, Goethe University, 60323 Frankfurt, Germany
4. Zimmer Biomet Dental, Palm Beach Gardens, FL 33410, USA
* Correspondence: haibo.wen@zimmerbiomet.com
† Author deceased.

Abstract: Porous tantalum trabecular metal biomaterial has a similar structure to trabecular bone, and was recently added to titanium dental implants as a surface enhancement. The purpose of this prospective pilot study was to describe 5-year survival results and crestal bone level changes around immediately-provisionalized Trabecular Metal Dental Implants. Eligible patients were adults in need of ≥1 implants in the posterior jaw. A non-occluding single acrylic provisional crown was in place for up to 14 days before final restoration. Clinical evaluations with radiographs were conducted at each follow-up visit (1 month, 3 months, 6 months, and 1 to 5 years). The primary endpoint was implant survival, characterized using the Kaplan-Meier method. The secondary endpoint was changes in crestal bone level, evaluated using a paired t-test to compare mean crestal bone levels between the baseline, 6-month, and annual follow-up values. In total, 30 patients (37 implants) were treated. Mean patient age was 45.5 years, and 63% were female. There was one implant failure; cumulative survival at 5 years was 97.2%. After the initial bone loss of 0.40 mm in the first 6 months, there were no statistically significant changes in crestal bone level over time up to 5 years of follow-up.

Keywords: dental implant; osseoincorporation; osseointegration; trabecular metal

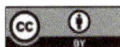

1. Introduction

Porous tantalum has been used in the orthopedic industry since the 1980s for joint arthroplasty, bone augmentation, and as an integral part of orthopedic implants to facilitate bone ingrowth [1]. Although tantalum is highly biocompatible and resistant to corrosion, its use in orthopedics was initially limited due to cost and difficulties in manipulating solid tantalum [2]. However, in the early 1990s porous tantalum trabecular metal (PTTM) was introduced [2]. Porous tantalum trabecular metal, known commercially as Trabecular Metal (TM) Material (Zimmer Trabecular Metal Technology, Inc., Parsippany, NJ, USA) is a highly porous biomaterial made from elemental tantalum, with a similar structure to trabecular bone by having a repeating pattern of regular, interconnecting pores, which provide a high volume (70% to 80%) of porosity [1–3]. Using a proprietary chemical deposition process, elemental tantalum is deposited onto a substrate, creating a nanotextured surface topography to build the TM material [4].

Early nonclinical (canine and bovine) research showed that the multi-dimensional enhancement of implant surfaces with PTTM allowed for excellent bone ingrowth within porous tantalum structures [1,3,5,6] and that the material was chemically stable and biocompatible [7,8]. Porous tantalum trabecular metal has excellent biocompatibility and high frictional characteristics, which make it conducive to biologic fixation [1,2], and it has been used in clinical applications for orthopedics for several decades. PTTM has been recently added to titanium dental implants as an enhancement to titanium implant surfaces [2].

As originally described by Bencharit et al., using PTTM as an enhancement for dental implants can potentially provide multiple advantages, including rapid endothelial budding, as well as ingrowth and endothelial neovascularization, both of which are critical for promoting new osseous tissue formation [2]. Based on the extensive prior clinical use of PTTM in orthopedics, a titanium alloy dental implant with a PTTM midsection was developed (Trabecular Metal Dental Implant, Zimmer Dental Inc., Carlsbad, CA, USA). The TM dental implant is manufactured from a combination of titanium alloy and trabecular metal and designed for integration into hard tissue through a process of bone apposition to the threaded implant surface and by bone ingrowth into the porous surface. These dental implants are indicated for delayed and immediate restoration.

There has been limited clinical research on TM dental implants, with a maximum of 1-year follow-up results reported. In 2013, the authors of the current report published the 1st year results of a 5-year descriptive, pilot study to evaluate TM dental implants which were immediately restored with a provisional restoration and fully loaded within two weeks. Their evaluation showed that during the first year of the study, PTTM-enhanced titanium dental implants had a 97.3% cumulative implant survival rate and appeared to be able to withstand the clinical demands of immediate loading [4]. The authors noted that longer-term follow-up was needed to better evaluate the performance and clinical characteristics of the TM dental implant. The present report describes the 5-year survival results and crestal bone loss associated with immediately-provisionalized and fully loaded (within two weeks) TM dental implants in a descriptive 5-year pilot study.

2. Materials and Methods

2.1. Study Design and Eligibility Criteria

This was a prospective, two-center, 5-year, nonrandomized, descriptive pilot study. Enrollment was open to all qualifying male or female patients of at least 18 years of age with adequate bone volume to support an implant in the posterior jaw. Other inclusion criteria included having residual facial and palatal/lingual plates at least 1.5 mm thick after osteotomy preparation, having a healed extraction site greater than six months post-extraction (with or without grafting), being able to provide informed consent, and ability to attend evaluation visits.

Exclusion criteria for enrollment into the study included bruxism, fresh extraction sites, smokers, uncontrolled systemic disease, bleeding disorders, use of biphosponates, and pregnancy. At the time of surgery, an additional exclusion criterion was employed; patients with type 4 bone or implants with <35 Ncm of insertion torque were also excluded. After a patient was deemed medically, dentally, psychologically, functionally, and anatomically to be a good candidate for dental implant therapy, informed consent was obtained, and the patient was enrolled. Up to 40 patients from two sites (one in Germany and one in the Netherlands) were planned for enrollment.

2.2. Data Collection

Before implant surgery, patient demographics, and medical and dental conditions were recorded. During the implant surgery, insertion torque values, implant size, and bone density were recorded. Radiographs were taken to evaluate mesial and distal bone levels. All data requested for this study were collected using electronic case report forms (eCRFs). Data collection and management were performed by the Sponsor.

2.3. Implant Procedure

Pre-operative photographs and radiographs were taken with an individualized imaging holder (Figure 1). All patients received pre-operative oral antibiotic therapy with either clindamycin or amoxicillin [9]. At the time of the surgical implant placement, the subject was administered anesthesia. As described in an earlier publication, implants of either 4.7 mm or 6.0 mm diameters were placed in either premolar or molar sites, in either jaw [4]. Implants were TM dental implants with a 0.5 mm machined collar, microtextured (MTX) surface, and microgrooves, and were placed according to the surgical manual using a one-stage (nonsubmerged) technique. Implant insertion torque and resonance-frequency analysis values were recorded at the time of placement. As noted earlier, if it was discovered that a patient had type 4 bone at the implant site, they were excluded from the study. Appropriate analgesics and postoperative physical therapy were prescribed as needed. Post-implantation antibiotic therapy was not prescribed unless indicated for infection. After the implant placement, a final impression was taken and sent to the dental lab for fabrication of the final restoration.

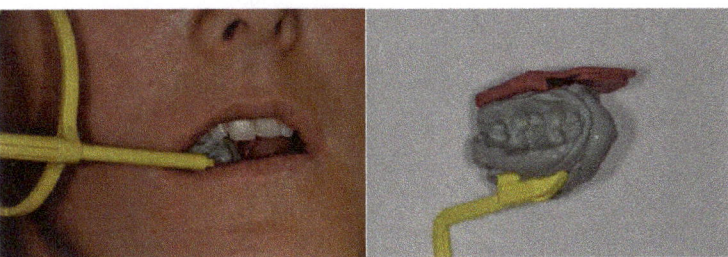

Figure 1. An individualized imaging holder was made and stored for each patient during the 5-year study period.

2.4. Immediate Provisional and Final Restoration

A standard contoured abutment was placed as the final abutment with 30 Ncm preload, as recommended. This was the abutment for both the provisional and final crown. A non-occluding single acrylic crown provisional prosthesis was immediately delivered and the soft tissues were sutured around the provisional restoration. All immediate provisional restorations were placed within 48 h of surgery. The provisional prosthesis was in place for 7 to 14 days to allow adequate time for soft tissue healing. Periapical radiographs were taken. Seven to 14 days after the implant procedure, the provisional prosthesis and sutures were removed. If the implant appeared stable, the final restoration was delivered (Figure 2). The final restorations were fully occluding, single-tooth ceramometal restorations. Any final occlusal adjustments were made at this visit.

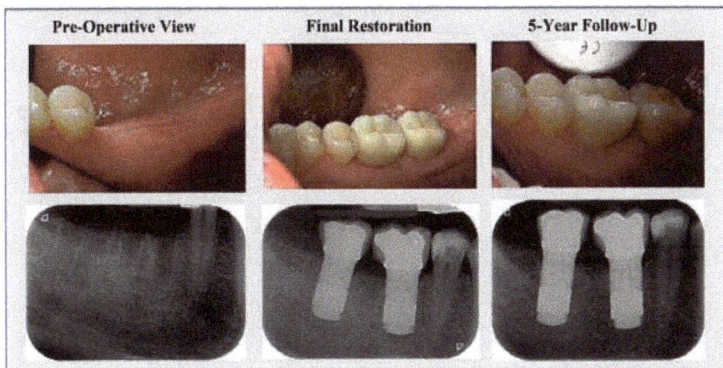

Figure 2. Shows the intraoral photos and periapical radiographs taken pre-operatively, at final restoration, and at 5-years follow-up. This female patient with missing posterior mandibular first and second molars received two TM implants (diameter 6.0 mm and length 10 mm for both). Final restoration was completed 13 days after implant placement consisting of two cement-retained crowns. The 5-year follow-up showed good soft tissue health and bone maintenance.

2.5. Follow-Up Visits

Subjects were scheduled to be re-evaluated at 1 month, 3 months, 6 months, and for annual visits for 5 years after delivery of the provisional restoration. During each follow-up visit, the study investigator took photographs in the facial, occlusal, and lingual views, assessed for any clinical complications, and took standardized periapical radiographs (Rinn, Dentsply, York, PA, USA) (Figure 1). An individualized imaging holder was made and stored for each patient during the 5-year study period. When mobility was suspected, opposing force from two hand instruments was applied to the post and any overt indication of mobility was recorded as a failure.

2.6. Study Endpoints

The primary endpoint was implant survival after 5 years of occlusal loading. Implant failure was defined as the presence of persistent pain, mobility, or loss or removal of the implant.

The secondary study endpoint was change in crestal bone level; mesial and distal levels were determined radiographically and a mean (per implant site) was calculated. Crestal bone loss was summarized as the mean of radiographic mesial and distal changes in bone height from baseline (implant surgery) values. Mean crestal bone loss served as the secondary endpoint, and was computed by averaging the mean bone loss per implant.

All periapical radiographs were evaluated by an independent radiologist using high-resolution uncompressed image files. As described in an earlier paper, crestal bone levels were measured by calculating the distance from the implant shoulder to the first bone-to-implant contact [4]. Both mesial and distal measurements were made on each periapical radiograph, and the mean value was used in the analyses. The known height of the implant's tantalum section (4.8 mm) was used as the standardized dimension for calibration. The height of the tantalum section was measured on the image in pixels, and the ratio between the length in pixels and tantalum height of 4.8 mm was calculated. Because the two study sites used different radiographic image sensors, each site was calibrated differently: 0.0234 mm/pixel (4.8 mm/205.5 px = 0.0234 mm) for the first site (Germany) and 0.0349 mm/pixel (4.8 mm/137.5 px = 0.0349 mm) for the second site (the Netherlands). Bone height values measured in pixels were then multiplied by the calculated calibration factors to arrive at the final data values in millimeters. Each image was opened using US FDA-cleared image analysis software (OsiriX MD, Pixmeo SARL, Bernex, Switzerland) on a personal computer [4]. Measurements were recorded in a spreadsheet (Excel, Microsoft Corp., Redmond, WA, USA).

2.7. Statistical Analyses

Descriptive statistics (N, %, mean ± SD, min, max, median) were used to summarize the data. The implant was the unit of analysis, except for patient demographics. Implant survival was summarized through the characterization of failure over time, using the Kaplan–Meier method. Cumulative survival of the implants was estimated at each time of assessment, with corresponding 95% confidence intervals. A paired t-test was performed to analyze the initial bone loss from implant placement/immediate provisional restoration to 6 months of follow-up, and the additional bone loss was analyzed by comparing crestal bone loss between annual follow-up values and the 6-month value. Statistical significance was declared if the 2-sided p-value was <0.05.

Because this was a descriptive pilot study with no control group and no prior hypothesis, no formal sample size calculations were conducted. This pilot study was conducted to gather initial, exploratory data; the sample size was not selected according to any statistical power calculation. Instead, the sample size was determined according to feasibility and was thought to provide sufficient exploratory results to inform the development of future confirmatory studies. Analyses were performed using SAS 9.4 TS (SAS Institute Inc., Cary, NC, USA) or Minitab 18 (Minitab, LLC, State College, PA, USA).

2.8. Human Subjects Protections

The research was conducted in compliance with applicable regulations, and according to the principles of the Declaration of Helsinki. The pilot study was conducted in accordance with the respective government regulatory authorities and the local regional Institutional Review Boards for two study sites in Germany and the Netherlands (Protocol CSU2010-07D Freiburger Ethik Kommission-an independent Ethics Committee-28 June 2010). All patient data were fully anonymized to safeguard patient confidentiality. All materials and procedures complied with local and international health and safety standards and good clinical practices. This report is structured in alignment with the Consolidated Standards of Reporting Trials (CONSORT) [10].

3. Results

After obtaining informed consent and verifying that potential subjects met the inclusion/exclusion criteria, 30 patients (37 implants) were treated per protocol. Each patient received one or two TM implants in premolar or molar sites (Figure 2). The mean patient age was 45.5 years (range 19 to 73 years), and the majority of patients were female (63.3%). Twenty-nine of the 30 patients were White, one patient was Asian. The most common comorbidity was hypersensitivity reactions/allergies (40%), followed by hypertension/hypotension (30%). Most of the implants (70.3%) were placed in the mandible. Regarding bone density, most implants (62.2%) were placed in type 2 bone, with the remaining placed in type 3 bone. The most common (and smallest) implant diameter that was used was 4.7 mm (64.9%), and the most common length was 10 mm (45.9%). The majority of implants (91.9%) received a provisional restoration on the final abutment at the time of surgery (Table 1). There were no surgical complications across the study cohort.

Table 1. Patient Demographics and Surgical Information.

Demographic and Surgical Information	
Age, mean (SD), years	45.5 (15.1)
Female, n (%)	19 (63.3)
Most Common Comorbid Conditions, N (%)	
Hypersensitivity Reactions/Allergies	12 (40.0)
Blood Pressure Disorder (Hypertension or Hypotension)	9 (30.0)
Thyroid Disorders	5 (16.7)
Bone Density Classification * at Surgery, n (%)	
Type 2	23 (62.2)
Type 3	14 (37.8)
Final Insertion Torque, n (%)	
30–44 Ncm	8 (21.6)
45–59 Ncm	25 (67.6)
>60 Ncm	4 (10.8)
Provisional Restoration at Surgery, n (%)	
No	3 (8.1)
Yes	34 (91.9)
Implant Site, n (%)	
Posterior Maxilla	11 (29.7)
Posterior Mandible	26 (70.3)
TM Implant Diameter, n (%)	
4.7 mm	24 (64.9)
6.0 mm	13 (35.1)
TM Implant Length, n (%)	
10 mm	17 (45.9)
11.5 mm	13 (35.1)
13 mm	7 (18.9)

SD = standard deviation. * Subjectively assessed by the clinician based on radiographic evaluations and tactile sensations during implant placement.

Radiographic evaluations of mean crestal bone levels over time (from baseline time of implant placement/provisional restoration to the 5-year follow-up evaluation) showed an initial bone loss of 0.40 mm in the first 6 months, after which there were no statistically significant changes in crestal bone level over time (Table 2). The mean crestal bone value levels changed minimally ($\leq$0.05 mm) from 6 months to any of the annual follow-up visits. Repeated Measures Analysis of Variance with Tukey Pairwise Comparison confirmed there is no statistical difference among the crestal bone level values of the 6-month and annual follow-up visits (details not shown). There was also no statistically significant difference in crestal bone level changes between those who had received 4.7 diameter versus 6 mm diameter implants (data not shown). Additionally, no implants were observed to have pain, mobility, or peri-implant radiolucency.

Table 2. Changes in Crestal Bone Levels Over the 5-Year Follow-Up Period.

Evaluation Timepoint	Crestal Bone Level	Mean ± SD Value in mm	p-Value [1]
Surgery/Provisional (N = 34)	Mean Bone Level	0.51 ± 0.49	
6 Months (N = 31)	Mean Bone Level Change from Provisional	−0.40 ± 0.48	$p = 0.00$
1 Year (N = 25)	Mean Bone Level Change from 6 Months	−0.05 ± 0.23	$p = 0.28$
2 Year (N = 25)	Mean Bone Level Change from 6 Months	−0.01 ± 0.34	$p = 0.89$
3 Year (N = 25)	Mean Bone Level Change from 6 Months	−0.03 ± 0.33	$p = 0.69$
4 Year (N = 22)	Mean Bone Level Change from 6 Months	−0.05 ± 0.36	$p = 0.56$
5 Year (N = 22)	Mean Bone Level Change from 6 Months	−0.01 ± 0.36	$p = 0.85$

[1] Analyses were conducted using a paired t-test. The study population for the bone loss value dataset had several missing values from follow-up visits, which is why there is a slight inconsistency in sample size between the crestal bone level dataset and the survival analysis dataset.

At the end of the 5-year follow-up period, 25 patients remained for evaluation (Table 3). The Kaplan-Meier cumulative survival rate of all implants in the study was 97.2% at the 3-month, 6-month, 1-year, 2-year, 3-year, 4-year, and 5-year evaluation visits; one implant failed to osseointegrate. The patient with a failed implant was a 46-year-old White male who had received a 6 × 10 implant in a mandibular molar site. The implant was placed into type 2 bone without complications. The implant failed to integrate and was removed 30 days after the implant surgery. The patient took no concomitant medications (outside of post-surgical analgesics) and had no recorded comorbidities.

Table 3. Kaplan-Meier Survival Analysis: 5-Years of Follow-Up.

Month of Follow-Up	No. of Implants at Risk	No. of Failed Implants	Survival Estimate	95% CI Survival Estimate [1]
1 Month	37	0	1.000	(1.0000, 1.0000)
2 Month	36	1	0.9722	(0.8187, 0.9960)
3 Month	35	0	0.9722	(0.8187, 0.9960)
6 Month	35	0	0.9722	(0.8187, 0.9960)
12 Month	31	0	0.9722	(0.8187, 0.9960)
18 Month	30	0	0.9722	(0.8187, 0.9960)
24 Month	30	0	0.9722	(0.8187, 0.9960)
36 Month	28	0	0.9722	(0.8187, 0.9960)
48 Month	26	0	0.9722	(0.8187, 0.9960)
60 Month	25	0	0.9722	(0.8187, 0.9960)

[1] The Kaplan-Meier method was used to calculate cumulative implant survival. One implant failed within 2 months after loading.

There were no other failures. All 25 implants that completed 5-years of follow-up were surviving and clinically stable, with no indicators of pain, mobility, radiolucency, or clinically meaningful crestal bone loss.

4. Discussion

The results from this descriptive pilot study of 37 implants showed that immediate provisional restoration (out of occlusion, with final restoration and loading within two weeks) of titanium dental implants with surfaces enhanced with PTTM were clinically effective, with a 5-year survival rate of 97.2%. As a comparison to non-TM systems, a recent systematic review and meta-analysis of 18 dental (non-TM) implant studies evaluated the 10-year survival of contemporary, two-piece titanium systems; the summary estimate for 10-year survival at the implant level was 96.4% (95% CI 95.2–97.5%) [11].

Professional consensus in dental implantology affirms that the success of implants is dependent on the presence and preservation of surrounding bone, particularly in the crestal area; however, a primary challenge of dental implant treatment is the bone resorption, particularly saucerization, that occurs after insertion [12]. Results from the present study showed an initial mean bone loss of 0.40 mm (SD = 0.48) after 6 months and minimal bone level changes over time up to 5 years in function. While the small sample size of this uncontrolled study limits direct comparisons to findings in other studies, these findings suggest that crestal bone loss around TM implants is lower than traditional titanium implant systems [13,14], and that the unique properties of PTTM may foster enhanced vital bone and surrounding tissue ingrowth and potentially reduce the amount of bone remodeling which occurs during the first year following implant surgery [15].

A recent 1-year retrospective case-control study by Edelmann et al. reported a 0.28-mm mean bone gain in a TM implant cohort, and multivariate logistic regression analysis demonstrated that the odds of having bone loss were 64% less in a TM group compared to a non-TM implant control group [16]. Another recent study by Bencharit et al. compared osteogenesis gene expression in a small group of patients who had received both TM and non-TM implants; the authors found that, compared to traditional titanium alloy, trephine samples from the TM implant group displayed higher expression of genes specific to neovascularization, growth factors, and osteogenesis [17].

To further contextualize these crestal bone level changes when compared to non-TM implants, contemporary literature was surveilled for studies with similar sample sizes and follow-up periods. An analysis by Payer et al. found that a cohort of 24 patients with 40 screw-type (non-TM) implants that were immediately provisionalized in molar and premolar sites experienced an overall survival rate of 95% at 5 years, with significant marginal bone loss (1.06 mm) in the first year [18].

To compare the crestal bone findings in this report with historical standards, longitudinal studies on the original Brånemark implant showed that one year after abutment connection, crestal bone loss frequently extended 1.5 mm to 2 mm below the implant-abutment junction [19]. This became the unofficial industry standard for acceptable crestal bone loss because most major implant systems experienced a similar bone loss phenomenon during the early years of their products. However, more contemporary implant surfaces typically include a rougher surface to foster better osseointegration, as improving the roughness of an implant surface has been correlated with less peri-implant bone loss [2]. Additionally, because the abutment was immediately placed with no intention of removal during the follow-up period, essentially the "one abutment/one-time" method was used in this study. The abutment was secured not only by the fixation screw, but also with a friction-fit connection. This type of "one-piece" implant has been shown to have less initial bone loss [20].

The TM implants used in this study have a PTTM shell that begins about 4.5 mm apical to the implant platform. A recent report by Fraser et al. compared osteogenic activity between titanium and TM-coated implants in a nonclinical study of rabbits. The authors reported higher vertical bone growth around TM implants compared to titanium implants, and increased activity in upregulation of key osteogenic genes. Furthermore, TM implants had greater bone-implant contact at 4, 8, and 12 weeks and significantly greater removal torque at 8 and 12 weeks [21]. It is not yet fully known how the TM shell impacts peri-implant bone healing and remodeling at the cervical aspect, though the current study shows promising results. The current clinical pilot study showed no statistically significant bone loss after the initial healing, which may in part be due to the high porosity and modulus of elasticity of the TM surface, which has similar properties to human cancellous bone. Prior studies have shown that these surface properties facilitate bone ingrowth and increased regions of bone-to-implant contact, potentially reducing stress on the coronal aspect of the implant due to rapid ingrowth of bone in the TM shell, though further confirmatory research with larger sample sizes is needed [1,3,5]. Taken together, these promising findings of increased osteogenesis indicators and crestal bone stability around TM implants warrant further study with larger study populations.

In this study, TM dental implants were clinically effective when fully loaded within two weeks in a small population with a variety of health risk factors that may be typically encountered in routine clinical practice.

Limitations

Patients were followed for 5 years post-restoration; during that interval, the number of evaluable implants went from 37 to 25, an attrition rate of 32%. This is an unfortunate challenge when obtaining long-term survival data, and may lead to a bias in the results [10]. Although the study investigators were aware of several patients moving away from the study site area, the reasons for other patients being lost-to-follow-up was unknown, as were their outcomes, which could potentially bias the study results and conclusions.

Additionally, because implants in this study were only placed in type 2 and 3 bone, the clinical response to TM implants in other bone types is unknown, possibly reducing the generalizability of the results.

5. Conclusions

Immediate provisional restoration (with final restoration within two weeks) of titanium dental implants with surfaces enhanced with PTTM were clinically effective in a small study population, with a 5-year survival rate of 97.2% and minimal crestal bone loss. These findings of potentially increased osteogenesis indicators and crestal bone stability around TM implants warrant further study with larger study populations.

Author Contributions: Conceptualization, P.v.d.S., M.S. and H.-B.W.; methodology, P.v.d.S., M.S. and H.-B.W.; investigation, P.v.d.S. and M.S.; data curation, P.v.d.S. and M.S.; writing—original draft preparation, P.v.d.S., M.S. and H.-B.W.; writing—review and editing, P.v.d.S., M.S. and H.-B.W.; project administration, P.v.d.S and M.S. All authors have read and agreed to the published version of the manuscript.

Funding: This research was funded by Zimmer Biomet Dental, Palm Beach Gardens, FL, USA.

Institutional Review Board Statement: The study was conducted in accordance with the Declaration of Helsinki and approved by an independent Ethics Committee (Freiburger Ethik Kommission) for two study sites in Germany and the Netherlands (Protocol CSU2010-07D, 28 June 2010).

Informed Consent Statement: Informed consent was obtained from all subjects involved in the study.

Data Availability Statement: The data presented in this study are not publicly available but can be requested from the corresponding author.

Acknowledgments: The authors are greatly indebted to Alexandra R M van der Schoor for her invaluable support in patient follow-up and clinical data collection and would also like to thank Na Ren and Cristina Matthews at Zimmer Biomet for their help in statistical analysis.

Conflicts of Interest: P.v.d.S. and M.S. declare no conflict of interest. H.-B.W. is an employee of Zimmer Biomet Dental.

References

1. Levine, B.; Della Valle, C.J.; Jacobs, J.J. Applications of porous tantalum in total hip arthroplasty. *J. Am. Acad. Orthop. Surg.* **2006**, *14*, 646–655. [CrossRef]
2. Bencharit, S.; Byrd, W.C.; Altarawneh, S.; Hosseini, B.; Leong, A.; Reside, G.; Morelli, T.; Offenbacher, S. Development and applications of porous tantalum trabecular metal-enhanced titanium dental implants. *Clin. Implant Dent. Relat. Res.* **2014**, *16*, 817–826. [CrossRef] [PubMed]
3. Bobyn, J.D.; Stackpool, G.J.; Hacking, S.A.; Tanzer, M.; Krygier, J.J. Characteristics of bone ingrowth and interface mechanics of a new porous tantalum biomaterial. *J. Bone Jt. Surg. Br.* **1999**, *81*, 907–914. [CrossRef]
4. Schlee, M.; van der Schoor, W.P.; van der Schoor, A.R. Immediate loading of trabecular metal-enhanced titanium dental implants: Interim results from an international proof-of-principle study. *Clin. Implant Dent. Relat. Res.* **2015**, *17* (Suppl. 1), e308–e320. [CrossRef] [PubMed]
5. Bobyn, J.D.; Toh, K.K.; Hacking, S.A.; Tanzer, M.; Krygier, J.J. Tissue response to porous tantalum acetabular cups: A canine model. *J. Arthroplast.* **1999**, *14*, 347–354. [CrossRef]
6. Battula, S.; Papanicolaou, S.; Wen, H.B.; Collins, M. Evaluation of a trabecular metal dental implant design for primary stability, structural integrity and abrasion. In Proceedings of the 27th Annual Meeting of the Academy of Osseointegration, Phoenix, AZ, USA, 1–3 March 2012.
7. Meneghini, R.M.; Ford, K.S.; McCollough, C.H.; Hanssen, A.D.; Lewallen, D.G. Bone remodeling around porous metal cementless acetabular components. *J. Arthroplast.* **2010**, *25*, 741–747. [CrossRef] [PubMed]
8. Li, H.; Yao, Z.; Zhang, J.; Cai, X.; Li, L.; Liu, G.; Liu, J.; Cui, L.; Huang, J. The progress on physicochemical properties and biocompatibility of tantalum-based metal bone implants. *SN Appl. Sci.* **2020**, *2*, 1–14. [CrossRef]
9. Sanchez, F.R.; Andres, C.R.; Arteagoitia, I. Which antibiotic regimen prevents implant failure or infection after dental implant surgery? A systematic review and meta-analysis. *J. Craniomaxillofac. Surg.* **2018**, *46*, 722–736. [CrossRef] [PubMed]
10. Schulz, K.F.; Altman, D.G.; Moher, D. CONSORT 2010 statement: Updated guidelines for reporting parallel group randomised trials. *BMJ* **2010**, *340*, c332. [CrossRef] [PubMed]
11. Howe, M.S.; Keys, W.; Richards, D. Long-term (10-year) dental implant survival: A systematic review and sensitivity meta-analysis. *J. Dent.* **2019**, *84*, 9–21. [CrossRef] [PubMed]
12. de Almeida, A.B.; Prado Maia, L.; Ramos, U.D.; de Souza, S.L.S.; Palioto, D.B. Success, survival and failure rates of dental implants: A cross-sectional study. *J. Oral Sci. Rehabil.* **2017**, *3*, 24–31.
13. Tadi, D.P.; Pinisetti, S.; Gujjalapudi, M.; Kakaraparthi, S.; Kolasani, B.; Vadapalli, S.H.B. Evaluation of initial stability and crestal bone loss in immediate implant placement: An in vivo study. *J. Int. Soc. Prev. Community Dent.* **2014**, *4*, 139–144. [CrossRef] [PubMed]
14. Baer, R.A.; Nolken, R.; Colic, S.; Heydecke, G.; Mirzakhanian, C.; Behneke, A.; Behneke, N.; Gottesman, E.; Ottria, L.; Pozzi, A.; et al. Immediately provisionalized tapered conical connection implants for single-tooth restorations in the maxillary esthetic zone: A 5-year prospective single-cohort multicenter analysis. *Clin Oral Investig.* **2022**, *Epub ahead of print*. [CrossRef]
15. Albrektsson, T.; Zarb, G.; Worthington, P.; Eriksson, A.R. The long-term efficacy of currently used dental implants: A review and proposed criteria of success. *Int. J. Oral Maxillofac. Implants* **1986**, *1*, 11–25. [PubMed]
16. Edelmann, A.R.; Patel, D.; Allen, R.K.; Gibson, C.J.; Best, A.M.; Bencharit, S. Retrospective analysis of porous tantalum trabecular metal-enhanced titanium dental implants. *J. Prosthet. Dent.* **2019**, *121*, 404–410. [CrossRef] [PubMed]
17. Bencharit, S.; Morelli, T.; Barros, S.; Seagroves, J.T.; Kim, S.; Yu, N.; Byrd, K.; Brenes, C.; Offenbacher, S. Comparing initial wound healing and osteogenesis of porous tantalum trabecular metal and titanium alloy materials. *J. Oral Implantol.* **2019**, *45*, 173–180. [CrossRef]
18. Payer, M.; Heschl, A.; Wimmer, G.; Wegscheider, W.; Kirmeier, R.; Lorenzoni, M. Immediate provisional restoration of screw-type implants in the posterior mandible: Results after 5 years of clinical function. *Clin. Oral Implants Res.* **2010**, *21*, 815–821. [CrossRef] [PubMed]
19. Branemark, P.I.; Hansson, B.O.; Adell, R.; Breine, U.; Lindstrom, J.; Hallen, O.; Ohman, A. Osseointegrated implants in the treatment of the edentulous jaw. Experience from a 10-year period. *Scand. J. Plast. Reconstr. Surg. Suppl.* **1977**, *16*, 1–132. [PubMed]
20. Canullo, L.; Omori, Y.; Amari, Y.; Iannello, G.; Pesce, P. Five-year cohort prospective study on single implants in the esthetic area restored using one-abutment/one-time prosthetic approach. *Clin. Implant Dent. Relat. Res.* **2018**, *20*, 668–673. [CrossRef] [PubMed]
21. Fraser, D.; Mendonca, G.; Sartori, E.; Funkenbusch, P.; Ercoli, C.; Meirelles, L. Bone response to porous tantalum implants in a gap-healing model. *Clin. Oral Implants Res.* **2019**, *30*, 156–168. [CrossRef] [PubMed]

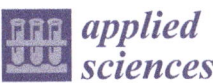

Review

Finding the Perfect Membrane: Current Knowledge on Barrier Membranes in Regenerative Procedures: A Descriptive Review

Sorina-Mihaela Solomon [1,†], Irina-Georgeta Sufaru [1,*,†], Silvia Teslaru [1,†], Cristina Mihaela Ghiciuc [2,†] and Celina Silvia Stafie [3,*,†]

1. Department of Periodontology, Grigore T. Popa University of Medicine and Pharmacy Iasi, 16 Universitatii Street, 700115 Iasi, Romania; sorina.solomon@umfiasi.ro (S.-M.S.); silvia.teslaru@umfiasi.ro (S.T.)
2. Department of Morpho-Functional Sciences II—Pharmacology and Clinical Pharmacology, Faculty of Medicine, Grigore T. Popa University of Medicine and Pharmacy of Iași, 16 Universitatii Street, 700115 Iasi, Romania; cristina.ghiciuc@umfiasi.ro
3. Department of Preventive Medicine and Interdisciplinarity—Family Medicine Discipline, Faculty of Medicine, Grigore T. Popa University of Medicine and Pharmacy of Iasi, 16 Universitatii Street, 700115 Iasi, Romania
* Correspondence: ursarescu.irina@umfiasi.ro (I.-G.S.); celina.stafie@umfiasi.ro (C.S.S.)
† These authors contributed equally to this work.

Abstract: Guided tissue regeneration (GTR) and guided bone regeneration (GBR) became common procedures in the corrective phase of periodontal treatment. In order to obtain good quality tissue neo-formation, most techniques require the use of a membrane that will act as a barrier, having as a main purpose the blocking of cell invasion from the gingival epithelium and connective tissue into the newly formed bone structure. Different techniques and materials have been developed, aiming to obtain the perfect barrier membrane. The membranes can be divided according to the biodegradability of the base material into absorbable membranes and non-absorbable membranes. The use of absorbable membranes is extremely widespread due to their advantages, but in clinical situations of significant tissue loss, the use of non-absorbable membranes is often still preferred. This descriptive review presents a synthesis of the types of barrier membranes available and their characteristics, as well as future trends in the development of barrier membranes along with some allergological aspects of membrane use.

Keywords: guided tissue regeneration; guided bone regeneration; barrier membranes; allergology

1. Introduction

Periodontitis is an infectious disease, often of multifactorial etiology, in which the perio-pathogenic bacterial biofilm plays an important role. The disease is characterized by an inflammatory reaction of the host to the bacterial aggression, reactions on which both local and systemic risk factors can be grafted. In the evolution of periodontitis, through the aggressive action of bacterial factors in the context of hyper-inflammatory status, there is a gradual destruction of the supporting periodontal tissues: periodontal ligaments, cementum and alveolar bone. To address this issue, periodontal therapy has evolved over time through regenerative therapy surgical methods that include guided tissue regeneration (GTR) and bone regeneration (GBR) techniques. Such guided techniques involve isolating the bone defect with the help of barrier membranes, allowing the regeneration of lost and damaged tissues [1]. The use of a barrier membrane, at the interface with the gingival/epithelial connective tissue and with periodontal ligaments and alveolar bone to promote the regeneration of periodontal tissues is called GTR, and the restoration of alveolar bone sites is called GBR.

The association of barrier membranes and biomaterials of infrabony periodontal lesions investigated in various clinical studies generated significantly better results in terms of attachment gain and reduction of probing depths than the open flap debridement alone [2–4].

In guided tissue regeneration, there is a number of four essential biological principles under the PASS acronym: (a) Primary closure of the surgical wound to allow uninterrupted healing; (b) Angiogenesis for adequate blood supply (supply of nutrients, as well as cell types that facilitate healing); (c) maintaining the Space for bone neo-formation, while blocking the proliferation of soft tissues and (d) wound Stability to allow blood clots to form [5].

The idea that the repopulation of cells on the root surface after periodontal surgery determines the nature of the attachment that will form is generally accepted. After the periodontal debridement, with or without open flap procedure, the root surface will be repopulated by the fastest cells, which were epithelial cells [6]. Barrier membranes placed over areas of tissue defect have as their main purpose the blocking of cell invasion from the gingival epithelium and connective tissue [7]. Barrier membranes require full in situ functionality for 4–6 weeks for periodontal tissue regeneration and 16–24 weeks for bone growth [8].

There are a number of mandatory requirements for a barrier membrane to be used successfully in guided regenerative therapies; these requirements include (a) good mechanical isolation, occlusion and blocking capabilities; (b) to be biologically active; (c) to be biocompatible; (d) to exhibit tolerance to exposure and (e) to be biodegradable [9]. Moreover, barrier membranes should have adequate porosity to prevent the excessive penetration of oral keratinocytes into the bone defect on one side but also to allow neovascularization and bone formation in the connective tissue part of the membrane [10]. It should also be easy to manipulate the membrane, to stabilize it at the site without damaging it [11].

To date, there is no commercially available membrane that meets all these parameters at optimum capacity, but recent developments in membrane production technology are trying, through various innovative forms, to meet as wide a range of characteristics as necessary to achieve predictable surgical results.

To meet some of these requirements, various techniques and materials have been developed to generate tissue neo-formation. They can be divided according to the biodegradability of the base material into absorbable membranes and non-absorbable membranes [12] (Figure 1). The use of absorbable membranes is extremely widespread due to their advantages, but in clinical situations of significant tissue loss, the use of non-absorbable membranes is often still preferred [13].

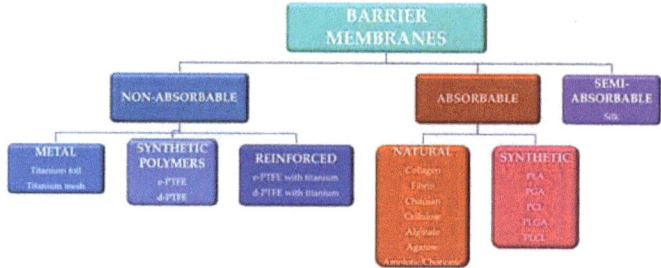

Figure 1. Main categories of barrier membranes used in guided tissue regeneration. e-PTFE: expanded polytetrafluoroethylene; d-PTFE: high density polytetrafluoroethylene; PLA: polylactic acid; PGA: polyglactic acid; PCL: polycaprolactone; PLGA: poly-lactic-co-glycolic acid PLCL: poly-lactic-co-caprolactone acid.

Another classification of barrier membranes includes the first generation of membranes (non-absorbable), second generation (absorbable) and third generation (membranes as a product of tissue engineering) [14].

We believe that a better understanding of the various types of membranes available and their properties is absolutely necessary in making clinical decisions. Thus, this review proposes a synthesis of the types of barrier membranes available and their characteristics; in addition, this paper presents future trends in the development of the field of barrier membranes, as well as some allergological aspects of membrane usage.

2. Non-Absorbable Membranes

Barrier membranes made of non-absorbable material are characterized by mechanical stability over time so that the by-products of degradation of the basic materials are not a cause for concern, and the period of fixation in place is easy to control [15]. Their setting to the anatomical substrate is usually done with the help of pins or mini-screws [16].

The major disadvantage of these membranes is the need for a second surgical time, removal from the site, after the completion of tissue neo-formation. This extra surgical time increases the risk of complications, such as infectious processes or healing disorders [12]. Moreover, non-absorbable membranes may present a higher risk of complications related to membrane exposure that include bacterial contamination or wound dehiscence [17,18]. Different types of non-absorbable membranes, with their advantages and disadvantages, are presented in Table 1.

Table 1. Types of non-absorbable membranes.

Composition		Commercial Variants	Observations
Titanium		Osteo-Mesh TM-300® Frios BoneShields	Very good mechanical properties Bio-inert High risk of oral exposure Requires setting pins Requires second surgical time
Silicone			Low cost Bio-inert Very low micro-porosity Requires second surgical time
Polytetrafluoroethylene (PTFE)	Expanded (e-PTFE)	Gore-Tex®	Good mechanical properties Good micro-porosity Bio-inert High risk of oral exposure, with bacterial loading
	High density (d-PTFE)	High density Gore-Tex® Cytoplast TXT-200® Cytoplast Regentex GBR-200®	Good mechanical properties Good micro-porosity Smooth surface (low risk of bacterial loading) Can be left partially exposed in the oral cavity High risk of oral exposure
	e-PTFE with titanium	Gore-Tex® Reinforced	Very good mechanical properties Bio-inert
	d-PTFE with titanium	Cytoplast Regentex Ti-250®	High risk of oral exposure

2.1. Non-Absorbable Metal Membranes

Titanium is the material of choice in making non-absorbable metal membranes. It is an inert, stable material with good mechanical strength; in addition, it has a high degree of biocompatibility [19,20]. These qualities of titanium make it usable in high-amplitude tissue defects, where it gives a constant shape over time [21]. An economic disadvantage is the high cost of these membranes compared to other common materials [12]. Titanium membranes may be available as all-metal membranes or metal mesh membranes.

In 2003, the Ultra-Ti® GTR titanium barrier membrane was introduced [22]. Ultra-Ti® membrane is a pure titanium membrane with a homogeneous structure, about 10 microns thick; due to its ultra-thin thickness, it is easy to handle and adapt to the receptor site [23]. Moreover, the surface roughness is reduced, which makes it less susceptible to bacterial contamination. In addition, it does not require setting with pins. Because it is radiolucent, it allows the monitoring of bone formation. As a disadvantage, being a non-porous membrane, it does not allow the perfect integration of tissues, which can lead to periodontal pocket formation [23].

In 1969, titanium mesh membranes were introduced to regenerate bone defects [24]. Titanium mesh has good mechanical properties in stabilizing bone regeneration materials. Its rigidity ensures the maintenance of the space and prevents the collapse of the defect; its elasticity prevents the compression of the mucosa, and its plasticity allows bending, contouring and adaptation to the bone defect [25]. Titanium mesh has been shown to maintain space with a higher degree of predictability, even in cases of extensive bone defects [26].

In general, titanium mesh membranes are characterized by macro-porosity; this quality is considered to play an important role in ensuring blood supply, allowing the diffusion of extracellular nutrients through the membrane [27]. Moreover, soft tissue attachment, favored by high porosity, facilitates the stabilization and restriction of epithelial cell migration [28]. Celletti et al. claimed in their study data that the use of a pore-free titanium membrane resulted in the exposure of all meshes in three weeks [29].

Of course, this type of membrane also has a number of disadvantages; due to its sharp edges, irritation of the soft tissue components can occur, which can lead to membrane exposure and even compromise therapeutic success [30]. However, titanium membranes can tolerate some degree of exposure. The exposure rate of titanium mesh membranes varies between 5.3% and 52% [31].

In a study of 44 patients who underwent titanium mesh-reinforced GTR, membrane exposure occurred in 23 cases, but graft failure occurred in only one patient [32]. In contrast, in another study, membrane exposure generated a bone resorption of 15–25% [33].

From the point of view of the predictability of the amount of newly formed bone, the studies generated discordant results, with growth values in vertical bone defects between 2.56 mm and 6 mm [32,34]. For increases in horizontal defects, the data indicate average values of 4 mm [32,35].

2.2. Non-Absorbable Membranes of Synthetic Polymers

From the category of synthetic polymers, polytetrafluoroethylene (PTFE) is an example of a material used in non-absorbable membranes. According to its structure, PTFE can be divided into two types: expanded PTFE (e-PTFE) and high density PTFE (d-PTFE) [24].

e-PTFE was developed in 1969 and became a standard material in the 1990s. Its structure is bi-layered, with pores between 5 and 20 microns in size. One side presents an open microstructure of 1 mm thickness, with 90% porosity, which delays epithelial growth, and on the other side there is a 0.15 mm thick membrane with 30% porosity, which generates space for new bone [36]. The main disadvantages of the e-PTFE membrane are the higher exposure rate and, of course, the need for a second surgical time to remove it from the site, a feature common to all non-absorbable membranes. Subsequently, in 1993, a high-density PTFE membrane (d-PTFE) was developed with pores smaller than 0.2 microns in diameter [36]. Research focused on d-PTFE has shown that surgical removal was easier for the d-PTFE membrane than for e-PTFE analogues, which could lead to fewer disruptions to the underlying tissue [12]. Due to its high density and micro-porosity, bacterial infiltration is much reduced [24]. Barber et al. reported that d-PTFE completely blocks the penetration of food and bacteria; thus, even if the membrane becomes exposed in the oral cavity, it maintains its functionality [37].

As both e-PTFE and d-PTFE had reduced mechanical stiffness, titanium mesh was introduced into their structure; this mesh or reinforcement is malleable for good adaptation to the receiving site [7]. Titanium-reinforced e-PTFE membranes have demonstrated higher space holding capacity and better stability than plain e-PTFE [38]. The Gore-Tex membrane (W.L. Gore & Associates, Flagstaff, AZ, USA), which is made of e-PTFE, has been widely used in clinical treatment and has become a first choice-material for GTR and GBR. It is also widely used for general surgery, neurosurgery and cardiovascular surgery [39].

2.3. Non-Absorbable Silk Membranes

Silk is a material produced by the *Bombyx mori* silkworm (*B. mori*). It is a natural biopolymer, composed mainly of fibroin and sericin [40]. Silk fibroin was used as a biomaterial after the removal of sericin [41]; it is a compound characterized by high capacity for biocompatibility and tissue integration [42]. Silk fibroin membranes can generate a favorable adhesion of osteogenic cells, favoring bone neo-formation [43]. The major disadvantage of these membranes is the difficult handling as well as the low mechanical properties [44,45].

An alternative to simple silk membranes is given by the silk pad; it is produced from the cocoon of silkworms by a simple peeling method [46]. The silk pad has a number of benefits; it has a higher tensile strength in wet conditions than collagen and/or d-PTFE membranes [47]. Moreover, the obtaining procedure is a simple one, and at a low cost [48]. In addition, the silk pad has a high amount of sericin, which promotes bone neoformation [49,50]; Ha et al. demonstrated, in an animal model study, a similar level of bone regeneration for the silk pad compared to collagen or d-PTFE membranes [47].

3. Absorbable Membranes

Absorbable (or second-generation) membranes were developed with the primary goal of avoiding the need for a second surgical time of guided regeneration for the barrier membrane removal from the site. Depending on the material from which the absorbable membrane is made, they can be of natural or synthetic origin (Table 2). In addition, absorbable membranes are characterized by lower costs than non-absorbable membranes, as well as reduced risks of complications [51,52]. Mechanical instability of absorbable membranes is a major disadvantage. Creating and maintaining the space needed for bone formation may be compromised; thus, it is recommended to associate the membranes with bone replacement material to fill the bone defect [12]. Moreover, membrane degradation products can affect the process of tissue regeneration [53]; in addition, there is a risk of cross-infection in membranes of animal origin [54].

3.1. Absorbable Membranes Made of Natural Polymers

The most commonly used natural polymers for barrier membranes are type I collagen and type III collagen. BioMend Membrane (Zimmer Biomet Dental, Warsaw, IN, USA) was the first collagen-based membrane produced for guided tissue and bone regeneration application. Natural collagen is obtained by a decellularization process followed by steps of removal of any antigenic components [55].

Sources for collagen include human skin (Alloderm®, LifeCell, Branchburg, NJ, USA), porcine skin (Bio-Gide®, Geistlich, Shirley, NY, USA), porcine peritoneum (MemGuide®, Ace, Boston, MA, USA) or Achilles' tendon (Cytoplast® RTM Collagen, Franklin Lakes, NJ, USA) [14,56]. After harvesting from the primary source, the product is subjected to decellularization, crosslinking and sterilization processes. The crosslinking treatment aims to increase the resistance of the membrane and can be achieved by different methods: UV irradiation or chemical processing. Glutaraldehyde, carbodiimide, hexamethylene diisocyanate, diphenyl-phosphoryl azide, formaldehyde or genipine can be used in chemical crosslinking [12,57]; other studies have also shown that crosslinking promoted prolonged biodegradation, reduced epithelial migration, decreased tissue integration and decreased vascularization [14,58].

The main concern related to the use of chemical agents is given by the potential toxic and inflammatory reactions produced in the recipient organism [59]. To overcome these disadvantages, other cross-linking agents with low cytotoxicity have been developed, such as (a) diphenylphosphorylazide, with biocompatibility and good handling characteristics, without cytotoxic effects [60]; (b) 1-ethyl-3-(3-dimethylaminopropyl) carbodiimide, with high resistance and low cytotoxicity [61] and (c) epigallocatechin-3-gallate, with better mechanical properties and anti-inflammatory effects [62].

Table 2. Types of absorbable barrier membranes.

Type				Commercial Variants	Absorption Time	Observations
Natural	Proteins	Collagen		BioGide®	24 weeks	From porcine dermis Composition: type I and III collagen
				Periogen®	4–8 weeks	
				RCM	26–38 weeks	
				BioMend®	6–8 weeks	From bovine tendon Composition: 100% type I collagen
				BioMend-Extend®	18 weeks	
				OSSIX®	6 months	
				Paroguide®	4–8 weeks	From calfskin Composition: 96% type I collagen, 4% chondroitin-4-sulfate
				Alloderm®	8–10 weeks	From human cadaver Composition: type I collagen
		Fibrin		Autologous	7–11 days	
				Etik-Patch®	4–6 weeks	Elastin and bovine fibrin with a polyglactin mesh
	Polysaccharides	Chitosan			16–20 weeks	
		Cellulose		Nanoskin®		
		Alginate				
		Agarose				
Synthetic	PGA/TMC			Resolut Adapt X®	16–24 weeks	
				Resolut Adapt LT®		
	PLA	Polylactic acid		Guidor®	10–12 weeks	
				Epi-guide®		
	PLA/PGA/TMC			Resolut Adapt®	8–10 weeks	

PGA: polyglactic acid; PLA: polylactic acid; TMC: trimethyl chitosan

Moreover, although crosslinked collagen membranes have prolonged degradation times, they also have significantly higher membrane exposure rates of up to 70.5% [63,64]. As already mentioned, premature exposure of membranes is often associated with bacterial invasion, as demonstrated by Becker [65].

Collagen membranes can perform hemostatic functions, allowing and stimulating the attachment and proliferation of fibroblasts and osteoblasts due to the presence of arginine-glycine-aspartic acid (Arg-Gly-Asp) and GFOGER sequences (glycine-phenylalanine-hydroxyproline-glycine-glycine) integrin-specific [66]; data suggest that cellular activity begins 3–5 days postoperatively [67]. At the same time, the membrane allows the signals from the cells associated with the membrane to be transferred to the cells in the bone defect, thus creating a favorable environment for bone neo-formation [68]. They can also be easily integrated with soft tissues and are permeable, so nutrient diffusion can be conducted easily [69,70].

There are data on the performance of non-crosslinked type I collagen membranes with non-absorbable PTFE membrane that claim that non-crosslinked collagen membranes promote a high rate of vascularization at two months postoperatively [71]. Other studies have compared the rate of bone formation of collagen membranes with e-PTFE membrane, both of which show similar results [26,72–74]; stromal cells attached to the collagen membrane promoted the production of fibroblast growth factor (FGF-2) and bone morphogenetic protein (BMP-2), stimulating bone regeneration. The influence of the use of collagen membrane in the regeneration of calvarial defects on Wistar rats was investigated; defects that were covered with collagen membranes demonstrated better bone regeneration than defects without membrane [75].

The resorption time differs for each membrane, from 8 to 38 weeks [76,77]. Accelerated resorption of the barrier membrane can compromise the success of surgery. In a study that looked at the degradation of uncoated collagen membranes, it was found that some membranes begin the resorption process in the first 8 h post-surgery [78].

Natural materials for making absorbable membranes include alginate and chitosan. Alginate is a dimeric polysaccharide with a structure composed of β-D-mannuronate and α-L-guluronate blocks. It is found in the walls of brown algae cells and in some bacterial capsules [79]. Alginate is biocompatible, non-toxic and does not cause inflammatory reactions, but has poor mechanical strength and adhesion. This material remains widely used in dentistry in impression techniques [80].

Chitosan is a copolymer of glucosamine and N-acetyl-D-glucosamine, produced from crustacean chitin [81]. Like alginate, it is a biocompatible and flexible material, the degree of resorption of which depends on its molecular weight [82]; membranes made of chitosan have demonstrated bacteriostatic properties [14] but, due to their fragility, are difficult to handle and to apply [83].

3.2. Absorbable Membranes of Synthetic Polymers

A stage in the development of membrane technologies was the artificial design of absorbable materials. These materials include biodegradable aliphatic polyesters: (a) polylactic acid (PLA); (b) polyglycolic acid (PGA) and (c) polycaprolactone (PCL) and their copolymers: poly-lactic-co-glycolic acid (PLGA) or poly-lactic-co-caprolactone acid (PLCL) [84,85]. PLA can be used alone or copolymerized with PGA. Polyester degradation is determined by hydrolysis and dependent on the hydrophobicity of the polymer [86]; PLA being more hydrophobic than PGA, degradation time is, thus, prolonged.

Aliphatic polyester membranes are bio-absorbable; the resorption of these membranes depends on the polyester types and ratio [87]. They also have good workability and maneuverability. Major disadvantages include lack of rigidity, stability but also concerns about the interactions of their degradation products with the recipient organism [88]; inflammatory reactions due to macrophages and leukocytes around the membrane were observed during absorption [89].

Improving mechanical properties using only biodegradable polyester can be difficult, which is why their main clinical indication is for small vertical bone defects, with the association of bone regeneration materials [12]. A combination of different porosity layers was proposed: the less porous side could act as a barrier, preventing epithelial cell infiltration, and the other side in contact with bone defect would allow tissue integration. Such techniques have been used in the Guidor Matrix Barrier (Sunstar Americas Inc., Schaumburg, IL, USA) and Resolut (W.L. Gore and Associates, Newark, DE, USA). Woven fibers technique (Vicryl Periodontal Mesh; Ethicon Inc., Cornelia, GA, USA), or polymer solution dissolved during the surgical procedure and molded in a cassette to form the Atrisorb membrane (Atrix Laboratories, Fort Collins, CO, USA) have also been adopted [55].

Poly-lactic-co-glycolic acid (PLGA) can be prepared in different copolymer forms depending on the ratio between PLA and PGA; its advantages include biocompatibility and biodegradability, and it is also easy to process [90]. Hoornaert et al. [91] developed a bi-layered PLGA membrane, composed of a dense, thin film that prevents the growth of epithelial cells and a thick, microfiber layer in order to stabilize the blood clot and promote cell colonization; the absorption rate was similar to the monolayer membrane of PLGA, but the rate of bone neo-formation was higher compared to the PLGA membrane [92]. Similar results were obtained by Abe et al. [93] with a bi-layered membrane from PLCL. The authors also observed that the two-layer PLCL membrane reduced bacterial adhesion and prevented bacterial invasion inside the membrane.

4. Enhanced Barrier Membranes

No polymer, natural or synthetic, seems to be sufficient alone. Therefore, the trends were either to combine materials or to enhance them with additives. New membranes have been developed, with additional functions such as the release of beneficial agents: antibiotics, growth factors and adhesion factors.

4.1. Membranes with Inorganic Compounds

In order to enhance the osteoconductive and osteoinductive effects, research has focused on the introduction into the structure of the barrier membrane of synthetic calcium phosphates (hydroxyapatite or β-tricalcium phosphate), single or combined in biphasic calcium phosphates. Such products allow vascular penetration, cell infiltration and attachment, cartilage formation and calcified tissue deposition [94,95]. Phipps et al. [95] showed that the membrane made of a mixture of particles of PCL, collagen and hydroxyapatite generated a rapid cell spread and a significant cell proliferation. Baek et al. [96] evaluated the effects of collagen membrane and a membrane of chitosan, fibroin and hydroxyapatite on calvarial defect in rats; the results were similar for both types of membranes, with the absence of inflammatory reactions [96].

Won et al. [97] compared the collagen membrane with a membrane made of PCL, PLGA and β-tricalcium phosphate; even if both membranes showed similar results in histological and histomorphometric analyses, the membrane made of PCL, PLGA and β-tricalcium phosphate generated a larger area of bone neo-formation [97].

Other studies have looked into potential effects of including zinc, magnesium, iron or strontium in the composition of the membrane. Zinc is an absolutely necessary mineral for skeletal growth and development [98], important in many physiological and metabolic processes [99]. The addition of ZnO in the structure of barrier membranes has generated improvements in the proliferation of osteoblasts, with an accelerated regenerative mechanism [100]; the use of zinc membranes has also demonstrated a faster healing process [101], as well as inhibiting the formation of bacterial biofilm [102,103]. In addition, Oh et al. [104] observed that PLA-Zn-bioactive glass membranes showed tensile strength, elongation and flexibility similar to those of zinc-free membranes [104].

Similar to zinc, magnesium is an important factor in bone metabolism, with both proliferative effects for osteoblasts and anti-osteoclastic effects [105]. The strength of the Mg alloy is higher than that of absorbable polymers, such as PLA; therefore, magnesium alloy can improve the mechanical properties of membranes. However, the rate of the degradation of magnesium alloy is too fast [106]. An in vitro study found that hydrofluoric acid coating can delay the corrosion of magnesium alloys [107]. Xin et al. [108] designed a barrier membrane made of PLA reinforced with a Mg alloy core, with a better loading capacity compared to membranes without Mg reinforcement; when fluorine-coated magnesium alloy was used, it showed better resistance to corrosion. The proliferation of fibroblasts and osteoblasts has also been easily achieved [109].

Strontium is involved in bone mineral metabolism by inducing osteogenesis, stimulating markers of differentiation and proliferation, and reducing apoptosis levels [109]. Kitayama et al. [110] studied the effect of covering rabbit calvarial defects with a collagen membrane with strontium and hydroxyapatite; after 24 weeks, they observed increased levels of newly mineralized bone and less residual grafting material compared to an unmodified collagen membrane [110].

Thus, membranes enhanced with inorganic compounds could offer a favorable alternative in GTR and GBR, but additional data are needed to optimize the protocols for the use of these membranes.

4.2. Membranes with Antimicrobial Factors

The inclusion of several antimicrobial substances, such as antibiotics or silver ions, has been investigated in the structure of barrier membranes. Metronidazole benzoate can be added to the layer in contact with the epithelial tissue, preventing bacterial adhesion and proliferation [111]. Favorable results of metronidazole supplementation were also obtained by Shi et al. [112] and Wang et al. [113]. Other studies have investigated the use of azithromycin [114], tetracyclines [115,116] or silver ions [117].

Techniques for loading silk fibroin with 4-hexylresorcinol have been developed; 4-hexylresorcinol is a natural phenolic compound, with antimicrobial, antioxidant and antimutagenic abilities [118]. Moreover, 4-hexylresorcinol has been shown to inhibit the pathways of nuclear factor-κB (NF-κB) [119], a molecule involved in osteoclast differentiation, with a resorptive role. Favorable results have been obtained in vivo and in other studies [120,121]. One of the obstacles to the practical applicability of these membranes is represented by their poor mechanical properties [45].

The disadvantages observed in the membranes with antimicrobial agents were the fact that most of them generally have a short release time of the drug; moreover, some periodontal tissue infections often occur after a relatively long period of time after surgery [112]. A number of studies have shown that the highest concentration of antibacterial substance is released in the first 3 days postoperatively, decreasing progressively in the following days and often becoming insufficient in situations of need [122–124]. Thus, the research focused on the development of techniques for making enriched membranes with slow and adequate release of microbial agent in order to prevent the so-called "waste" of the agent in unnecessary situations. Xue et al. [125] managed to extend the release time of the antimicrobial agent to 15 days, using fibers with encapsulated nanotubes that were loaded with metronidazole.

Trying to obtain the "release as needed" of metronidazole incorporated into the barrier membrane, Shi et al. [112] investigated the effects of esterified and grafted metronidazole on the surface of PCL nanofiber pads modified with ester bonds as a barrier membrane; ester bonds can be selectively hydrolyzed by cholesterol esterase. Cholesterol esterase is an enzyme secreted by macrophages accumulated at the site of infection, the concentration of which is positively related to the severity of the infection. Increased cholesterol esterase results in an increased release of metronidazole from the membrane, with antibacterial action [112].

One of the major problems with the use of membranes with antimicrobial agent is the risk of generating resistant bacterial species [126]; thus, there is an absolute need for clear guidelines and protocols for the use of such membranes.

4.3. Membranes with Growth Factors

Growth factors have been the subject of numerous studies, being included both in bone addition material and in the structure of barrier membranes. These factors include the group of bone morphogenetic proteins (BMP), stromal cell derived factor 1 alpha (SDF-1α), transforming growth factor beta (TGF-β), platelet-derived growth factor (PDGF), growth factor rich in platelets (PRGF) or fibroblast growth factor-2 (FGF-2) [55].

Bone morphogenetic proteins are among the most powerful osteoinductive proteins; they have modulatory effects on the differentiation and functionality of cells involved in bone formation [127]. Jones et al. [128] and Hsu et al. [129] investigated the treatment of ePTFE and titanium membranes, respectively, with BMP-2, both studies providing favorable data on new bone formation. One study reported beneficial results of BMP-9 incorporation into the collagen barrier membrane; BMP-9 stimulated alkaline phosphatase activity as well as osteoblastic gene expression [130].

A number of studies have shown that BMP-6 induces bone neo-formation, favoring bone augmentation procedures [8,131]. Gümüşderelioğlu et al. [127] developed a biodegradable chitosan membrane whose porous surface that comes in contact with the bone surface was enriched with hydroxyapatite and BMP-6; in order to improve the resistance of chitosan, the membrane was treated with glycerol solution. The authors concluded that this membrane demonstrated osteogenic activity and prevented the migration of epithelial cells [127]. In another study, Soran et al. [132] showed that the application of BMP-6 improved the osteoblastic differentiation of mesenchymal stem cells derived from bone marrow in vivo. A polymeric membrane loaded with BMP-6 on the hydroxyapatite coated membrane surface was patented (WO2016186594A1) [133], with the aim of providing memory and osteogenic activity, supporting bone regeneration, preventing epithelial cell migration and eliminating inflammation.

Incorporation of BMP-9 into the collagen membrane in vivo has also generated favorable results for bone neoformation in horizontal defects [134]. Shalumon et al. [135]

demonstrated favorable results regarding the differentiation of osteogenic cells in GTR therapies with chitosan-fibroin-hydroxyapatite membrane in which BMP was incorporated.

PDGF-enriched PLA membranes have been associated with improved regenerative effects [136,137]. Other studies investigating PLA membranes with TGF-β in alginate/nanofiber hybrid mesh have found effective regeneration in bone defects [138]. In another in vivo study, a six-fold increase in bone volume was observed when using a PCL/gelatin membrane enriched with SDF-1α compared to the use of titanium membrane [139].

Major disadvantages of growth factors supplementation in the structure of barrier membranes include the high production cost, but also the fact that the doses are usually over-physiological, with potential adverse effects [55,140].

5. Trends in the Development of Barrier Membranes

5.1. Amniotic and Chorionic Membranes

Amniotic and chorionic membranes are biological membranes, which means that they are bio-absorbable and compatible with tissues. The human placenta is essential in the development and survival of the fetus, ensuring physical and biological protection [141]. The amniotic membrane consists of a thick basal membrane and an avascular stromal matrix; this is the innermost layer of the placenta. Chorion forms the outer end of the sac and is made up of several types of collagen and bioactive components of cell adhesion [142]. Amniotic and chorionic membranes have been used in transplant surgery, proving healing, anti-inflammatory and antibacterial properties [143].

Membrane harvesting is usually done from healthy pregnant patients; caesarean section is preferred because vaginal birth placentas may be contaminated [141]. After harvesting, the collected placenta is placed in a sterile transport medium; to obtain the amniotic membrane, the amnion is separated from the underlying chorion along their natural plane of cleavage. Subsequently, the amniotic membrane is abundantly irrigated with a saline solution containing streptomycin, penicillin, neomycin and amphotericin prior to storage [143]. Methods of preserving the amniotic membrane include cryopreservation, lyophilization or air drying. Cryopreservation results in an improved retention of proteins and growth factors compared to lyophilization [144], but cryopreservation can affect the viability of cells in the amniotic membrane [145]. After lyophilization or air drying, it is necessary to sterilize the membrane with the help of gamma radiation [146] or with peracetic acid [147].

The amniotic membrane contains type IV, V and VI collagen as well as proteins (fibronectin, laminin, proteoglycans, glycosaminoglycans) [148]. The amniotic membrane contains laminin 5, a protein that stimulates the cell adhesion of gingival epithelial cells, collagen types I, II, IV, V and VI, platelet-derived growth factor, fibroblast growth factor and TGF-β [149]. Perlecan found in the amniotic membrane plays an important role in binding growth factors and interacts with various cell adhesion molecules [150].

Histologically, the chorionic membrane consists of three layers: reticulate, basal membrane and trophoblastic. Collagen types I, III, IV, V, VI and VII, as well as proteoglycans are found in the crosslinked layer; the basal membrane contains type IV collagen, fibronectin and laminin [151]. Inhibitors of matrix metalloproteinases have been identified in the chorion, factors that can inhibit inflammatory status and stop collagen degradation [152].

Given these aspects, amniotic and chorion structures offer potential for use as barrier membranes in GTR and GBR. Such membranes have antibacterial and antifungal properties, minimize wound inflammation and provide a protein-rich matrix that allows cells to migrate more easily [153]. Moreover, the harvesting technique is relatively simple; by hydration with the blood, the membrane becomes malleable [142]. Major limitations include the risk of cross-contamination, as well as their fragility [151].

Amniotic and chorionic membranes have been shown to be effective in bone neoformation in periodontal defects, on canine [154] and human [155] subjects. Venkatesan et al. used an amniotic membrane in combination with an alloplastic biphasic bone substitute

(60% hydroxyapatite, 40% tricalcium phosphate) to treat infrabony defects; this membrane generated similar results to porcine-derived collagen membrane in terms of postoperative healing and the amount of newly formed bone [155]. Holtzclaw et al. [156] used an amnio-chorionic membrane to treat infrabony defects, observing significant improvements of clinical parameters (probing depth and loss of periodontal clinical attachment) at 12 months [156]. Another study compared the effects of lyophilized amniotic membrane and collagen membrane on newly formed bone density; the bone density of defects treated with amniotic membrane was higher than the sites where no barrier membrane was used and equivalent to the density obtained with collagen membrane ($p < 0.05$) at 3 weeks [157].

The amniotic membrane has also been used successfully in periodontal muco-gingival surgery; the association of the amniotic membrane with repositioned flaps has generated favorable results in covering the gingival recessions and in increasing the thickness of the attached gingiva [158,159].

An amniotic membrane with different potential areas of use was patented (US6326019B1) [160], but its usage was directed mainly in skin and mucosal grafting. Actishield™ (Wright Medical, Memphis, TN, USA) was also developed, but with main indication for orthopedic surgery. Up to date, there is no approved commercial amniotic/chorionic membrane for periodontal tissue regeneration. Nevertheless, in all types of membranes, Quality by Design principles and regulations have been introduced in order to obtain benefits of an integrated and risk-free approach to the industrialization process in membranes manufacturing [55].

5.2. Barrier Membranes from PRF

Platelet concentrates have been a research topic for more than 20 years; platelet-rich plasma, discovered in the late 1990s, was the result of centrifugation of blood harvested on the spot from the patient, offering good advantages in oral and maxillofacial surgery [161]. This procedure, on the other hand, had disadvantages related to the use of anticoagulants that could interfere with the healing process. Subsequently, a new product without anticoagulant was developed, platelet-rich fibrin (PRF). PRF has been shown to significantly increase the potential for tissue regeneration, favoring the slow and gradual release of growth factors trapped in its fibrin matrix [162].

PRP has been used primarily for soft tissue regeneration rather than osteogenesis and requires more blood than PRF. PRP is centrifuged at a higher rate, causing all heavy white blood cells and stem cells to sink to the base of the tube, not being collected in the sample [163]. Further research has found that a higher platelet concentration with the inclusion of white blood cells and stem cells in the sample would be even more therapeutic. The inclusion of white blood cells helped prevent postoperative infection, and the presence of stem cells generated an obvious capacity for regeneration. PRF is centrifuged at a slower rate, which causes a higher concentration of white blood cells, stem cells and platelets to remain in the middle plasma layer. Thus, PRF has a platelet concentration almost double that of blood. Platelets are involved in the release of growth and clotting factors. If the release of the growth factor occurs rapidly in the case of PRP, it is slow for PRF, with an average duration of 7–10 days postoperatively [164].

Lekovic et al. [165] investigated the association of PRF with bovine xenograft in filling periodontal infrabony defects in patients with bilateral defects, evaluating treatment with PRF alone or with PRF combined with bovine bone. Results after 6 months were more favorable when PRF was combined with bovine bone; they noticed a decrease in probing depth and gains in periodontal attachment and bone height. Lekovic et al. concluded that increased efficacy during bone defect regeneration treatment is achieved by the combination of PRF and xenograft, rather than by PRF alone [165]. Mathur et al. [166] compared the efficacy of PRF and autologous bone graft to increase attachment and reduce infrabony defects. Subjects showed infrabony defects that were treated with either an access flap associated with PRF or an access flap supplemented with an autologous bone graft; the third control group followed only the access flap procedure. Plaque index, the gingival index, the loss of attachment, the gingival recession and the depth of the periodontal pockets were analyzed on the day of surgery and 9 months later. The use of PRF had a more efficient result than the access flap alone, but the combination of the regenerating material allowed for obtaining an even more efficient treatment [166].

PRF has also proven effective in treating gingival recessions. Anilkumar et al. [167] compared PRF and connective tissue grafting with lateral repositioned flap to cover Miller class II recessions. Recession coverage was complete for 91% of patients treated with PRF, compared with 66% for those treated with a connective graft [167]. Jankovic et al. [168], in a treatment of Miller class I or II recessions, compared the results of the use of PRF membranes and connective tissue graft, combined with coronally repositioned flaps and connective tissue graft. The parameters studied were the size of the recession, attachment gain, the height of the keratinized gingiva, the pocket depth, the quality and speed of wound healing and the patient's discomfort; clinical parameters were evaluated at baseline and after 12 months. The results were similar between the use of a PRF membrane and a connective graft. The authors noted that although the amount of acquired keratinized tissue is higher with the connective graft, PRF provided better healing and less discomfort to the patient [168]. Thus, PRF may be an interesting, effective and relatively low-cost option, but further studies are needed on larger study groups in order to establish accurate protocols.

5.3. 3D Printed Membranes

Three-dimensional printing aims to generate an individualized 3D object, according to a design developed by software (computer aided design—CAD), by depositing the chosen material layer by layer. Three-dimensional technology already has applications in various fields, such as the production of anatomical models and surgical guides or regenerative medicine. There are multiple methods of 3D printing, including fusion deposition modeling (FDM), stereolithography (SLA) or selective laser sintering (SLS), but FDM remains the technique of choice for bioprinting [169]. The biomaterials used include hydrogels in combination with living cells and/or growth factors, natural and synthetic bioplastics, proteins, polymer biomolecules and ceramics [170].

Natural biomaterials used in 3D printing techniques include collagen, agarose, alginate, chitosan, silk, gelatin, cellulose, hyaluronic acid and fibrin [171], and synthetic biomaterials include PLA, PGA, PLGA and PCL [172,173]. Decellularized matrix components containing both conserved cellular elements and specific signaling factors of high importance in regenerative processes can also be used, because the latter can guide the cells of the resident tissue or provide the host cells with the necessary instructions for tissue regeneration [174].

Tayebi et al. tested a 3D-printed membrane of sodium elastin/gelatin/hyaluronate in vitro; the membrane has shown good mechanical properties as well as a stimulation of fibroblast proliferation [10]. Bai et al. [175] developed an individualized membrane with 3D-printed titanium mesh; various types of titanium mesh designed with different diameters, and thicknesses were tested based on their mechanical strength by a three-point bending test and FEA. According to the authors, the mechanical properties of the titanium mesh increased when the thickness decreased (0.5 mm to 0.3 mm); by increasing mesh diameter (3 mm to 5 mm), the mechanical properties of the mesh decreased [175].

A time dimension was added to 3D technology, with the appearance of being 4D; 3D printed construction thus changes, resulting in a transition in shape, structure and function [176]. This technology is based on intelligent biomaterials that have the ability to undergo changes as a result of exposure to various stimuli (temperature, pH, humidity, electric or magnetic fields, light, sound or a combination thereof) [177]. Thus, 4D bioprinting offers new directions for the development of tissue reconstruction techniques.

6. Allergological Considerations

The most common allergic reactions to various implants, reported in the literature, were with nickel, cobalt and even titanium, although the latter has a high biocompatibility [178]. The titanium test was patch-type and was conducted later and not before the implant. Authors who tried a lymphoblastic transformation test (LLT) are cited, but did not have success. However, these reactions are very rare [108].

The implantation of biomembranes can give two types of reactions: type I reactions (non IgE dependent) and IV (delayed type). A type I immune-allergic reaction is manifested by immediate angioedema and type IV by late reactions, which occur after a few days, even weeks, from the implant [179].

Regarding biological biomembranes (platelet concentrate, amniotic and chorionic concentrate) the high risk is rejection, as well as type IV reactions, such as contact dermatitis or mucositis, due to the additives with which they are impregnated, and which have been previously described [180].

Prophylactic testing would not be indicated, as it has no real clinical predictive benefit. Especially in the case of titanium, the time of penetration into the tissues is long. If the patient develops an immediate allergic reaction, which occurs in a few minutes, it would require a prior sensitization of the patient so that he already has cellular memory, with a specific IgE dosage, such as the situation of another implant, and not necessarily in the dental field or for the patient to work in an industry that uses titanium or other metals invoked in biomembranes. Type IV reactions would occur within weeks or even 2 months after membrane insertion.

The only test that would be eloquent is the patch test (with reading at 30 min, 1 h, 24 h, 72 h and 7 days), but only if after the placement of these membranes the suspicion of an allergic reaction arises. Additionally, if the reaction is not severe, such as anaphylactic shock, difficult to control generalized urticaria, or a Stevens Johnson-type reaction, it would be worthwhile to treat the reaction and keep the membrane in place, even if the test is positive.

What is the profile of a risk patient? This is best illustrated by the patient who has had an implant, such as knee, hip, etc., the patient who works in industries that handle these materials and may associate contact dermatitis and, practically, a patient who could have been professionally sensitized prior to a dental implant.

Would immunosuppressive treatment be justified or not, in the case of these delayed type allergic reaction implants? This might depend on the severity of the periodontal disease, the severity of the rejection reaction and the patient's choice (since these implants are not cheap and the immunosuppressive therapy might not be subsidized by the state in this situation).

7. Conclusions

There is a wide range of technologies and materials used in guided tissue regeneration, some of which are still in the in vitro or in vivo testing phase. The use of the barrier membrane associated with bone grafting materials has shown better results than its single use. Further studies are needed to develop treatment algorithms and protocols to obtain predictable, case-specific regenerative results. In order to respond to our aim, it is more than clear that the perfect barrier membrane is not quite here, but the choice of the most appropriate membrane relies on the particular case, as well as on the medical experience of the operator.

Author Contributions: Conceptualization, S.-M.S. and C.S.S.; methodology, S.-M.S., C.S.S. and S.T.; validation, S.-M.S., I.-G.S. and C.S.S.; formal analysis, I.-G.S., S.T. and C.M.G.; investigation, I.-G.S., S.T. and C.M.G.; resources, S.-M.S. and C.S.S.; data curation, I.-G.S., S.T., C.M.G.; writing—original draft preparation, I.-G.S., C.S.S. and C.M.G.; writing—review and editing, S.-M.S., C.M.G. and S.T.; visualization, S.-M.S.; supervision, S.-M.S. and C.S.S.; project administration, C.S.S. All authors have read and agreed to the published version of the manuscript.

Funding: This research received no external funding.

Institutional Review Board Statement: Not applicable.

Informed Consent Statement: Not applicable.

Conflicts of Interest: The authors declare no conflict of interest.

References

1. Cheng, X.; Yang, F. More than just a barrier-challenges in the development of guided bone regeneration membranes. *Matter* **2019**, *1*, 550–644. [CrossRef]
2. Trombelli, L.; Heitz-Mayfield, L.; Needleman, I.; Moles, D.; Scabbia, A. A systematic review of graft materials and biological agents for periodontal intraosseous defects. *J. Clin. Periodontol.* **2002**, *29* (Suppl. S3), 117–135. [CrossRef] [PubMed]
3. Murphy, K.G.; Gunsolley, J.C. Guided tissue regeneration for the treatment of periodontal intrabony and furcation defects. A systematic review. *Ann. Periodontol.* **2003**, *8*, 266–302. [CrossRef]
4. Needleman, I.G.; Worthington, H.V.; Giedrys-Leeper, E.; Tucker, R.J. Guided tissue regeneration for periodontal infra-bony defects. *Cochrane Database Syst. Rev.* **2006**, *19*, CD001724. [CrossRef]
5. Wang, H.L.; Boyapati, L. "PASS" principles for predictable bone regeneration. *Implant. Dent.* **2006**, *15*, 8–17. [CrossRef] [PubMed]
6. Melcher, A.H. On the repair potential of periodontal tissues. *J. Periodontol.* **1976**, *47*, 256–260. [CrossRef] [PubMed]
7. Liu, J.; Kerns, D.G. Mechanisms of guided bone regeneration: A review. *Open Dent. J.* **2014**, *8*, 56–65. [CrossRef]
8. Caballe-Serano, J.; Abdeslam-Mohammed, Y.; Munar-Frau, A.; Fujioka-Kobayashi, M.; Hernandez-Alfaro, F.; Miron, R. Adsorption and release kinetics of growth factors on barrier membranes for guided tissue/bone regeneration: A systematic review. *Arch. Oral Biol.* **2019**, *100*, 57–68. [CrossRef]
9. Sanz, M.; Dahlin, C.; Apatzidou, D.; Artzi, Z.; Bozic, D.; Calciolari, E.; De Bruyn, H.; Dommisch, H.; Donos, N.; Eickholz, P.; et al. Biomaterials and regenerative technologies used in bone regeneration in the craniomaxillofacial region: Consensus report of group 2 of the 15th European Workshop on Periodontology on Bone Regeneration. *J. Clin. Periodontol.* **2019**, *46*, 82–91. [CrossRef]
10. Tayebi, L.; Rasoulianboroujeni, M.; Moharamzadeh, K.; Almela, T.K.D.; Cui, Z.; Ye, H. 3D-printed membrane for guided tissue regeneration. *Mater. Sci. Eng. C Mater. Biol. Appl.* **2018**, *84*, 148–158. [CrossRef]
11. Dimitriou, R.; Mataliotakis, G.I.; Calori, G.M.; Giannoudis, P.V. The role of barrier membranes for guided bone regeneration and restoration of large bone defects: Current experimental and clinical evidence. *BMC Med.* **2012**, *10*, 81. [CrossRef] [PubMed]
12. Sasaki, J.I.; Abe, G.L.; Aonan, L.; Thongthai, P.; Tsuboi, R.; Kohno, T.; Imazato, S. Barrier membranes for tissue regeneration in dentistry. *Biomater. Investig. Dent.* **2021**, *8*, 54–63. [CrossRef] [PubMed]
13. Kaushal, S.; Kumar, A.; Khan, M.A.; Lal, N. Comparative study of nonabsorbable and absorbable barrier membranes in periodontal osseous defects by guided tissue regeneration. *J. Oral Biol. Craniofac. Res.* **2016**, *6*, 111–117. [CrossRef] [PubMed]
14. Lee, H.S.; Byun, S.H.; Cho, S.W.; Yang, B.E. Past, present, and future of regeneration therapy in oral and periodontal tissue: A review. *Appl. Sci.* **2019**, *9*, 1046. [CrossRef]
15. Soldatos, N.K.; Stylianou, P.; Koidou, V.P.; Angelov, N.; Yukna, R.; Romanos, G.E. Limitations and options using resorbable versus nonresorbable membranes for successful guided bone regeneration. *Quintessence Int.* **2017**, *48*, 131–147. [PubMed]
16. Wadhawan, A.; Gowda, T.M.; Mehta, D.S. Gore-tex® versus resolut adapt® GTR membranes with perioglas® in periodontal regeneration. *Contemp. Clin. Dent.* **2012**, *3*, 406–411. [CrossRef]
17. Machtei, E.E. The effect of membrane exposure on the outcome of regenerative procedures in humans: A meta-analysis. *J. Periodontol.* **2001**, *72*, 512–516. [CrossRef] [PubMed]
18. Verardi, S.; Simion, M. Management of the exposure of e-PTFE membranes in guided bone regeneration. *Pract. Proced. Aesthetic Dent.* **2007**, *19*, 111–117.
19. Ottria, L.; Lauritano, D.; Andreasi, B.M.; Palmieri, A.; Candotto, V.; Tagliabue, A.; Tettamanti, L. Mechanical, chemical and biological aspects of titanium and titanium alloys in implant dentistry. *J. Biol. Regul. Homeost. Agents* **2018**, *32*, 81–90.
20. Hanawa, T. Titanium-tissue interface reaction and its control with surface treatment. *Front. Bioeng. Biotechnol.* **2019**, *17*, 170. [CrossRef]
21. Hasegawa, H.; Masui, S.; Ishihata, H. New microperforated pure titanium membrane created by laser processing for guided regeneration of bone. *Br. J. Oral Maxillofac. Surg.* **2018**, *56*, 642–643. [CrossRef]
22. Wong, C. Guided Tissue Regeneration with Ultra-ti Titanium Membrane. 2003. Available online: http://www.oralimplant.orghk/newsletter/8no3.html (accessed on 20 December 2021).
23. Khanna, R.; Khanna, R.; Pardhe, N.D.; Srivastava, N.; Bajpai, M.; Gupta, S. Pure titanium (Ultra–Ti) in the treatment of periodontal osseous defects: A split-mouth comparative study. *J. Clin. Diagn. Res.* **2016**, *10*, ZC47–ZC51. [CrossRef]
24. Rakhmatia, Y.D.; Ayukawa, Y.; Furuhashi, A.; Koyano, K. Current barrier membranes: Titanium mesh and other membranes for guided bone regeneration in dental applications. *J. Prosthodont. Res.* **2013**, *57*, 3–14. [CrossRef]
25. Her, S.; Kang, T.; Fien, M.J. Titanium mesh as an alternative to a membrane for ridge augmentation. *J. Oral Maxillofac. Surg.* **2012**, *70*, 803–810. [CrossRef]
26. Zitzmann, N.U.; Naef, R.; Scharer, P. Resorbable versus nonresorbable membranes in combination with Bio-Oss for guided bone regeneration. *Int. J. Oral Maxillofac. Implant.* **1997**, *12*, 844–852.
27. Weng, D.; Hurzeler, M.B.; Quinones, C.R. Contribution of the periosteum to bone formation in guided bone regeneration. *Clin. Oral Implant. Res.* **2000**, *11*, 546–554. [CrossRef]
28. Shanaman, R.; Filstein, M.R.; Danesh-Meyer, M.J. Localized ridge augmentation using GBR and platelet-rich plasma: Case reports. *Int. J. Periodont. Restor. Dent.* **2001**, *21*, 345–355.

29. Celletti, R.; Davarpanah, M.; Etienne, D.; Pecora, G.; Tecucianu, J.F.; Djukanovic, D.; Donath, K. Guided tissue regeneration around dental implants in immediate extraction sockets: Comparison of e-PTFE and a new titanium membrane. *Int. J. Periodontics Restor. Dent.* **1994**, *14*, 243–253.
30. Watzinger, F.; Luksch, J.; Millesi, W. Guided bone regeneration with titanium membranes: A clinical study. *Br. J. Oral Maxillofac. Surg.* **2000**, *38*, 312–315. [CrossRef] [PubMed]
31. Briguglio, F.; Falcomata, D.; Marconcini, S.; Fiorillo, L.; Briguglio, R.; Farronato, D. The use of titanium mesh in guided bone regeneration: A systematic review. *Int. J. Dent.* **2019**, *2019*, 9065423. [CrossRef] [PubMed]
32. Louis, P.J.; Gutta, R.; Said-Al-Naief, N.; Bartolucci, A.A. Reconstruction of the maxilla and mandible with particulate bone graft and titanium mesh for implant placement. *J. Oral Maxillofac. Surg.* **2008**, *66*, 235–245. [CrossRef]
33. Maiorana, C.; Santoro, F.; Rabagliati, M.; Salina, S. Evaluation of the use of iliac cancellous bone and anorganic bovine bone in the reconstruction of the atrophic maxilla with titanium mesh: A clinical and histologic investigation. *Int. J. Oral Maxillofac. Implant.* **2001**, *16*, 427–432.
34. Corinaldesi, G.; Pieri, F.; Sapigni, L.; Marchetti, C. Evaluation of survival and success rates of dental implants placed at the time of or after alveolar ridge augmentation with an autogenous mandibular bone graft and titanium mesh: A 3- to 8-year retrospective study. *Int. J. Oral Maxillofac. Implant.* **2009**, *24*, 1119–1128.
35. Miyamoto, I.; Funaki, K.; Yamauchi, K.; Kodama, T.; Takahashi, T. Alveolar ridge reconstruction with titanium mesh and autogenous particulate bone graft: Computed tomography-based evaluations of augmented bone quality and quantity. *Clin. Implant. Dent. Relat. Res.* **2011**, *14*, 304–311. [CrossRef] [PubMed]
36. Madhuri, S.V. Membranes for Periodontal Regeneration. *Int. J. Pharm. Sci. Invent.* **2016**, *5*, 19–24.
37. Barber, H.D.; Lignelli, J.; Smith, B.M.; Bartee, B.K. Using dense PTFE membrane without primary closure to achieve bone and tissue regeneration. *J. Oral Maxillofac. Surg.* **2007**, *65*, 748–752. [CrossRef]
38. Canullo, L.; Malagnino, V.A. Vertical ridge augmentation around implants by e-PTFE titanium- reinforced membrane and bovine bone matrix: A 24- to 54-month study of 10 consecutive cases. *Int. J. Oral Maxillofac. Implant.* **2008**, *23*, 858–866.
39. Lee, J.Y.; Kim, Y.K.; Yun, P.Y.; Oh, J.S.; Kim, S.G. Guided bone regeneration using two types of non-resorbable barrier membranes. *J. Korean Assoc. Oral Maxillofac. Surg.* **2010**, *36*, 275–279. [CrossRef]
40. Cao, Y.; Wang, B. Biodegradation of silk biomaterials. *Int. J. Mol. Sci.* **2009**, *10*, 1514–1524. [CrossRef]
41. Khan, M.M.R.; Tsukada, M.; Gotoh, Y.; Morikawa, H.; Freddi, G.; Shiozaki, H. Physical properties and dyeability of silk fibers degummed with citric acid. *Bioresour. Technol.* **2010**, *101*, 8439–8445. [CrossRef]
42. Vepari, C.; Kaplan, D.L. Silk as a biomaterial. *Prog. Polym. Sci.* **2007**, *32*, 991–1007. [CrossRef]
43. Yoo, C.K.; Jeon, J.Y.; Kim, Y.J.; Kim, S.G.; Hwang, K.G. Cell attachment and proliferation of osteoblast-like mg63 cells on silk fibroin membrane for guided bone regeneration. *Maxillofac. Plast. Reconstr. Surg.* **2016**, *38*, 17. [CrossRef]
44. Song, J.Y.; Kim, S.G.; Lee, J.W.; Chae, W.S.; Kweon, H.; Jo, Y.Y.; Lee, K.G.; Lee, Y.C.; Choi, J.Y.; Kim, J.Y. Accelerated healing with the use of a silk fibroin membrane for the guided bone regeneration technique. *Oral Surg. Oral Med. Oral Pathol. Oral Radiol.* **2011**, *112*, e26–e33. [CrossRef] [PubMed]
45. Kwon, K.J.; Seok, H. Silk protein-based membrane for guided bone regeneration. *Appl. Sci.* **2018**, *8*, 1214. [CrossRef]
46. Jo, Y.Y.; Kweon, H.Y.; Kim, D.W.; Baek, K.; Kim, M.K.; Kim, S.G.; Chae, W.S.; Choi, J.Y.; Rotaru, H. Bone regeneration is associated with the concentration of tumour necrosis factor-alpha induced by sericin released from a silk mat. *Sci. Rep.* **2017**, *7*, 15589. [CrossRef] [PubMed]
47. Ha, Y.Y.; Park, Y.W.; Kweon, H.; Jo, Y.Y.; Kim, S.G. Comparison of the physical properties and in vivo bioactivities of silkworm-cocoon-derived silk membrane, collagen membrane, and polytetrafluoroethylene membrane for guided bone regeneration. *Macromol. Res.* **2014**, *22*, 1018–1023. [CrossRef]
48. Kweon, H.Y.; Jo, Y.Y.; Seok, H.; Kim, S.G.; Chae, W.S.; Sapru, S.; Kundu, S.; Kim, D.W.; Park, N.R.; Xiangguo, C.; et al. In vivo bone regeneration ability of different layers of natural silk cocoon processed using an eco-friendly method. *Macromol. Res.* **2017**, *25*, 806–816. [CrossRef]
49. Nayak, S.; Dey, T.; Naskar, D.; Kundu, S.C. The promotion of osseointegration of titanium surfaces by coating with silk protein sericin. *Biomaterials* **2013**, *34*, 2855–2864. [CrossRef] [PubMed]
50. Jo, Y.Y.; Oh, J.H. New resorbable membrane materials for guided bone regeneration. *Appl. Sci.* **2018**, *8*, 2157. [CrossRef]
51. Bottino, M.C.; Pankajakshan, D.; Nor, J.E. Advanced scaffolds for dental pulp and periodontal regeneration. *Dent. Clin. N. Am.* **2017**, *61*, 689–711. [CrossRef]
52. Eliaz, N. Corrosion of metallic biomaterials: A review. *Materials* **2019**, *12*, 407. [CrossRef] [PubMed]
53. Hoogeveen, E.J.; Gielkens, P.F.; Schortinghuis, J.; Ruben, J.L.; Huysmans, M.C.D.J.M.; Stegenga, B. Vivosorb as a barrier membrane in rat mandibular defects. An evaluation with transversal microradiography. *Int. J. Oral Maxillofac. Surg.* **2009**, *38*, 870–875. [CrossRef] [PubMed]
54. Wang, J.; Wang, L.; Zhou, Z.; Lai, H.; Xu, P.; Liao, L.; Wei, J. Biodegradable polymer membranes applied in guided bone/tissue regeneration. A review. *Polymers* **2016**, *8*, 115. [CrossRef] [PubMed]
55. Aprile, P.; Letourneur, D.; Simon-Yarza, T. Membranes for guided bone regeneration: A road from bench to bedside. *Adv. Healthc. Mater.* **2020**, *9*, 2000707. [CrossRef] [PubMed]

56. Felipe, M.E.M.; Andrade, P.F.; Grisi, M.F.; Souza, S.L.; Taba, M., Jr.; Palioto, D.B.; Novaes, A.B., Jr. Comparison of two surgical procedures for use of the acellular dermal matrix graft in the treatment of gingival recession: A randomized controlled clinical study. *J. Periodontol.* **2007**, *78*, 1209–1217. [CrossRef]
57. Sbricoli, L.; Guazzo, R.; Annunziata, M.; Gobbato, L.; Bressan, E.; Nastri, L. Selection of collagen membranes for bone regeneration: A literature review. *Materials* **2020**, *13*, 786. [CrossRef] [PubMed]
58. Schwarz, F.; Rothamel, D.; Herten, M.; Sager, M.; Becker, J. Angiogenesis pattern of native and cross-linked collagen membranes: An immunohistochemical study in the rat. *Clin. Oral Implant. Res.* **2006**, *17*, 403–409. [CrossRef] [PubMed]
59. Ferreira, A.M.; Gentile, P.; Chiono, V.; Ciardelli, G. Collagen for bone tissue regeneration. *Acta Biomater.* **2012**, *8*, 3191–3200. [CrossRef]
60. Zahedi, C.S.; Miremadi, S.A.; Brunel, G.; Rompen, E.; Bernard, J.P.; Benque, E. Guided tissue regeneration in human Class II furcation defects using a diphenylphosphorylazide-cross-linked collagen membrane: A consecutive case series. *J. Periodontol.* **2003**, *74*, 1071–1079. [CrossRef]
61. Park, J.Y.; Jung, I.H.; Kim, Y.K.; Lim, H.C.; Lee, J.S.; Jung, U.W.; Choi, S.H. Guided bone regeneration using 1-ethyl-3-(3-dimethylaminopropyl) carbodiimide (EDC)-cross-linked type-I collagen membrane with biphasic calcium phosphate at rabbit calvarial defects. *Biomater. Res.* **2015**, *19*, 15. [CrossRef]
62. Chu, C.; Deng, J.; Hou, Y.; Xiang, L.; Wu, Y.; Qu, Y.; Man, Y. Application of PEG and EGCG modified collagen-base membrane to promote osteoblasts proliferation. *Mater. Sci. Eng. C Mater. Biol. Appl.* **2017**, *76*, 31–36. [CrossRef] [PubMed]
63. Friedmann, A.; Gissel, K.; Soudan, M.; Kleber, B.M.; Pitaru, S.; Dietrich, T. Randomized controlled trial on lateral augmentation using two collagen membranes: Morphometric results on mineralized tissue compound. *J. Clin. Periodontol.* **2011**, *38*, 677–685. [CrossRef]
64. Bouguezzi, A.; Debibi, A.; Chokri, A.; Sioud, S.; Hentati, H.; Selmi, J. Cross-linked versus Natural Collagen Membrane for Guided Bone Regeneration? A Literature Review. *Am. J. Med. Biol. Res.* **2020**, *8*, 12–16.
65. Becker, J.; Al-Nawas, B.; Klein, M.O.; Schliephake, H.; Terheyden, H.; Schwarz, F. Use of a new cross-linked collagen membrane for the treatment of dehiscence-type defects at titanium implants: A prospective, randomized-controlled double blinded clinical multicenterstudy. *Clin. Oral Implant. Res.* **2009**, *20*, 742–749. [CrossRef] [PubMed]
66. Sun, D.; Song, B.; Sun, D. Cytocompatibility of collagen membranes with bladder transitional cells of rabbit in vitro. *Zhongguo Xiu Fu Chong Jian Wai Ke Za Zhi* **2004**, *18*, 217–219. [PubMed]
67. Pokrywczynska, M.; Jundzill, A.; Rasmus, M.; Adamowicz, J.; Balcerczyk, D.; Buhl, M.; Warda, K.; Buchholl, L.; Gagat, M.; Grzanka, D.; et al. Understanding the role of mesenchymal stem cells in urinary bladder regeneration-a preclinical study on a porcine model. *Stem Cell Res. Ther.* **2018**, *9*, 328. [CrossRef] [PubMed]
68. Omar, O.; Elgali, I.; Dahlin, C.; Thomsen, P. Barrier membranes: More than the barrier effect? *J. Clin. Periodontol.* **2019**, *46*, 103–123. [CrossRef]
69. Kirpatovskii, V.I.; Efimenko, A.Y.; Sysoeva, V.Y.; Mudraya, I.S.; Kamalov, D.M.; Akopyan, Z.A.; Kamalov, A.A. Collagen-1 membrane for replacing the bladder wall. *Bull. Exp. Biol. Med.* **2016**, *162*, 102–106. [CrossRef]
70. Brum, I.S.; Elias, C.N.; de Carvalho, J.J.; Pires, J.L.S.; Pereira, M.J.S.; de Biasi, R.S. Properties of a bovine collagen type I membrane for guided bone regeneration applications. *e-Polymers* **2021**, *21*, 210–221. [CrossRef]
71. Ghanaati, S. Non-cross-linked porcine-based collagen I–III membranes do not require high vascularization rates for their integration within the implantation bed: A paradigm shift. *Acta Biomater.* **2012**, *8*, 3061–3072. [CrossRef]
72. Bunyaratavej, P.; Wang, H.L. Collagen membranes: A review. *J. Periodontol.* **2001**, *72*, 215–229. [CrossRef] [PubMed]
73. Turri, A.; Elgali, I.; Vazirisani, F.; Johansson, A.; Emanuelsson, L.; Dahlin, C.; Thomsen, P.; Omar, O. Guided bone regeneration is promoted by the molecular events in the membrane compartment. *Biomaterials* **2016**, *84*, 167–183. [CrossRef]
74. Gueldenpfennig, T.; Houshmand, A.; Najman, S.; Stojanovic, S.; Korzinskas, T.; Smeets, R.; Gosau, M.; Pissarek, J.; Emmert, S.; Jung, O.; et al. The condensation of collagen leads to an extended standing time and a decreased pro-inflammatory tissue response to a newly developed pericardiumbased barrier membrane for guided bone regeneration. *In Vivo* **2020**, *34*, 985–1000. [CrossRef] [PubMed]
75. Fadel, R.A.; Samarani, R.; Chakar, C. Guided bone regeneration in calvarial critical size bony defect using a double-layer resorbable collagen membrane covering a xenograft: A histological and histomorphometric study in rats. *Oral Maxillofac. Surg.* **2018**, *22*, 203–213. [CrossRef]
76. Raz, P.; Brosh, T.; Ronen, G.; Tal, H. Tensile properties of three selected collagen membranes. *BioMed Res. Int.* **2019**, *2019*, 5163603. [CrossRef] [PubMed]
77. Roca-Millan, E.; Jané-Salas, E.; Estrugo-Devesa, A.; López-López, J. Evaluation of bone gain and complication rates after guided bone regeneration with titanium foils: A systematic review. *Materials* **2020**, *13*, 5346. [CrossRef]
78. Toledano, M.; Asady, S.; Toledano-Osorio, M.; García-Godoy, F.; Serrera-Figallo, M.A.; Benítez-García, J.A.; Osorio, R. Differential biodegradation kinetics of collagen membranes for bone regeneration. *Polymers* **2020**, *12*, 1290. [CrossRef]
79. Draget, K.I.; Smidsrød, O.; Skjåk-Bræk, G. Alginates from Algae. In *Biopolymers Online*; Steinbüchel, A., Ed.; Wiley-VCH Verlag GmbH & Co. KGaA: Weinheim, Germany, 2005.
80. Catoira, M.C.; Fusaro, L.; Di Francesco, D.; Ramella, M.; Boccafoschi, F. Overview of natural hydrogels for regenerative medicine applications. *J. Mater. Sci. Mater. Med.* **2019**, *30*, 115. [CrossRef] [PubMed]

81. Tharanathan, R.N.; Kittur, F.S. Chitin–the undisputed biomolecule of great potential. *Crit. Rev. Food Sci. Nutr.* **2003**, *43*, 61–87. [CrossRef]
82. Lauritano, D.; Limongelli, L.; Moreo, G.; Favia, G.; Carinci, F. Nanomaterials for periodontal tissue engineering: Chitosan-based scaffolds. A systematic review. *Nanomaterials* **2020**, *10*, 605. [CrossRef]
83. Shah, A.T.; Zahid, S.; Ikram, F.; Maqbool, M.; Chaudhry, A.A.; Rahim, M.I.; Schmidt, F.; Goerke, O.; Khan, A.S.; Rehman, I.U. Tri-layered functionally graded membrane for potential application in periodontal regeneration. *Mater. Sci. Eng. C Mater. Biol. Appl.* **2019**, *103*, 109812. [CrossRef] [PubMed]
84. Annunziata, M.; Nastri, L.; Cecoro, G.; Guida, L. The use of Poly-d,l-lactic acid (PDLLA) devices for bone augmentation techniques: A systematic review. *Molecules* **2017**, *22*, 2214. [CrossRef] [PubMed]
85. Yoshimoto, I.; Sasaki, J.I.; Tsuboi, R.; Yamaguchi, S.; Kitagawa, H.; Imazato, S. Development of layered PLGA membranes for periodontal tissue regeneration. *Dent. Mater.* **2018**, *34*, 538–550. [CrossRef]
86. Woodard, L.N.; Grunlan, M.A. Hydrolytic degradation and erosion of polyester biomaterials. *ACS Macro Lett.* **2018**, *7*, 976–982. [CrossRef]
87. Zamboulis, A.; Nakiou, E.A.; Christodoulou, E.; Bikiaris, D.N.; Kontonasaki, E.; Liverani, L.; Boccaccini, A.R. Polyglycerol hyperbranched polyesters: Synthesis, properties and pharmaceutical and biomedical applications. *Int. J. Mol. Sci.* **2019**, *20*, 6210. [CrossRef]
88. Elgali, I.; Omar, O.; Dahlin, C.; Thomsen, P. Guided bone regeneration: Materials and biological mechanisms revisited. *Eur. J. Oral Sci.* **2017**, *125*, 315–337. [CrossRef]
89. Hutmacher, D.; Hurzeler, M.B.; Schliephake, H. A review of material properties of biodegradable and bioresorbable polymers and devices for GTR and GBR applications. *Int. J. Oral Maxillofac. Implant.* **1996**, *11*, 667–678.
90. Gentile, P.; Chiono, V.; Carmagnola, I.; Hatton, P.V. An overview of poly(lactic-co-glycolic) acid (PLGA)-based biomaterials for bone tissue engineering. *Int. J. Mol. Sci.* **2014**, *15*, 3640–3659. [CrossRef]
91. Hoornaert, A.; d'Arros, C.; Heymann, M.F.; Layrolle, P. Biocompatibility, resorption and biofunctionality of a new synthetic biodegradable membrane for guided bone regeneration. *Biomed. Mater.* **2016**, *11*, 045012. [CrossRef] [PubMed]
92. Abe, G.L.; Sasaki, J.I.; Katata, C.; Kohno, T.; Tsuboi, R.; Kitagawa, H.; Imazato, S. Fabrication of novel poly(lactic acid/caprolactone) bilayer membrane for GBR application. *Dent. Mater.* **2020**, *36*, 626–634. [CrossRef]
93. Yuan, H.; Fernandes, H.; Habibovic, P.; de Boer, J.; Barradas, A.M.; de Ruiter, A.; Walsh, W.R.; van Blitterswijk, C.A.; de Bruijn, J.D. Osteoinductive ceramics as a synthetic alternative to autologous bone grafting. *Proc. Natl. Acad. Sci. USA* **2010**, *107*, 13614–13619. [CrossRef]
94. Tang, Z.; Li, X.; Tan, Y.; Fan, H.; Zhang, X. The material and biological characteristics of osteoinductive calcium phosphate ceramics. *Regen. Biomater.* **2018**, *5*, 43–59. [CrossRef]
95. Phipps, M.C.; Clem, W.C.; Catledge, S.A.; Xu, Y.; Hennessy, K.M.; Thomas, V.; Jablonsky, M.J.; Chowdhury, S.; Stanishevsky, A.V.; Vohra, Y.K.; et al. Mesenchymal stem cell responses to bone-mimetic electrospun matrices composed of polycaprolactone, collagen I and nanoparticulate hydroxyapatite. *PLoS ONE* **2011**, *8*, e16813. [CrossRef] [PubMed]
96. Baek, Y.Y.; Kim, J.H.; Song, J.M.; Yoon, S.Y.; Kim, H.S.; Shin, S.H. Chitin-fibroin-hydroxyapatite membrane for guided bone regeneration: Micro-computed tomography evaluation in a rat model. *Maxillofac. Plast. Reconstr. Surg.* **2016**, *38*, 14. [CrossRef] [PubMed]
97. Won, J.Y.; Park, C.Y.; Bae, J.H.; Ahn, G.; Kim, C.; Lim, D.H.; Cho, D.W.; Yun, W.S.; Shim, J.H.; Huh, J.B. Evaluation of 3D printed PCL/PLGA/β-TCP versus collagen membranes for guided bone regeneration in a beagle implant model. *Biomed. Mater.* **2016**, *7*, 055013. [CrossRef] [PubMed]
98. Raj Preeth, D.; Saravanan, S.; Shairam, M.; Selvakumar, N.; Selestin Raja, I.; Dhanasekaran, A.; Vimalraj, S.; Rajalakshmi, S. Bioactive zinc(II) complex incorporated PCL/gelatin electrospun nanofiber enhanced bone tissue regeneration. *Eur. J. Pharm. Sci.* **2021**, *160*, 105768. [CrossRef] [PubMed]
99. Fraga, C.G.; Oteiza, P.I.; Keen, C.L. Trace elements and human health. *Mol. Asp. Med.* **2005**, *26*, 233–234. [CrossRef] [PubMed]
100. Toledano-Osorio, M.; Manzano-Moreno, F.J.; Ruiz, C.; Toledano, M.; Osorio, R. Testing active membranes for bone regeneration: A review. *J. Dent.* **2021**, *105*, 103580. [CrossRef] [PubMed]
101. Toledano, M.; Gutierrez-Pérez, J.L.; Gutierrez-Corrales, A.; Serrera-Figallo, M.A.; Toledano-Osorio, M.; Rosales-Leal, J.I.; Aguilar, M.; Osorio, R.; Torres-Lagares, D. Novel non-resorbable polymeric-nanostructured scaffolds for guided bone regeneration. *Clin. Oral Investig.* **2020**, *24*, 2037–2049. [CrossRef]
102. Bueno, J.; Sánchez, M.C.; Toledano-Osorio, M.; Figuero, E.; Toledano, M.; Medina-Castillo, A.L.; Osorio, R.; Herrera, D.; Sanz, M. Antimicrobial effect of nanostructured membranes for guided tissue regeneration: An in vitro study. *Dent. Mater.* **2020**, *36*, 1566–1577. [CrossRef]
103. Osorio, R.; Carrasco-Carmona, Á.; Toledano, M.; Osorio, E.; Medina-Castillo, A.L.; Iskandar, L.; Marques, A.; Deb, S.; Toledano- Osorio, M. Ex Vivo Investigations on bioinspired electrospun membranes as potential biomaterials for bone regeneration. *J. Dent.* **2020**, *98*, 103359. [CrossRef] [PubMed]
104. Oh, S.A.; Won, J.E.; Kim, H.W. Composite membranes of poly(lactic acid) with zinc-added bioactive glass as a guiding matrix for osteogenic differentiation of bone marrow mesenchymal stem cells. *J. Biomater. Appl.* **2012**, *27*, 413–422. [CrossRef]
105. Pang, K.M.; Lee, J.W.; Lee, J.Y.; Lee, J.B.; Kim, S.M.; Kim, M.J.; Lee, J.H. Clinical outcomes of magnesium-incorporated oxidised implants: A randomised double-blind clinical trial. *Clin. Oral Implant. Res.* **2014**, *25*, 616–621. [CrossRef]

106. Li, X.; Qi, C.; Han, L.; Chu, C.; Bai, J.; Guo, C.; Xue, F.; Shen, B.; Chu, P.K. Influence of dynamic compressive loading on the in vitro degradation behavior of pure PLA and Mg/PLA composite. *Acta Biomater.* **2017**, *64*, 269–278. [CrossRef] [PubMed]
107. Tian, P.; Liu, X. Surface modification of biodegradable magnesium and its alloys for biomedical applications. *Regen. Biomater.* **2015**, *2135*, 151. [CrossRef] [PubMed]
108. Xie, Y.; Hu, C.; Feng, Y.; Li, D.; Ai, T.; Huang, Y.; Ai, T.; Huang, Y.; Chen, X.; Huang, L.; et al. Osteoimmunomodulatory effects of biomaterial modification strategies on macrophage polarization and bone regeneration. *Regen. Biomater.* **2020**, *7*, 233–245. [CrossRef]
109. Ehret, C.; Aid-Launais, R.; Sagardoy, T.; Siadous, R.; Bareille, R.; Rey, S.; Pechev, S.; Etienne, L.; Kalisky, J.; de Mones, E.; et al. Strontium-doped hydroxyapatite polysaccharide materials effect on ectopic bone formation. *PLoS ONE* **2017**, *14*, e0184663. [CrossRef]
110. Kitayama, S.; Wong, L.O.; Ma, L.; Hao, J.; Kasugai, S.; Lang, N.P.; Mattheos, N. Regeneration of rabbit calvarial defects using biphasic calcium phosphate and a strontium hydroxyapatite-containing collagen membrane. *Clin. Oral Implant. Res.* **2016**, *27*, e206–e214. [CrossRef]
111. Sam, G.; Pillai, B.R.M. Evolution of barrier membranes in periodontal regeneration—"Are the third generation membranes really here?". *J. Clin Diagn. Res.* **2014**, *8*, ZE14. [CrossRef]
112. Shi, R.; Ye, J.; Li, W.; Zhang, J.; Li, J.; Wu, C.; Xue, J.; Zhang, L. Infection-responsive electrospun nanofiber mat for antibacterial guided tissue regeneration membrane. *Mater. Sci. Eng. C* **2019**, *100*, 523. [CrossRef]
113. Wang, Y.; Jiang, Y.; Zhang, Y.; Wen, S.; Wang, Y.; Zhang, H. Dual functional electrospun core-shell nanofibers for anti-infective guided bone regeneration membranes. *Mater. Sci. Eng.* **2019**, *100*, 134. [CrossRef]
114. Mathew, A.; Vaquette, C.; Hashimi, S.; Rathnayake, I.; Huygens, F.; Hutmacher, D.W.; Ivanovski, S. Antimicrobial and immunomodulatory surface-functionalized electrospun membranes for bone regeneration. *Adv. Healthc. Mater.* **2017**, *6*, 10. [CrossRef]
115. Kütan, E.; Duygu-Çapar, G.; Özçakir-Tomruk, C.; Dilek, O.C.; Özen, F.; Erdoğan, Ö.; Özdemir, I.; Korachi, M.; Gürel, A. Efficacy of doxycycline release collagen membrane on surgically created and contaminated defects in rat tibiae: A histopathological and microbiological study. *Arch. Oral Biol.* **2016**, *63*, 15–21. [CrossRef]
116. Lian, M.; Sun, B.; Qiao, Z.; Zhao, K.; Zhou, X.; Zhang, Q.; Zou, D.; He, C.; Zhang, X. Bi-layered electrospun nanofibrous membrane with osteogenic and antibacterial properties for guided bone regeneration. *Colloids Surf. B Biointerfaces* **2019**, *176*, 219–229. [CrossRef] [PubMed]
117. Ye, J.; Yao, Q.; Mo, A.; Nie, J.; Liu, W.; Ye, C.; Chen, X. Effects of an antibacterial membrane on osteoblast-like cells in vitro. *Int. J. Nanomed.* **2011**, *6*, 1853–1861. [CrossRef]
118. Kang, Y.J.; Noh, J.E.; Lee, M.J.; Chae, W.S.; Lee, S.Y.; Kim, S.G. The effect of 4-hexylresorcinol on xenograft degradation in a rat calvarial defect model. *Maxillofac. Plast. Reconstr. Surg.* **2016**, *38*, 29. [CrossRef] [PubMed]
119. Kim, S.G.; JeonG, J.H.; Park, Y.W.; SonG, J.Y.; Kim, A.S.; CHoI, J.Y.; Chae, W.S. 4-hexylresorcinol inhibits transglutaminase-2 activity and has synergistic effects along with cisplatin in KB cells. *Oncol. Rep.* **2011**, *25*, 1597–1602. [CrossRef] [PubMed]
120. Kim, M.K.; Park, Y.T.; Kim, S.G.; Park, Y.W.; Lee, S.K.; Choi, W.S. The effect of a hydroxyapatite and 4-hexylresorcinol combination graft on bone regeneration in the rabbit calvarial defect model. *Maxillofac. Plast. Reconstr. Surg.* **2012**, *34*, 377–383.
121. Seok, H.; Lee, S.W.; Kim, S.G.; Seo, D.H.; Kim, H.S.; Kweon, H.Y.; Jo, Y.Y.; Kang, T.Y.; Lee, M.J.; Chae, W.S. The effect of silk membrane plus 3% 4-hexylresorcinol on guided bone regeneration in a rabbit calvarial defect model. *Int. J. Ind. Entomol.* **2013**, *27*, 209–217. [CrossRef]
122. Xue, J.; He, M.; Liang, Y.; Crawford, A.; Coates, P.; Chen, D.; Shi, R.; Zhang, L. Fabrication and evaluation of electrospun PCL–gelatin micro-/nanofiber membranes for anti-infective GTR implants. *J. Mater. Chem. B* **2014**, *2*, 6867–6877. [CrossRef]
123. Xue, J.; Shi, R.; Niu, Y.; Gong, M.; Coates, P.; Crawford, A.; Chen, D.; Tian, W.; Zhang, L. Fabrication of drug-loaded anti-infective guided tissue regeneration membrane with adjustable biodegradation property. *Colloids Surf. B Biointerfaces* **2015**, *135*, 846–854. [CrossRef] [PubMed]
124. Shi, R.; Xue, J.; Wang, H.; Wang, R.; Gong, M.; Chen, D.; Zhang, L.; Tian, W. Fabrication and evaluation of a homogeneous electrospun PCL–gelatin hybrid membrane as an anti-adhesion barrier for craniectomy. *J. Mater. Chem. B* **2015**, *3*, 4063–4073. [CrossRef] [PubMed]
125. Xue, J.; Niu, Y.; Gong, M.; Shi, R.; Chen, D.; Zhang, L.; Lvov, Y. Electrospun microfiber membranes embedded with drug-loaded clay nanotubes for sustained antimicrobial protection. *ACS Nano* **2015**, *9*, 1600–1612. [CrossRef] [PubMed]
126. Campoccia, D.; Montanaro, L.; Speziale, P.; Arciola, C.R. Antibiotic-loaded biomaterials and the risks for the spread of antibiotic resistance following their prophylactic and therapeutic clinical use. *Biomaterials* **2010**, *31*, 6363–6377. [CrossRef] [PubMed]
127. Gümüşderelioğlu, M.; Sunal, E.; Tolga Demirtaş, T.; Kiremitçi, A.S. Chitosan-based double-faced barrier membrane coated with functional nanostructures and loaded with BMP-6. *J. Mater. Sci. Mater. Med.* **2020**, *31*, 4. [CrossRef] [PubMed]
128. Jones, A.A.; Buser, D.; Schenk, R.; Wozney, J.; Cochran, D.L. The effect of rhBMP-2 around endosseous implants with and without membranes in the canine model. *J. Periodontol.* **2006**, *77*, 1184–1193. [CrossRef]
129. Hsu, Y.T.; Al-Hezaimi, K.; Galindo-Moreno, P.; O'Valle, F.; Al-Rasheed, A.; Wang, H.L. Effects of recombinant human bone morphogenetic protein-2 on vertical bone augmentation in a canine model. *J. Periodontol.* **2017**, *88*, 896–905. [CrossRef]

130. Fujioka-Kobayashi, M.; Sawada, K.; Kobayashi, E.; Schaller, B.; Zhang, Y.; Miron, R.J. Recombinant human bone morphogenetic protein 9 (rhBMP9) induced osteoblastic behavior on a collagen membrane compared with rhBMP2. *J. Periodontol.* **2016**, *87*, e101–e107. [CrossRef]
131. Akman, A.C.; Tığlı, R.S.; Gümüşderelioğlu, M.; Nohutcu, R.M. Bone morphogenetic protein-6-loaded chitosan scaffolds enhance the osteoblastic characteristics of MC3T3-E1 cells. *Artif. Organs* **2010**, *34*, 65–74. [CrossRef]
132. Soran, Z.; Tığlı Aydın, R.S.; Gümüşderelioğlu, M. Chitosan scaffolds with BMP-6 loaded alginate microspheres for periodontal tissue engineering. *J. Microencapsul.* **2012**, *29*, 770–780. [CrossRef]
133. Lee, D.Y.; Lee, S.B.; Park, K.J.; Park, J.J. A Barrier Membrane Used in Periodontitis Treatment and a Production Method Thereof. WO2016186594A1, 24 November 2016.
134. Fujioka-Kobayashi, M.; Kobayashi, E.; Schaller, B.; Mottini, M.; Miron, R.J.; Saulacic, N. Effect of recombinant human bone morphogenic protein 9 (rhBMP9) loaded onto bone grafts versus barrier membranes on new bone formation in a rabbit calvarial defect model. *J. Biomed. Mater. Res. A* **2017**, *105*, 2655–2661. [CrossRef] [PubMed]
135. Shalumon, K.; Lai, G.J.; Chen, C.H.; Chen, J.P. Modulation of bone-specific tissue regeneration by incorporating bone morphogenetic protein and controlling the shell thickness of silk fibroin/chitosan/nanohydroxyapatite core–shell nanofibrous membranes. *ACS Appl. Mater. Interfaces* **2015**, *7*, 21170–21181. [CrossRef] [PubMed]
136. Park, Y.J.; Ku, Y.; Chung, C.P.; Lee, S.J. Controlled release of platelet-derived growth factor from porous poly(L-lactide) membranes for guided tissue regeneration. *J. Control. Release* **1998**, *51*, 201–211. [CrossRef]
137. Raja, S.; Byakod, G.; Pudakalkatti, P. Growth factors in periodontal regeneration. *Int. J. Dent. Hyg.* **2009**, *7*, 82–89. [CrossRef]
138. Chen, F.M.; Shelton, R.M.; Jin, Y.; Chapple, I.L.C. Localized delivery of growth factors for periodontal tissue regeneration: Role, strategies, and perspectives. *Med. Res. Rev.* **2009**, *29*, 472–513. [CrossRef]
139. Ji, W.; Yang, F.; Ma, J.; Bouma, M.J.; Boerman, O.C.; Chen, Z.; van den Beucken, J.J.; Jansen, J.A. Incorporation of stromal cell-derived factor-1α in PCL/gelatin electrospun membranes for guided bone regeneration. *Biomaterials* **2013**, *34*, 735–745. [CrossRef]
140. Herford, A.S.; Miller, M.; Lauritano, F.; Cervino, G.; Signorino, F.; Maiorana, C. The use of virtual surgical planning and navigation in the treatment of orbital trauma. *Chin. J. Traumatol.* **2017**, *20*, 9–13. [CrossRef]
141. Fénelon, M.; Catros, S.; Meyer, C.; Fricain, J.-C.; Obert, L.; Auber, F.; Louvrier, A.; Gindraux, F. Applications of Human Amniotic Membrane for Tissue Engineering. *Membranes* **2021**, *11*, 387. [CrossRef]
142. Shankar, P.; Kumar, A.; Kumari, C.B.N.; Mahendra, J.; Ambalavanan, N. Amnion and chorion membrane in periodontal regeneration. *Ann. Rom. Soc. Cell Biol.* **2020**, *24*, 435–441.
143. Riau, A.K.; Beuerman, R.W.; Lim, L.S.; Mehta, J.S. Preservation, sterilization and de-epithelialization of human amniotic membrane for use in ocular surface reconstruction. *Biomaterials* **2010**, *31*, 216–225. [CrossRef]
144. Rodríguez-Ares, M.T.; López-Valladares, M.J.; Touriño, R.; Vieites, B.; Gude, F.; Silva, M.T.; Couceiro, J. Effects of lyophilization on human amniotic membrane. *Acta Ophthalmol.* **2009**, *87*, 396–403. [CrossRef] [PubMed]
145. Laurent, R.; Nallet, A.; Obert, L.; Nicod, L.; Gindraux, F. Storage and qualification of viable intact human amniotic graft and technology transfer to a tissue bank. *Cell Tissue Bank.* **2014**, *15*, 267–275. [CrossRef]
146. Jirsova, K.; Jones, G.L.A. Amniotic membrane in ophthalmology: Properties, preparation, storage and indications for grafting—A review. *Cell Tissue Bank.* **2017**, *18*, 193–204. [CrossRef] [PubMed]
147. Shortt, A.J.; Secker, G.A.; Lomas, R.J.; Wilshaw, S.-P.; Kearney, J.N.; Tuft, S.J.; Daniels, J.T. The effect of amniotic membrane preparation method on its ability to serve as a substrate for the ex-vivo expansion of limbal epithelial cells. *Biomaterials* **2009**, *30*, 1056–1065. [CrossRef]
148. Mamede, A.C.; Carvalho, M.J.; Abrantes, A.M.; Laranjo, M.; Maia, C.J.; Botelho, M.F. Amniotic membrane: From structure and functions to clinical applications. *Cell Tissue Res.* **2012**, *349*, 447–458. [CrossRef]
149. Takashima, S.; Yasuo, M.; Sanzen, N.; Sekiguchi, K.; Okabe, M.; Yoshida, T.; Toda, A.; Nikaido, T. Characterization of laminin isoforms in human amnion. *Tissue Cell* **2008**, *40*, 75–81. [CrossRef]
150. Niknejad, H.; Peirovi, H.; Jorjani, M.; Ahmadiani, A.; Ghanavi, J.; Seifalian, A.M. Properties of the amniotic membrane for potential use in tissue engineering. *Eur. Cell Mater.* **2008**, *15*, 88–99. [CrossRef]
151. Lei, J.; Priddy, L.B.; Lim, J.J.; Koob, T.J. Dehydrated human amnion/chorion membrane (dHACM) allografts as a therapy for orthopedic tissue repair. *Tech. Orthop.* **2017**, *32*, 149–157. [CrossRef]
152. Nishihara, S.; Someya, A.; Yonemoto, H.; Ota, A.; Itoh, S.; Nagaoka, I.; Takeda, S. Evaluation of the expression and enzyme activity of matrix metalloproteinase-7 in fetal membranes during premature rupture of membranes at term in humans. *Reprod. Sci.* **2008**, *15*, 156–165. [CrossRef]
153. Chen, E.; Tofe, A. A literature review of the safety and biocompatibility of amnion tissue. *J. Implant. Adv. Clin. Dent.* **2010**, *2*, 67–75.
154. Ben Ali, L.M.S.; Mostafa Elazab, S. Amniotic membrane as a biodegradable barrier in technique of guided tissue regeneration in advanced periodontal disease in dogs: Histopathological assessment. *Tissue Reg. Stem. Cell* **2020**, *2020*, 1–16.
155. Venkatesan, N.; Lavu, V.; Balaji, S.K. Clinical efficacy of amniotic membrane with biphasic calcium phosphate in guided tissue regeneration of intrabony defects- a randomized controlled clinical trial. *Biomater. Res.* **2015**, *25*, 15. [CrossRef]
156. Holtzclaw, D.J.; Toscano, N.J. Amnion–chorion allograft barrier used for guided tissue regeneration treatment of periodontal intrabony defects: A retrospective observational report. *Clin. Adv. Periodontics* **2013**, *3*, 131–137. [CrossRef]

157. Ríos, L.K.; Espinoza, C.V.; Alarcón, M.; Huamaní, J.O. Bone density of defects treated with lyophilised amniotic membrane versus collagen membrane: A tomographic and histomorfogenic study in rabbit's femur. *J. Oral Res.* **2014**, *3*, 143–149. [CrossRef]
158. Sharma, A.; Yadav, K. Amniotic membrane—A Novel material for the root coverage: A case series. *J. Indian Soc. Periodontol.* **2015**, *19*, 444–448. [CrossRef]
159. Shetty, S.S.; Chatterjee, A.; Bose, S. Bilateral multiple recession coverage with platelet-rich fibrin in comparison with amniotic membrane. *J. Indian Soc. Periodontol.* **2014**, *18*, 102–106. [CrossRef] [PubMed]
160. Tseng, S.C.G. Grafts Made from Amniotic Membrane; Methods of Separating, Preserving and Using Such Grafts in Surgeries. U.S. Patent US6326019B1, 4 December 2001.
161. Miron, R.J.; Pikos, M.A. PRF as a barrier membrane in guided bone regeneration. *Dent. Today* **2017**, *216*, 36.
162. Miron, R.J.; Bosshardt, D.D. OsteoMacs: Key players around bone biomaterials. *Biomaterials* **2016**, *82*, 1–19. [CrossRef]
163. Giannini, S.; Cielo, A.; Bonanome, L.; Rastelli, C.; Derla, C.; Corpaci, F.; Falisi, G. Comparison between PRP, PRGF and PRF: Lights and shadows in three similar but different protocols. *Eur. Rev. Med. Pharmacol. Sci.* **2015**, *19*, 927–930.
164. Kobayashi, E.; Flückiger, L.; Fujioka-Kobayashi, M.; Sawada, K.; Sculean, A.; Schaller, B.; Miron, R.J. Comparative release of growth factors from PRP, PRF, and advanced-PRF. *Clin. Oral Investig.* **2016**, *20*, 2353–2360. [CrossRef]
165. Lekovic, V.; Milinkovic, I.; Aleksic, Z.; Jankovic, S.; Stankovic, P.; Kenney, E.B.; Camargo, P.M. Platelet-rich fibrin and bovine porous bone mineral vs. platelet-rich fibrin in the treatment of intrabony periodontal defects. *J. Periodontal. Res.* **2012**, *47*, 409–417. [CrossRef] [PubMed]
166. Mathur, A.; Bains, V.K.; Gupta, V.; Jhingran, R.; Singh, G.P. Evaluation of infrabony defects treated with platelet-rich fibrin or autogenous bone graft: A comparative analysis. *Eur. J. Dent.* **2015**, *9*, 100–108. [PubMed]
167. Anilkumar, K.; Geetha, A.; Umasudhakar, T.R.; Vijayalakshmi, R.; Pameela, E. Platelet-rich-fibrin: A novel root coverage approach. *J. Indian Soc. Periodontol.* **2009**, *13*, 50–54. [CrossRef]
168. Jankovic, S.; Aleksic, Z.; Klokkevold, P.; Lekovic, V.; Dimitrijevic, B.; Kenney, E.B.; Camargo, P. Use of platelet-rich fibrin membrane following treatment of gingival recession: A randomized clinical trial. *Int. J. Periodontics Restor. Dent.* **2012**, *32*, e41–e50.
169. Yeong, W.Y.; Chua, C.K.; Leong, K.F.; Chandrasekaran, M. Rapid prototyping in tissue engineering: Challenges and potential. *Trends Biotechnol.* **2004**, *22*, 643–652. [CrossRef] [PubMed]
170. Skardal, A.; Atala, A. Biomaterials for integration with 3-D bioprinting. *Ann. Biomed. Eng.* **2015**, *43*, 730–746. [CrossRef] [PubMed]
171. Sears, N.A.; Seshadri, D.R.; Dhavalikar, P.S.; Cosgriff-Hernandez, E. A review of three-dimensional printing in tissue engineering. *Tissue Eng. B Rev.* **2016**, *22*, 298–310. [CrossRef]
172. Tamay, D.G.; Dursun Usal, T.; Alagoz, A.S.; Yucel, D.; Hasirci, N.; Hasirci, V. 3D and 4D printing of polymers for tissue engineering applications. *Front. Bioeng. Biotechnol.* **2019**, *7*, 164. [CrossRef]
173. Mobaraki, M.G.; Yazdanpanah, M.A.; Luo, Y.; Mills, D.K. Bioinks and bioprinting: A focused review. *Bioprinting* **2020**, *2020*, e00080. [CrossRef]
174. Hospodiuk, M.; Dey, M.; Sosnoski, D.; Ozbolat, I.T. The bioink: A comprehensive review on bioprintable materials. *Biotechnol. Adv.* **2017**, *35*, 217–239. [CrossRef]
175. Bai, L.; Ji, P.; Li, X.; Gao, H.; Li, L.; Wang, C. Mechanical characterization of 3D-printed individualized Ti-mesh (membrane) for alveolar bone defects. *J. Healthc. Eng.* **2019**, *2019*, 4231872. [CrossRef] [PubMed]
176. Vanderburgh, J.; Sterling, J.A.; Guelcher, S.A. 3D printing of tissue engineered constructs for in vitro modeling of disease progression and drug screening. *Ann. Biomed. Eng.* **2017**, *45*, 164–179. [CrossRef] [PubMed]
177. Groll, J.; Burdick, J.A.; Cho, D.W.; Derby, B.; Gelinsky, M.; Heilshorn, S.C.; Jüngst, T.; Malda, J.; Mironov, V.A.; Nakayama, K.; et al. A definition of bioinks and their distinction from biomaterial inks. *Biofabrication* **2018**, *11*, 013001. [CrossRef] [PubMed]
178. Pacheco, K.A. Allergy to surgical implants. *Clin. Rev. Allergy Immunol.* **2019**, *56*, 72–85. [CrossRef] [PubMed]
179. Sicilia, A.; Cuesta, S.; Coma, G.; Arregui, I.; Guisasola, C.; Ruiz, E.; Maestro, A. Titanium allergy in dental implant patients: A clinical study on 1500 consecutive patients. *Clin. Oral Implant. Res.* **2008**, *19*, 823–835. [CrossRef] [PubMed]
180. Demoly, P.; Michel, F.; Bousquet, J. *Allergy, Principles and Practice*, 5th ed.; Mosby-Year Book: St. Louis, MO, USA, 1998; pp. 430–439.

MDPI
St. Alban-Anlage 66
4052 Basel
Switzerland
Tel. +41 61 683 77 34
Fax +41 61 302 89 18
www.mdpi.com

Applied Sciences Editorial Office
E-mail: applsci@mdpi.com
www.mdpi.com/journal/applsci

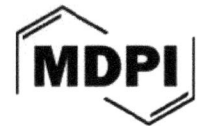

www.ingramcontent.com/pod-product-compliance
Lightning Source LLC
LaVergne TN
LVHW070438100526
838202LV00014B/1620